ADOLESCENT PSYCHIATRY

DEVELOPMENTAL AND CLINICAL STUDIES

VOLUME 14

Annals of the American Society for Adolescent Psychiatry

ADOLESCENT PSYCHIATRY

DEVELOPMENTAL AND CLINICAL STUDIES

VOLUME 14

Edited by
SHERMAN C. FEINSTEIN
Editor in Chief

Senior Editors
AARON H. ESMAN
JOHN G. LOONEY
GEORGE H. ORVIN
JOHN L. SCHIMEL
ALLAN Z. SCHWARTZBERG
ARTHUR D. SOROSKY
MAX SUGAR

The University of Chicago Press
Chicago and London

The University of Chicago Press, Chicago 60637
The University of Chicago Press, Ltd., London

International Standard Book Number: 0-226-24060-6
Library of Congress Catalog Card Number: 70-147017

The paper used in this publication meets the minimum requirements of American National Standard for Information Sciences—Permanence of Paper for Printed Library Materials, ANSI Z39.48-1984. ∞™

CONTENTS

PART II. DEVELOPMENTAL ISSUES IN ADOLESCENT PSYCHIATRY

PART III. PSYCHOPATHOLOGICAL ISSUES IN ADOLESCENT PSYCHIATRY

PART IV. PSYCHOTHERAPEUTIC ISSUES IN ADOLESCENT PSYCHIATRY

PART V. PERSONALITY FUNCTIONING DURING ADOLESCENCE: A LONGITUDINAL STUDY
HARVEY GOLOMBEK, Special Editor

uptill here

PART VI. EDUCATIONAL ISSUES IN ADOLESCENT PSYCHIATRY

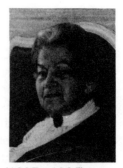

IN MEMORIAM
Dedication to Margaret S. Mahler (1897–1985)

This volume is respectfully and lovingly dedicated to the memory of Margaret S. Mahler, M.D., psychoanalyst, researcher, teacher, and author. Dr. Mahler was the 1983 recipient of the William A. Schonfeld Award of the American Society for Adolescent Psychiatry, in recognition of the invaluable contributions she made to the understanding of adolescence.

Margaret Schoenberger (Mahler) was born in Sopron, Hungary, in 1897. She knew as a young girl that she wanted to become a physician like her father. At the age of fourteen she read an article by Sandor Ferenczi and then met him at the home of her friend, Alice Kovaks, later Alice Balint. Dr. Mahler once said, "Meeting Ferenczi sealed my fate. Right then and there I decided I would become an analyst." She did her undergraduate studies at the University of Budapest. She studied medicine in Germany during and after World War I, graduating cum laude from the University of Jena, in spite of strong prejudices against female students, Jews, and Eastern Europeans. She took training in pediatrics in Vienna and began research work with children. Her earlier interest in psychoanalysis soon led her into analytic training in Vienna during the formative years of Freudian conceptualizations. She had a partial analysis with Helene Deutsch, a training analysis with August Aichhorn, and a classical analysis with Willi Hoffer. Her colleagues included Anna Freud, Heinz Hartmann, Ernst and Marianne Kris, Robert and Jenny Waelder, Anna Maenchen, Jeanne Lampl-de-Groot, and Grete Bibring. A few years after acceptance into the Vienna Society for Psychoanalysis in 1933 she married Paul Mahler, a Viennese chemist with a doctorate in philosophy. The increasing Nazi threat caused the Mahlers to emigrate to the United States in 1938. Dr. Mahler became associated with the New York State Psychiatric Institute of the Columbia University College of Physicians and Surgeons. Her first work was with children suffering from tics. Follow-up studies showed that several of the children who had lost their tic symptoms became psychotic during adolescence. In the early 1940s, Dr. Mahler turned her attention to the study of childhood psychosis. Her brilliant insights into autistic and symbiotic psychoses eventually led her to the study of normal developmental stages of infancy and early childhood—the area of her most far-reaching discoveries and psychoanalytic contributions.

Dr. Mahler always made it very clear that her formulations about the first three years of life, based on meticulous analytic observations of infants and toddlers and their parents, were rooted in, and extensions of, Freud's thinking. Using ego psychology and object relations theory as a framework, Dr. Mahler outlined the by now well-known stages and substages of separation-individuation. She emphasized the importance of the symbiotic union with the mother out of which the infant emerges during the "psychological birth." After "hatching" and the "practicing" stage came the crucial "rapprochement" stage before the toddler could be "on the way to object constancy." Dr. Mahler's ideas and descriptions of developmental phases were quickly accepted into the body of psychoanalysis, and they continue to grow, interdigitate with earlier concepts, and cross-fertilize newer thinking. Peter Blos soon formulated the idea of "the second individuation phase of adolescence." The American Psychoanalytic Association held a series of panels exploring the reverberations of separation-individuation throughout the life cycle. Terms that Dr. Mahler introduced have become standard in our lexicon, for example, "separation-individuation," "separation anxiety," "emotional refueling," and "rapprochement." At a time when ideas about the self preoccupy our field, Dr. Mahler's concepts have much to offer. In an earlier time when it was fashionable to blame mothers for many difficulties with children, Dr. Mahler steadfastly opposed such ill-founded, harmful notions. She was always aware of, and sympathetic to, the need for helping young parents with child-rearing. Her films and videotapes, culled from thousands of feet of film made during her research studies, which now are preserved as her archives at Yale University, are available for rental or purchase for instruction of child mental health professionals through the Mahler Psychiatric Research Foundation.

Dr. Mahler will always occupy a place of honor among the great pioneers in psychoanalysis who extended research into the direct observation of infants and young children. Among the many honors she received, she cherished being named, along with Erik Erikson, an honorary president of the World Association for Infant Psychiatry and Allied Disciplines. Equally important to her have been the setting up of infant research and infant care centers named in her honor. Teaching child and adolescent analysis and the training of candidates were likewise interests in which she excelled. The setting up of an outstanding child analysis curriculum in the Philadelphia Psychoanalytic Institute by her and her teaching at the New York Psychoanalytic Institute and at the Albert Einstein College of Medicine were close to her heart. It was especially in direct, interpersonal contact with her that her enormous effect could be felt; one would marvel at her intuitive ability to get right to the crux of the issue, the unusual way in which she actually "lived the unconscious"—not merely paying lip service to it but using it to sense the truth and to communicate. Her students and colleagues would always marvel too at her uncanny ability to select the precisely right word to use in a keen interpretation or in a clinical paper.

In many ways, Dr. Mahler could be said to have had a hard life. She overcame great difficulties to become a doctor in Germany in the early 1920s. She coped with much danger and turmoil in escaping from the Nazi regime and in resettling in New York, adopting a new language and culture. She was beset with a variety of serious illnesses in the latter part of her life but again showed herself to be a true survivor until she finally succumbed to the sequelae of surgery for abdominal adhesions on October 2, 1985, at the age of eighty-eight. It was not until her funeral services that it was revealed how much she and her family had suffered at the hands of the Nazis; she asked that her gravestone should read: "One of the Holocaust."

Because of the nature of her discoveries and formulations, Dr. Mahler's influence will always illuminate thinking about adolescents and older people as well as infants and young children; normal development as well as psychopathology; the fields of social work, child care, and education as well as the fields of psychoanalysis and child psychiatry. As long as there are children and those who care for them, Dr. Mahler will be remembered—and missed.

HERMAN D. STAPLES

IN MEMORIAM

Dana L. Farnsworth (1905–1986)

Dana L. Farnsworth, a pioneer in the development of college student psychiatry, died Saturday, August 2, 1986, at the age of eighty-one, following a long illness. At the time of his death Dr. Farnsworth was the Henry K. Oliver Professor Emeritus at Harvard University, where he had held joint appointments as professor of hygiene and director of the university health services from 1954 to 1971, when he retired.

Dr. Farnsworth was the recipient of the William A. Schonfeld Distinguished Service Award of the American Society for Adolescent Psychiatry in 1971. He is generally credited with the idea that adolescence is extended into the early twenties for those young people who attend college. His extensive writings, which include two books, numerous chapters, editorials, book reviews, and over 200 journal articles, have contributed extensively to the adolescent psychiatric literature.

Dr. Farnsworth's long and productive career dates from 1935, when he was appointed assistant director of health at Williams College. In 1941 he left Williams for the U.S. Navy, where he served during World War II as a commander in the Medical Corps. Following the war and a brief return to head the Health Department at Williams, Dr. Farnsworth became medical director of the Massachusetts Institute of Technology in 1946, a position he held until 1954, when he was appointed Henry K. Oliver Professor of Hygiene and Director, University Health Services, Harvard University. Since his retirement in 1971, he served as editorial director for *Psychiatric Annals* and as chairman of the Board of Directors, Medicine in the Public Interest.

Dr. Farnsworth received honorary degrees from ten colleges and universities, and, in addition to the 1971 Schonfeld Award, he has been the recipient of eleven different distinguished awards from professional organizations and academic institutions. He held office as president of the Group for the Advancement of Psychiatry and the American College Health Association, chaired numerous national and international conferences, and served on the Joint Commission on Mental Health of Children from 1966 to 1970.

   With Dana Farnsworth's passing, psychiatry has lost one of its true giants. A man of good humor and kindness, dedicated physician, distinguished educator, noble friend, and true gentleman, Dana Farnsworth was surely one of the twentieth century's most significant psychiatrists. In mourning our loss we must also rejoice in the rich legacy he has conferred on us.

M. ROBERT WILSON

PREFACE

This volume of the *Annals of the American Society for Adolescent Psychiatry* is being published at a time of unusual stress in the field of psychiatry generally, and specifically in the subspecialty of adolescent psychiatry. Unfortunately, much of the stress concerns the financial aspects of psychiatry in the clinical, research, and training areas.

It is not that there is any dearth of patients. The proportion of adolescents among our patient population has been increasing steadily. The American Medical Association recently announced a demonstration project to improve the health of the nation's 45 million adolescents, targeting the areas of substance abuse, teen pregnancy, psychiatric disorder, and violent or vulnerable subgroups (runaways and the homeless).

The problem is that, in a period of general physician oversupply, there is a shortage of adequately trained child and adolescent psychiatrists. The gap between child and adolescent patients and the availability of child psychiatrists and adolescent psychiatrists to treat them will continue to expand. We are concerned that the shortage will lead to expansion of nonmedical, behavioral approaches to psychiatric problems with inadequate medical supervision.

The American Society for Adolescent Psychiatry has been in the forefront of activities to improve treatment facilities and techniques for the care of adolescent patients. The Society has collaborated with a wide variety of agencies, institutions, and societies to foster these goals.

With all the problems besetting the profession, it is, nevertheless, a matter of pride for us that professionals continue their struggle to advance our knowledge of adolescent development and the vicissitudes of this most fascinating stage of life. This volume is a testimonial to the broad-ranging interests and creativity of members of our profession.

Two of our most creative authors and Schonfeld Award Fellows died in 1986, Margaret Mahler and Dana Farnsworth. Herman Staples and Robert Wilson have written about these two pioneers in adolescent psychiatry, to whom this volume is dedicated.

SHERMAN C. FEINSTEIN

PART I

ADOLESCENCE: GENERAL CONSIDERATIONS

EDITORS' INTRODUCTION

Adolescents continue to be a touchstone to the culture and society in which they live and to which, in a variety of ways, they seek to adapt. More than those of any other stage of development, the adolescent seems to serve as a repository for the conflicts of the culture and as a bearer of its mythic projections. The more complex society becomes, the more perplexing, troubling, and problematic their role appears to be, at least to those adults who require an external focus for their own sense of anomie. The chapters in this part address a number of contemporary issues affecting adolescents, including psychosocial dimensions of adolescent health, the myths and needs of adolescents, and the impact of early sexual identification on subsequent career choice and adaptation.

Daniel Offer, in the William A. Schonfeld Memorial Lecture, explores "The Mystery of Adolescence," a phase of development that Sigmund Freud saw as puzzling and obscure. Offer, on the other hand, sees adolescence as an understandable period that has, probably, not changed much over the centuries. He reviews his studies of the normal adolescent's self-image and describes the psychological self, the social self, the sexual self, the familial self, and the coping self as revealed by his epidemiological studies. Offer concludes that normal adolescents are hopeful, positive, and future oriented. The vast majority function well, enjoy good relationships with their families and friends, and accept the values of the larger society. On the other hand, among 20 percent of adolescents, turmoil and maladaption exist and require psychiatric care. It is a disservice to dismiss deviant and disturbed adolescents as just "going through a stage."

Carol C. Nadelson, as president of the American Psychiatric Association, discusses developmental aspects of leadership roles for women in academic medicine and elsewhere. She reviews the history and current status of women and concludes, pessimistically, that the discrepancy in men's and women's career paths is influenced by early feminine characteristics of responsiveness, accommodation and nurturance, training programs, a lack of female mentors, and even by the tax structure. Douglas B. Hansen provides a discussion of Dr. Nadelson's chapter.

Saul V. Levine discusses a series of myths and attitudes concerning adolescence, derived from his experience as author of a syndicated column on the teenager. He provides an overview of the needs of youth from a developmental and experiential perspective.

David A. Halperin examines the brief but vigorous period of creativity during the adolescence of the poet Arthur Rimbaud. A quasi-cult figure, who had a maximum impact on contemporary artistic movements (mysticism, occultism), Rimbaud self-consciously renounced any artistic concerns at the age of nineteen and thereafter lived the life of an adventurer and explorer. Halperin traces this act of renunciation during Rimbaud's transitional phase to adulthood and documents the affective responses and identity diffusion that were prevalent. (He also considers the diagnosis of bipolar affective disorder.) The author concludes that certain dynamic themes dominated Rimbaud's adolescence: the absence of a consistent father figure; his efforts to escape a rigid, puritanical, hypocritical mother; and the presence of affective disorder about age seventeen. Halperin discusses the therapeutic elements in his brief but intense creative period.

Bonnie E. Litowitz and Robert A. Gundlach look at the writings of adolescents (diaries, letters, and notes) that were shared with their therapists during treatment. They examine the semiotic function (communication through material expression) and social aspect (interpersonal relationship) of writing. They explore three uses of writing by adolescents: to externalize and objectify an inner feeling or content; to continue a process begun by speech; and to experiment with various relationships. Using examples of adolescents' writing, the authors illustrate that writing affords adolescents yet another means to address the particular developmental tasks they face and to present the self and its inner world with greater distance from and control over the audience.

4

Sadi Bayrakal sees the emotionally disturbed adolescent as caught in a vicious cycle as a result of intrapsychic and interpersonal conflict. The psychic energy consumed fosters borderline, narcissistic personality formation, which is critically affected by current sociocultural atmosphere. The author considers the interplay between the adolescent and his society, the gradual loss of strength and influence by the family, the general crisis of American culture, the compartmentalization of sexuality, the denigration and abdication of authority, and the failure of schools. Bayrakal concludes that the total impact of these sociocultural factors engenders a basic core of anxiety.

Lucia Villela and Richard Markin further explore the psychodynamics of adolescence through a study of mythmaking. Considering film preferences as modern forms of myths, which may provide clues to the conscious and unconscious of the adolescent group, Villela and Markin examine the assumption that myths, fairy tales, and narratives are metaphorical attempts to understand and explain the perceived realities of our own selves—our origins, our future, our world. The authors analyze *Purple Rain,* a recent film, to demonstrate that one of the functions of myths and narratives is to narrow the gap between experience and expectations.

1   THE MYSTERY OF ADOLESCENCE

DANIEL OFFER

The title of my talk reflects unending concerns of most aging individuals: What is happening to our youth? What have we done wrong? and The future is doomed if these youth will one day run the country. It is of great interest that, excluding technological advances, little change has actually occurred during the past 2,000 years. We subscribe to similar ethical standards, practice the same religions, and still have the family as the anchor of the socialization process. Indeed, it is a mystery how the more things change, the more they remain the same.

Mystery is defined as "something that has not been, or cannot be, explained; hence something beyond human (i.e., adult) comprehension" (*Webster's Collegiate Dictionary* 1951).

Traditionally, mysteries are harder to solve than we first believe. Everyone has an opinion as to the culprit or culprits, and everyone has a relatively quick solution. We shall not solve the mystery of adolescence today, but I hope to leave you with a few clues that may bring us closer to solving it eventually.

The purpose of this chapter is to share with you some of the recent empirical findings concerning adolescents (ages fourteen to eighteen). Most of us get our experience and impressions from seeing individual adolescent patients and their families in a clinical setting, be it the hospital, the clinic, or private practice. We try to understand why a particular person has specific problems and help him or her resolve them. Waddington's (1957) epigenetic landscape (see fig. 1) shows the conceptual relationship between the ball, representing the course of

William A. Schonfeld Distinguished Service Award Address, presented to the American Society for Adolescent Psychiatry, Dallas, Texas, May 18, 1985.

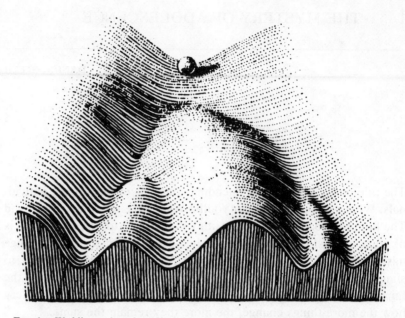

F<small>IG</small>. 1.—Waddington's epigenetic landscape: a model of genetic canalization in development (Waddington 1957).

life of an individual, and the terrain, representing genetic templates and environmental influences. It is very difficult to predict the course of a specific ball downhill. You have to know every grass blade, every stone, the wind's strength, the sun, and the speed of the ball. Even if you are able to keep almost everything constant, a second ball rolls down differently. Similarly, the course of a particular individual is difficult, if not impossible, to predict. So many unforeseen things may happen; unexpected crises, good fortunes, and so forth. In our field, we have all too often tried to map the course in reverse order: Why did the ball go down a particular course? Who helped the person? Who stood in his way? How was he brought up?

Overview

Adolescence is not, as has been previously assumed, a developmental stage that began after the Industrial Revolution. There is plenty of historical evidence to suggest that adolescence as a stage was known to the ancient Romans, Greeks, and even Egyptians. It seemed to have

8

almost disappeared during the Dark Ages, although there are countless medieval texts that mention adolescence. For example, in *Le Grand Proprietaire* (1556), it states that "the third age, which is called adolescence . . . ends in the twenty-first year . . . and it can go on till thirty or thirty-five. This age is called adolescence because the person is big enough to beget children. In this age the limbs are soft and able to grow and receive strength and vigor from natural heat" (Ariès 1962, p. 21).

In the last eighty years, in Western cultures, adolescence, particularly in the middle class, has become a progressively longer stage (Kett 1977). The concept of reasonable independence has been translated into financial independence and marriage. If this criterion is accepted, a high school student who, on graduation, begins to work and marries at nineteen experiences a shorter period of parental dependence and hence adolescence than the individual who attends college and graduate school, is supported by his or her parents until the age of twenty-seven, and marries at twenty-eight. The latter person will tend to have a much longer adolescence. The lowering of the age at which puberty takes place has dramatically decreased during the past three decades. Recently, it has stabilized for girls at the age of twelve, and boys go through puberty approximately eighteen months later.

A vast and ever-expanding literature exists describing characteristics of adolescents studied in clinical or correctional settings. Adolescents studied clinically are described as being in "emotional turmoil" most of the time (Blos 1961; A. Freud 1946, 1958). The term "adolescent turmoil" has been used freely by psychiatrists, psychoanalysts, and other mental health professionals for both describing disturbed adolescents and discussing the developmental process of normal adolescence. It is defined as an emotional condition that represents significant disruption in psychological equilibrium leading to fluctuation in moods, confusion in thought, rebellion against one's parents, and changeable and unpredictable behavior. Typical—or normal—adolescents, it has been thought, need to experience "adolescent turmoil." If they do not, they stay overdependent on their parents, have trouble developing their sense of identity, and have difficulties relating well to male and female peers. The studies of nonpatient adolescents show that, in general, this statement cannot be supported. The studies of normal adolescents show that these teenagers are well adjusted and get along well with their peers, teachers, and families (Block 1971; Csikszentmihalyi and

9

Larson 1984; Douvan and Adelson 1966; Offer and Offer 1975; Offer, Ostrov, and Howard 1981a; Vaillant 1977; Westley and Epstein 1969).

Studies of Normal Adolescents' Self-Image

METHOD

The Offer Self-Image Questionnaire (OSIQ) is a self-descriptive personality test that assesses the adjustment of teenage boys and girls between the ages of thirteen and nineteen. It measures the teenager's feelings about his own psychological world in eleven content areas (for the background of the OSIQ, its reliability, validity, and standard scoring methodology, see Offer et al. 1981a and Offer, Ostrov, and Howard 1984).

Since 1962, the questionnaire has been used in more than 400 samples, and it has been administered to more than 30,000 teenagers in the United States alone. The samples included males and females; younger and older teenagers; normal, delinquent, psychiatrically disturbed, and physically ill adolescents; and urban, suburban, and rural adolescents in the United States. The questionnaire has been translated into fifteen languages, and normative data have been collected in Australia, Israel, West Germany, Italy, Bangladesh, Taiwan, Japan, Hungary, and Turkey.

Our particular operational approach rests on two basic assumptions. First, it is necessary to evaluate the functioning of the adolescents in multiple areas, since they can master one aspect of their world while failing to adjust in another. Second, the psychological sensitivity of adolescents is sufficiently acute to allow us to use their self-descriptions as a basis for reliable selection of subgroups. Empirical work with the questionnaire has supported both assumptions (Offer et al. 1981a, 1984).

We used standard scoring methodology to analyze and interpret the OSIQ data. Normal is, therefore, a standard score of 50, with a standard deviation of 15. Our 1979 and 1980 samples were used to establish norms ($N = 1,385$). Any adolescent whose score in any scale is below 46 has a significantly poorer self-image in the area the scale covers. The opposite, though, in the positive side, is true for any adolescent whose score in any scale is above 54. Norms were derived separately for thirteen- to fifteen-year-old males, thirteen- to fifteen-year-old females, sixteen- to nineteen-year-old males, and sixteen- to nineteen-year-old females (for a detailed description, see Offer et al. 1981a).

There were no statistically significant differences between the 1979 and 1983 studies.

The 130 items on the questionnaire cover eleven content areas and five different "selves":

Psychological self 1—impulse control;
Psychological self 2—emotional tone (mood);
Psychological self 3—body image;
Social self 1—social relations;
Social self 2—morals;
Social self 3—vocational and educational goals;
Sexual self—sexual attitudes and behavior;
Familial self—family relations;
Coping self 1—mastery of the external world;
Coping self 2—psychopathology (symptoms);
Coping self 3—superior adjustment.

In 1983, as part of a larger epidemiological study, data were gathered from 356 adolescents in a suburban high school in the Chicago area and two Roman Catholic parochial high schools in Chicago's inner city. The students in the Chicago suburban high school were a random sample from the entire high school; they were tested in their homes in the community. Eighty-seven percent of the students sampled took part in the research. The Roman Catholic parochial high school students, sampled in 1983, were drawn from representative classes in those high schools, and almost every student asked to cooperate did so. One was an all-white, and the other one was an all-black, high school.

In 1983, the study also included a survey on drug abuse, mental health utilization, delinquent activities, relations with parents, demographic data, and open-ended questions. I will report only on results utilizing the OSIQ and mental health utilization.

RESULTS: GENERAL FINDINGS

The psychological self of the normal adolescent.—The results from our study clearly indicate that it is normal among young people in our culture to enjoy life and be happy with themselves most of the time. The adolescents do not feel inferior to others (peers included), and

11

they do not feel that others treat them adversely. The normal adolescent also reports him- or herself to be relaxed under usual circumstances. They believe that they can control themselves in ordinary life situations and have confidence that, when presented with novel situations, they will find themselves prepared.

In another area—body image—the data indicate that normal adolescents feel proud of their physical development, and the vast majority of them believe that they are strong and healthy. The implication is that positive psychological self goes along with a feeling of physical health. We did find that adolescent girls were less satisfied with their body image than the boys; they also were more sensitive to the feelings of others.

The social self of the normal adolescent.—The highest endorsed item in the whole test—"A job well done gives me pleasure"—shows the work ethic in its purest form. Judging by the adolescents' responses, in our culture, it is a universal value. The adolescents are unreservedly work oriented. They say they will be proud of their future profession. It is as if they believe that there is a job waiting for them, ready to be taken when they are ready to take it. Work is part of their everyday world. Similarly, they also state that they do not wish to be supported for the rest of their lives. As a group these adolescents see themselves as making friends easily and believe that they will be as likely to be successful both socially and vocationally in the future.

The sexual self of the normal adolescent.—In general, our findings show that normal adolescents state that they are not afraid of their sexual feelings and impulses. Seven out of ten adolescents state that they like the recent changes in their bodies. Both boys and girls strongly reject the statement that their bodies are poorly developed. The majority of the boys and girls indicate that they had a relatively smooth transition to more active sexuality. Eight out of ten subjects say no to the statement, "The opposite sex finds me a bore." A majority of the subjects state that it is important for them to have a friend of the opposite sex.

The familial self of the normal adolescent.—The normal adolescents surveyed do not perceive any major problems between themselves and their parents. The adolescents do not present any evidence that there is a major intergenerational conflict. The generation gap so often written about is not in evidence among the vast majority of these subjects. Not

12

DANIEL OFFER

only do these teenagers have positive feelings toward their parents, but their parents share the good feelings. In addition, both sides expect that these positive feelings will persist in the future.

The coping self of the normal adolescent.—The normal adolescents are hopeful about their future, and they believe that they can actively participate in activities that will lead to their success. They seem to have the inner strength to motivate them and to put their belief in themselves into constructive action. They are optimistic, and they enjoy challenges; they try to learn in advance about novel situations. The normal adolescents have the willingness to do the work necessary to achieve. They like to put things in order. Moreover, even if they fail, they believe that they can learn from it. The normal adolescents deny having psychiatric signs and symptoms.

On the whole, the adolescents see themselves without major problems. However, that does not mean that everybody in our normal samples said he or she did not have problems. There is a significant minority who do not feel as secure about their coping abilities. Our data indicate that about one out of five normal adolescents feels empty emotionally and finds life an endless series of problems without solution in sight. A similar number of adolescents state that they are confused most of the time.

DISTURBED ADOLESCENTS' SELF-IMAGE

For contrast, we would like to present the self-image of anorectic girls. We do have self-image profiles for the majority of the psychiatric syndromes and want to present these data only as illustrating the range of differences between the normal and disturbed adolescents that we have found in one specific group.

The anorectic girls have a considerably disturbed self-system, although the younger girls seem healthier than the older ones (see figs. 2 and 3). The reasons for these differences are beyond the scope of this paper but are discussed in Casper and Offer (1981) and Koenig, Howard, Offer, and Cremerius (1984).

In a recent study, Offer, Ostrov, and Howard (1981b) have shown that mental health professionals, including psychiatric residents, psychiatric nurses, psychiatric social workers, and clinical psychologists, who work with adolescents (ages thirteen to fifteen), tend to think that

13

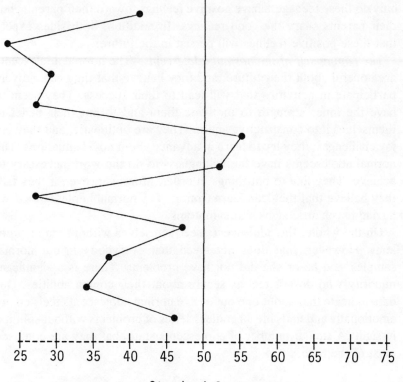

Standard Scores

FIG. 2.—Offer Self-Image Questionnaire (OSIQ) standard score profile: older female anorectics. *PS*, psychological self; *SS*, social self; *S × S*, sexual self; *FS*, familial self; *CS*, coping self. *PS*-1, Impulse Control (41); *PS*-2, Emotional tone (23); *PS*-3, body and self-image (29); *SS*-1, social relationships (27); *SS*-2, morals (55); *SS*-3, vocational-educational goals (52); *S × S*, sexual attitudes (27); *FS*, family relationships (47); *CS*-1, mastery of external world (37); *CS*-2, psychopathology (34); *CS*-3, superior adjustment (46). Numbers in parentheses are standard score values for each scale. Data collected by Drs. Casper and Swift, 1977–1983.

normal teenagers are as disturbed and as unhappy as hospitalized, psychiatrically ill teenagers (see figs. 4, 5). The perception of the mental health professionals was remarkably similar to that of investigators who adhere to the turmoil theory of adolescence. To quote Oldham (1978), "The clinician who views adolescence as a period of inevitable turbulence and disruption will approach the problem differently from colleagues who regard normal adolescence as characterized by stability."

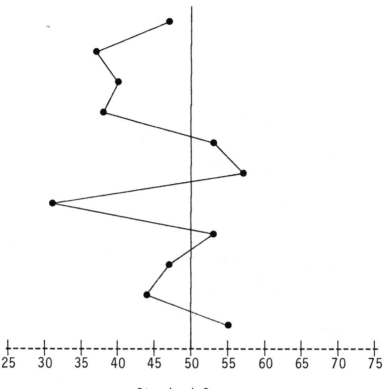

Standard Scores

Fig. 3.—Offer Self-Image Questionnaire (OSIQ) standard score profile: younger female anorectics. *PS*, psychological self; *SS*, social self; *S × S*, sexual self; *FS*, familial self; *CS*, coping self. *PS*-1, impulse control (47); *PS*-2, emotional tone (37); *PS*-3, body and self-image (40); *SS*-1, social relationships (38); *SS*-2, morals (53); *SS*-3, vocational-educational goals (57); *S × S*, sexual attitudes (31); *FS*, family relationships (53); *CS*-1, mastery of external world (47); *CS*-2, psychopathology (44); *CS*-3, superior adjustment (55). Numbers in parentheses are standard score values for each scale. Data collected by Drs. Casper and Swift, 1977–1983.

MENTAL HEALTH UTILIZATION

The question arises of what proportion of psychiatrically ill youths seek or obtain professional help. A review of the literature revealed only two studies of help-seeking behavior among adolescents. One study (Leslie 1974) was conducted in Britain; it concluded that "the parents of twenty-four out of the sixty-seven children with psychiatric

15

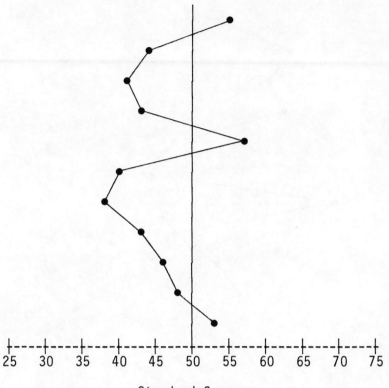

Standard Scores

Fɪɢ. 4.—Offer Self-Image Questionnaire (OSIQ) standard score profile: mental health professionals' concept of the normal younger adolescent male. *PS*, psychological self; *SS*, social self; *S × S*, sexual self; *FS*, familial self; *CS*, coping self. *PS*-1, impulse control (55); *PS*-2, emotional tone (44); *PS*-3, body and self-image (41); *SS*-1, social relationships (43); *SS*-2, morals (57); *SS*-3, vocational-educational goals (40); *S × S*, sexual attitudes (38); *FS*, family relationships (43); *CS*-1, mastery of external world (46); *CS*-2, psychopathology (48); *CS*-3, superior adjustment (53). Numbers in parentheses are standard score values for each scale. Data collected by Dr. Offer, Chicago, 1979.

disorder (or 36 percent) had not sought advice at any time; some did not perceive abnormality, but others did not know of anyone who would help with such problems." The other study (Kellam, Branch, Brown, and Russell 1981) presents even more dramatic results. According to these authors, an adolescent's acceptance of an offer of help through counseling was associated not with how disturbed the adolescent was

16

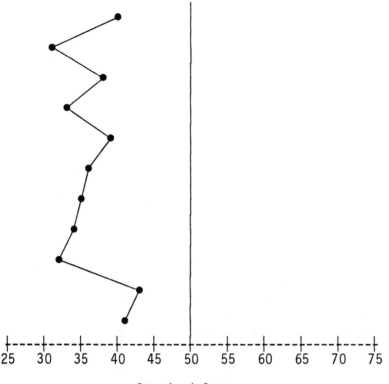

Standard Scores

Fig. 5.—Offer Self-Image Questionnaire (OSIQ) standard score profile: mental health professionals' concept of the normal younger female adolescent. *PS*, psychological self; *SS*, social self; *S* × *S*, sexual self; *FS*, familial self; *CS*, coping self. *PS*-1, impulse control (40); *PS*-2, emotional tone (31); *PS*-3, body and self image (38); *SS*-1, social relationships (33); *SS*-2, morals (39); *SS*-3, vocational-educational goals (36); *S* × *S*, sexual attitudes (35); *FS*, family relationships (34); *CS*-1, mastery of external world (32); *CS*-2, psychopathology (43); *CS*-3, superior adjustment (41). Numbers in parentheses are standard score values for each scale. Data collected by Dr. Offer, Chicago, 1979.

but with the characteristics of the persons offering the help. The implication seems to be that many adolescents in need of help probably do not receive it, particularly when it is left up to them to initiate and carry through on the help-seeking behavior.

In the 1983 study, we discovered that approximately 20 percent of the adolescents had a significantly disturbed self-image (see table 1).

TABLE 1

PERCENT OF MALE AND FEMALE ADOLESCENTS IN
THREE CHICAGO COMMUNITY HIGH SCHOOLS WHO
WERE DISTURBED (1983 Study)

	Disturbed (%)
Male ($N = 156$)	17
Female ($N = 170$)	21

NOTE.—Disturbed was defined in terms of an adolescent's being 1 SD or more lower than the norming group average on three or more of eleven Offer Self-Image Questionnaire (OSIQ) scales. All other adolescents were considered normal. The numbers of subjects throughout the tables differ slightly among the tables because of problems with missing data.

It is of interest to note that recent studies of adults (Freedman 1984) have found a similar percent of disturbed adults. Only half of those who said that they were emotionally troubled had ever consulted a mental health professional. Psychiatrists constituted only 24 percent of those delivering mental health service to adolescents (see table 2).

The 1983 study demonstrates that a significant minority (20 percent) of adolescents in our culture are psychiatrically disturbed. This figure is a general one that cuts across gender, ethnic, and social class factors. Viewed nationally, though, that percentage represents a very large

TABLE 2

THE MENTAL HEALTH PROFESSIONAL:
WHO DELIVERS THE CARE IN THREE CHICAGO
COMMUNITY HIGH SCHOOLS?
(1983 Study)

Profession	Of the Students Who Do Receive Care, Who Delivers the Care? (%)
Psychiatrist	24
Psychologist	15
Social worker	66
Alcoholism or drug abuse counselor	5
Other (i.e., minister)	7
Total	117
Overlapping usage*	17

* Students who used more than one type of help or who were referred from one professional to another.

number of teenagers. Currently, there are approximately 17 million adolescents (fourteen to eighteen years old) in the United States. If 20 percent are disturbed, nearly 3.4 million may require some kind of intervention. Our results suggest that of those, 1.7 million have received mental health care at some time during high school. This includes teenagers who consulted a mental health professional only once or twice plus those who received extensive therapy. The remaining 1.7 million adolescents have not received any mental health care or have not been disturbing enough to attract attention during the adolescent years. Thus, 1.7 million adolescents are in need of mental health care and do not receive it. Future research should determine why some adolescents receive help and others with identical symptoms and psychopathology do not. We are also studying the value systems of adolescents and their parents in the communities described above. Thus, we should be able to map out a meaningful intervention approach for disturbed adolescents in the future.

Another way of looking at the problem of mental health care delivery is cross-sectionally. Using the recent study by Taube et al. (1984), we find that, at any one time, 800,000 adolescents in the United States are receiving outpatient mental health care from either private mental health practitioners or from organized (public) clinics. This is 4.7 percent of the total adolescent population and considerably below the percentage of adolescents who are in need of mental health care.

SEXUAL BEHAVIOR

In a study on sexual behavior done by us in the spring of 1984, we randomly selected a group from among adolescents present in two suburban high schools on a particular day (for a description on the methodology of this study plus further details about the results of the project refer to Ostrov, Offer, Howard, Kaufman, and Meyer [1985]). The major findings were that, by their seventeenth birthdays, 37 percent of the girls and 53 percent of the boys have had sexual intercourse (see table 3).

Sexual activity in adolescence is strongly related to aspects of the teenager's home life and scholastic status. Teenagers who live with both natural parents are less likely to have had sexual intercourse (43 percent) than are other teenagers (64 percent). This finding is especially true for girls. Teenagers who are growing up with both natural parents

19

TABLE 3
ADOLESCENT SEXUAL ACTIVITY: PERCENT OF
ADOLESCENTS WHO HAVE HAD SEXUAL
INTERCOURSE IN 1984 BY AGES THIRTEEN,
FOURTEEN, FIFTEEN, SIXTEEN, AND SEVENTEEN

	% HAVING HAD SEXUAL INTERCOURSE	
AGE	Boys	Girls
13* ...	9	1
14* ...	15	2
15* ...	29	8
16† ...	39	16
17‡ ...	54	37

* Based on the full sample of 202 boys and 255 girls who were all fifteen years old or older.

† Based on the subsample of 147 boys and 170 girls who were sixteen years old or older.

‡ Based on the subsample of 81 boys and 105 girls who were seventeen years old or older.

are more likely to look to their family for gratification and support than are other teenagers. They also are more likely to have internalized the values of their parents with respect to their own behavior. Findings with regard to perceived parental harmony reinforce this impression. Of teenagers who perceive their parents as getting along very well, 47 percent have had intercourse, while among those perceiving their parents as not getting along well, 68 percent had intercourse. It is evident that adolescents' home environment has an important effect on their sexual behavior.

The data also show that only about one-third of the teenagers who are performing at an above-average level in school have had sexual intercourse. In contrast, 60 percent of the teenagers who are performing at an average level or below report having had intercourse. For teenagers to do well in school requires a substantial commitment of time. Consequently, in the suburban middle-class environment, achieving students may have less available time to engage in the amount and kind of social activity that would be required to develop a sexual relationship or are more socially isolated. It may also be the case that scholastically achieving teenagers are more reluctant to engage in behavior that might result in adverse social consequences, such as pregnancy or the contraction of a venereal disease.

ADOLESCENT SUICIDE

Between 1956 and 1976, adolescent suicide has increased dramatically in the United States. There has been a 300 percent increase in adolescent male suicide and 200 percent in adolescent female suicide. In the same period, there has been a decrease in suicide among people over sixty-five. It has been the opinion of some epidemiologists that this increase in adolescent suicide will continue to soar. This has not, however, been the case. Holinger and Offer, in a series of studies over the past five years, had predicted in 1980 that the suicide rate among youths would slowly decline over the coming decade (Holinger and Offer 1981, 1982, 1984, 1986). As data from the *Vital Statistics of the United States* have shown, the suicide rate among youths (ages fifteen to twenty-four) between 1977 and 1982 has indeed decreased (see table 4). Holinger and Offer developed a population-model hypothesis to explain these changes.

Focusing on the proportion of adolescents relative to the remainder of the population, they have looked at the cohort theories of Murphy and Wetzel (1980) from a different perspective by showing that the post–World War II baby boom has provided us with an unusually large

TABLE 4
SUICIDE RATES AMONG THE YOUNG, 1977–1983:
FIFTEEN- TO TWENTY-FOUR-YEAR-OLDS

Year	Rate
1977	13.6
1978	12.4
1979	12.3
1980	12.3
1981	12.3
1982	12.1
1983	11.7

SOURCE.—Holinger and Offer (1985).
NOTE.—Rates are calculated per 100,000 population.

adolescent population over the past twenty years and that both social and economic distress and, consequently, higher suicide rates in this group have resulted. Now that this group has moved on to young adulthood, the suicide rates for adolescents (and the crime rates from juvenile delinquency) have begun to fall.

Holinger and Offer's theory lends itself to a more flexible approach to suicide rates within a given cohort as it ages, rather than a fixed view, such as the one espoused by Hendin (1982). Whereas Hendin's view predicts continued increases as the baby-boom cohort moves into old age, Holinger and Offer's view by contrast is consonant with the observed data (namely, decreasing suicide rates in the elderly) by explaining that an increased proportion of the elderly—relative to the rest of the population—can bring about better legislation (e.g., Medicare, Medicaid), and thereby the quality of life for the elderly is improving sufficiently to cause decreased suicide rates.

Holinger and Offer's emphasis on "period effects" (i.e., events impinging on a cohort at any given time) rather than on "cohort effects," as though they were static over a given cohort's lifetime, provides a theoretical view that fits the data. Hence, we should expect to see further decline in suicide rates among youth during the next decade.

Although the rate has decreased slightly in the past few years, it is important to remember that adolescent suicide is extremely devastating from the point of view of years lost to the person and in the tragic impact it has on the families of the adolescents.

Our data are related to Brenner's (1971, 1979) and Easterlin's (1980) work. Brenner demonstrated that indicators of economic instability and insecurity, such as unemployment, were associated over time with higher mortality rates, including suicide and homicide rates. His explanation for this association was that the lack of economic security is stressful—social and family structures break down, and habits that are harmful to health are adopted. Some data show that suicide, homicide, and accident rates run parallel over time and may all reflect self-destructive tendencies to some extent. Brenner's model suggests a reason for the parallel rates—economic cycles. Easterlin has related population increases and decreases in economic conditions among adolescents, which correspond clearly to the decreases and increases, respectively, of the youthful population data.

It should be noted that these epidemiologic data appear to be consistent with data from questionnaires and interviews with samples of the normal adolescents presented above. In studying thousands of adolescents, Offer et al. (1981a, 1984) noted that the self-image of adolescents was better in the early 1960s than in the late 1970s for every category tested except the sexual sphere. These differences correspond closely to the smaller numbers of adolescents in the late 1950s and early 1960s and the larger numbers of adolescents in the mid to late 1970s. The cycle began to change in the 1980s as the self-image began improving again.

Discussion

A variety of developmental theories explain the psychosocial development of adolescence. Differences in tone among these theories should not obscure important theoretical differences among the various systems. For example, Piaget (1968) wrote about the adolescent as a philosopher who ponders his place in the world and struggles with his attempts to make sense of life. In contrast, psychoanalysts (Blos 1961; H. Deutsch 1967; Erikson 1959; A. Freud 1946) describe the adolescent as an ascetic, introspective, idealistic person who challenges the "truths" of his elders and suffers from inner turmoil.

Our data support none of these interpretations. We believe, instead, that each theory explains aspects of the psychology of certain adolescents but that none is universal enough to explain the psychology of adolescence in general. In another study (Offer and Offer 1975), we have found three developmental routes describing "normal" middle-class American adolescents, and our findings thus stress diversity rather than one common route for development common to all mentally healthy or normal adolescents.

Some questions concerning adolescent development have to be considered more broadly. What are the crucial childhood variables that predict functioning during adolescence? Similarly, what factors during adolescence hold the key to correct predictions later in adulthood? The etiology of both mental health and mental illness is multifactorial and multidimensional. No one factor, or even group of factors, can be singled out in isolation as causing one or the other. The factors are part of the biopsychosocial system, and they continually interact with one another. The relationship of the factors change as their relative values change over time. Furthermore, no two generations or cultures can reasonably be expected to be identical with one another, so that

23

it is imperative that we compare the adjustment of different groups of adolescents along the time dimension as well as the social, psychological, and biological ones.

The normal adolescents we studied are hopeful, positive, and future oriented. The vast majority of these teenagers function well, enjoy good relationships with their families and friends, and accept the values of the larger society. In addition, most report having adapted without undue conflict to the bodily changes and emerging sexuality brought on by puberty. The only notable symptom that we encountered among normals was a situation-specific anxiety that normal adolescents can handle without undue trauma. Once the biological-genetic factors have been controlled for, the best psychological innoculation against possible future psychiatric problems is a mentally healthy and well-functioning family system. As we have seen in our studies, this aspect of adolescent life best differentiates normal adolescents from the variety of disturbed adolescents (Offer et al. 1984).

Conclusions

There is no question but that extremely stressed teenagers who are in the midst of severe adolescent turmoil do exist. By their own self-report, 20 percent were among our group of normal adolescents. These 20 percent are disturbed and in need of help. These figures indicate that turmoil and maladaptation are a real and important part of many teenagers' lives. A disturbed youngster is not helped when his mood swings are inaccurately seen as predictable, his negative affect as typical, and his extreme rebellion as understandably normal. It is a disservice to the deviant and disturbed adolescents who are in need of psychiatric care and are denied this help by mental health professionals who blithely assert that these adolescents are just "going through a stage."

Diagnostic work with adolescents has always been difficult. In part, the difficulty has been in distinguishing serious psychopathology from mild crisis. But the facts are that a severe identity crisis or emotional turmoil is not just a part of "normal" growing up. By further understanding the behavioral and psychosocial complexities of normal and disturbed adolescents, we should be able to get one step closer to solving the mystery of adolescence.

REFERENCES

Ariès, P. 1962. *Centuries of Childhood*. New York: Vintage.

Block, J. 1971. *Lives through Time*. Berkeley, Calif.: Bancroft.

Blos, P. 1961. *On Adolescence*. New York: Free Press of Glencoe.

Brenner, M. H. 1971. *Time Series Analysis of Relationships between Selected Economic and Social Indicators*. Springfield, Va.: National Technical Information Service.

Brenner, M. H. 1979. Mortality and the national economy: a review, and the experience of England and Wales, 1936–76. *Lancet* 2:568–573.

Casper, R. C.; Offer, D.; and Ostrov, E. 1981. The self-image of adolescents with acute anorexia nervosa. *Journal of Pediatrics* 98(4): 656–661.

Csikszentmihalyi, M., and Larson, R. 1984. *Being Adolescent*. New York: Basic.

Deutsch, H. 1967. *Selected Problems of Adolescence*. New York: International Universities Press.

Douvan, E., and Adelson, J. 1966. *The Adolescent Experience*. New York: Wiley.

Easterlin, R. A. 1980. *Birth and Fortune*. New York: Basic.

Erikson, E. H. 1959. Identity and the life cycle. *Psychological Issues* 1:1–171.

Freedman, D. X. 1984. Psychiatric epidemiology counts. *Archives of General Psychiatry* 41:931–933.

Freud, A. 1946. *The Ego and the Mechanism of Defense*. New York: International Universities Press.

Freud, A. 1958. Adolescence. *Psychoanalytic Study of the Child* 16:225–278.

Hendin, H. 1982. *Suicide in America*. New York: Norton.

Holinger, P. C., and Offer, D. 1981. Perspectives on suicide in adolescence. *Social and Community Mental Health* 2:139–157.

Holinger, P. C., and Offer, D. 1982. Prediction of adolescent suicide: a population model. *American Journal of Psychiatry* 139:302–307.

Holinger, P. C., and Offer, D. 1984. Toward the prediction of violent deaths among the young. In H. S. Sudak, A. B. Ford, and N. B. Rushforth, eds. *Suicide in the Young*. Boston: Wright.

Holinger, P. C., and Offer, D. 1986. The epidemiology of suicide, homicide and accidents among adolescents: 1900–1980. In R. Feldman, ed. *Advancements in Adolescent Mental Health*. Greenwich, Conn.: JAI.

Kellam, S. G.; Branch, J. D.; Brown, C. H.; and Russell, G. 1981. Why teenagers come for treatment: a ten-year prospective epidemiological study in Woodlawn. *Journal of the American Academy of Child Psychiatry* 20:477–495.

Kett, J. F. 1977. *Rites of Passage: Adolescence in America, 1790 to the Present*. New York: Basic.

Koenig, L.; Howard, K. I.; Offer, D.; and Cremerius, M. 1984. Psychopathology and adolescent self-image. In D. Offer, E. Ostrov, and K. I. Howard, eds. *Patterns of Adolescent Self-Image*. San Francisco: Jossey-Bass.

Leslie, S. A. 1974. Psychiatric disorder in the young adolescents of an industrial town. *British Journal of Psychiatry* 125:113–124.

Murphy, G. E., and Wetzel, R. D. 1980. Suicide risk by birth cohort in the United States, 1949–1974. *Archives of General Psychiatry* 37:519–523.

Offer, D., and Offer, J. B. 1975. *From Teenage to Young Manhood: A Psychological Study*. New York: Basic.

Offer, D.; Ostrov, E.; and Howard, K. I. 1981a. *The Adolescent: A Psychological Self-Portrait*. New York: Basic.

Offer, D.; Ostrov, E.; and Howard, K. I. 1981b. The mental health professional's concept of the normal adolescent. *Archives of General Psychiatry* 38:149–152.

Offer, D.; Ostrov, E.; and Howard, K. I. 1984. *Patterns of Adolescent Self-Image*. San Francisco: Jossey Bass.

Oldham, D. G. 1978. Adolescent turmoil: a myth revisited. *Adolescent Psychiatry* 6:267–282.

Ostrov, E.; Offer, D.; Howard, K. I.; Kaufman, B.; and Meyer, H. 1985. Adolescent sexual feelings and behavior. *Medical Aspects of Human Sexuality* 19(5): 28–44.

Piaget, J. 1968. *Six Psychological Studies*. New York: Vintage.

Taube, C. A.; Burns, B. J.; and Kessler, L. 1984. Patients of psychiatrists and psychologists in office-based practice: 1980. *American Psychologist* 39(12): 1435–1447.

Vaillant, G. E. 1977. *Adaptation to Life*. Boston: Little, Brown.

Waddington, C. H. 1957. *The Strategy of the Genes*. London: Allen & Unwin.

Webster's New Collegiate Dictionary. 1951. 2d ed. Springfield, Mass.: Merriam.

Westley, W. A., and Epstein, N. B. 1969. *The Silent Majority.* San Francisco: Jossey-Bass.

CAROL C. NADELSON

While women have made great strides in obtaining access to careers in male-dominated fields, including medicine, in the past few decades, they have had a long history of active participation. Women were known to have been physicians in ancient Egypt, Greece, and Rome. They founded hospitals during the Crusades, and by the tenth and eleventh centuries women formally studied medicine at the University of Salerno, Italy. They did not, however, receive an official medical degree until the fifteenth century (Corner 1937).

The history of these early women physicians is not well known. During the eleventh century, a woman "physician," Trotula, wrote texts on obstetrics and gynecology and headed a department of diseases of women. She was regarded as one of the finest academicians of her time. Hildegard of Bingen was another notable medieval medical woman who wrote textbooks for the nurses in charge of Benedictine monasteries and in them demonstrated an understanding of normal and abnormal psychology.

The beginning of the fifteenth century saw the birth of a new "feminism." A group of literary women, who were critical of traditional views of femininity and female roles, challenged male authority on that subject. The fact that most of us have not heard about Christine de Pisan and her eloquent discourse in *The Book of the City of Ladies* perhaps reveals more about those who write history than those who make it.

By the end of the fifteenth century, as formal medical training became established in various centers in Europe, the movement to exclude women gained momentum, and women were specifically limited to functioning as midwives. This reflected wider societal attitudes that were made explicit in the *Malleus Maleficarum* (A.D. 1486), a document that essentially sanctioned witch hunting and emphasized the "spiritual and mental" inferiority of women. Even when this movement subsided, women found themselves eliminated from roles in medical care, other than traditional caretaking ones or those that involved the treatment of women.

In the seventeenth and eighteenth centuries in the colonial United States, the healing role of women was critical to survival. At this time, there were relatively few formally trained physicians. The first American medical school, founded in 1765 at the University of Pennsylvania, excluded women. By the nineteenth century, although women were barred from "regular" medical training, many were trained and practiced in the homeopathic or eclectic traditions.

When Elizabeth Blackwell (1821–1910), the first woman to be admitted to a regular medical school in the United States, was awarded her medical degree from the Geneva Medical School, the New York State Medical Association censured the school. In 1850, Harriet K. Hunt (1805–1875), who had established herself in an "irregular" practice in Boston, applied for admission to Harvard Medical School. She was accepted but denied her seat after the class threatened to leave if she were admitted. It was not until almost 100 years later, in 1946, that Harvard Medical School began to admit women (Nadelson and Notman 1978).

The resistance to women in medicine is not surprising if we consider prevailing attitudes about women at the time. An 1848 obstetrics textbook stated, "She [woman] has a head almost too small for the intellect but just big enough for love" (Shryock 1966). The president of the Oregon State Medical Society in 1905 noted that "hard study killed sexual desire in women, took away their beauty, brought on hysteria, neuroasthenia, dyspepsia, astigmatism, and dysmenorrhea." "Educated women," he added, "could not bear children with ease because study arrested the development of the pelvis at the same time it increased the size of the child's brain and therefore its head. This caused extensive suffering in childbirth" (Bullough and Voght 1973).

The founding of three all-female, "irregular," proprietary medical colleges in the United States by the middle of the nineteenth century was based more on concern about "female delicacy" than on equality of opportunity. The road continued to be difficult, even for those women who managed to obtain medical training. Women were refused admission to medical societies, and hospitals denied them appointments. The effect of this exclusion was to stimulate the development of a separatist movement. Many female physicians opened and ran their own hospitals and clinics, including Drs. Elizabeth and Emily Blackwell. In 1857 they founded the New York Infirmary for Women, which cared largely for indigent women. These separate institutions flourished until women acquired positions at male institutions and began to leave the female institutions. Many women were philosophically opposed to separatism. Many also believed that equality had been attained so there was no need for separate institutions. The view that male institutions were of higher quality also prevailed.

The role and productivity of women in medicine continued to be a topic of debate. In 1881, Rachel Bodley, dean of the Women's Medical College of Pennsylvania, surveyed the 224 living graduates of the school and found that the overwhelming majority continued to practice. Those who had married reported that their profession had no adverse effect on their marriages nor had marriage interfered with work. By 1900 over 50 percent of the students at Boston University and over 40 percent at Tufts University were women. The figures changed rapidly, however, over the next decade.

The Flexner Report of 1910 consolidated the changes that had begun in the prior fifty years and pushed medicine to become an established academic discipline, with high standards for training and practice (Flexner 1910; Ludmerer 1985). A number of proprietary and irregular medical schools were closed. Among these were many of the schools that admitted women. The number of women physicians declined and remained between 4 and 6 percent for the next half century. Between 1970 and 1975, when overt efforts were made to attract and admit women, the number of women entering medical school accelerated very rapidly (Dube 1973, 1977), and today women make up almost 40 percent of medical students (Turner 1981).

As these changes have been occurring in medicine, higher female enrollments have also been reported for other traditionally male-dominated professions such as architecture, engineering, the sciences, and law. What is evident, however, is that despite these increases, there is a wide gap between the proportion of women in professional training and those who have attained positions of prominence and leadership in their fields (Epstein 1975; Kilson 1976; Suter and Miller 1973).

One of the reasons cited for the discrepancy is that younger women may not have developed the experience necessary for leadership positions. Before we accept this explanation and become overly optimistic, we must understand historical lessons. Where women have had a significant influence, external factors often have been influential. For example, wars, physician shortages, or major cultural reorganizations have enabled women to enter medicine. This change, however, has not produced permanent attitudinal alteration in medicine or other fields. Those changes brought about by expedience or pragmatics are often erased when environmental factors shift.

The Current Status of Women Leaders: What Are the Facts?

This brief review underscores the need for us to look more closely at the current status of women in leadership positions. In academic medicine, the number of these women remains low, particularly as one ascends the academic ladder. Women also take longer than men to reach higher ranks. By 1981, 16.2 percent of medical school faculties were women physicians. They comprised 5.4 percent of professors, 13 percent of associate professors, and 19.8 percent of assistant professors (Braslow and Heins 1981). Although the number of women in medicine nearly tripled between 1968 and 1978, the proportion of women on medical school faculties increased only from 13.3 percent to 15.2 percent.

Few women serve on specialty boards or are department chairmen. Until five years ago, there were no women deans of coeducational medical schools, and currently there are none. In 1978, thirty-three women chaired academic departments out of approximately 2,400 positions; by 1980, fifty-six chairs were occupied by women, but the number of positions had also increased. More women hold chairs in pediatrics than in any other specialty; 7 percent of pediatric departments are headed by women, although 28 percent of pediatric faculty are women. Today, sixty-five chairs of medical school departments are women, but fifteen are acting or interim chairmen (Association of American Medical Colleges 1985).

31

There are parallels to medicine in other fields. In the last decade, the proportion of women in college and university administration declined both in women's institutions that have become coeducational and in women's colleges that have remained single-sex institutions (Kilson 1976). While approximately 26 percent of all college professors are women, women represent only 10 percent of full professors. The overall proportion of women faculty rose slightly in four-year institutions; however, the proportion of tenured women dropped from 17 percent in 1971–1972 to 13 percent in 1974–1975. Further, the salary differential between women and men faculty is increasing, not decreasing (Rinke 1981).

The picture is not very different in other fields. Less than 8 percent of judges, 15 percent of local elected officials, 5 percent of the U.S. House of Representatives, and 2 percent of the Senate are women. In 1984 there were 16,000 men on major corporate boards, while there were only 400 women. In spite of the dramatic influx of women into the corporate world, barely 5 percent of middle and 1 percent of top management are women.

What about women's scholarly productivity? If measured in terms of numbers of papers published, the data indicate that female scientists publish fewer papers than their male counterparts (Braslow and Heins 1981). This quantitative measure does not consider quality and scope of contribution. The number of women scientists, however, has been increasing; they have been awarded a comparably greater proportion of research grants and are represented on grant review committees, although not as much in research policy areas.

With regard to organizational positions in medicine, women have not been very actively involved in organized medicine; when they are, it is rarely as leaders. The proportion of women physicians joining the American Medical Association is about half that of men, and there have been no women American Medical Association officers. Only a handful of women have been officers of any medical specialty organizations (American Medical Association 1979).

Within medical specialization there are differences in the numbers of men and women who are board certified. This has clear implications for career advancement and leadership. Fewer than 40 percent of women physicians who finish residencies are board certified in their specialties, compared to almost 60 percent of male physicians (Rinke 1981). Further, of the officers and directors of the American Board of Medical Specialties, less than 5 percent are women (Braslow and Heins 1981).

Women's Experience in Leadership Roles

With these data in mind, let us look more closely at the issues confronting women when they pursue leadership positions. Women are generally aware, from early in life, that unanticipated and even surprising responses occur by virtue of gender-related expectations, even on the part of those who are manifestly egalitarian. Gender-related distinctions are so ingrained in our culture and in our colleagues—male and female—that change is slow. We grow up with internalized values, attitudes, and expectations that do not foster equal access.

Many authors have suggested that the socialization of males is more akin to management training than that of females. Block (1982) emphasized the importance of the fact that, in childhood, boys participate in team sports, often with those they dislike, and compete with those they like, but girls rarely do this. Girls generally play with those they like and exclude those they do not like, unless involved in active athletic participation. They feel conflicted about competition with friends.

Kagan and Moss (1962) found that childhood passivity and dependence predicted passivity and dependence in adulthood for women but not for men. They suggested that a passive, dependent boy would experience greater social pressure to suppress those behaviors, but a girl would not. Kagan noted that behavior that deviated markedly from sex-role standards would be inhibited because of a child's desire to avoid social rejection and to model himself or herself after positively valued role models.

Douvan and Adelson (1966) reported in the 1960s that boys were more likely than girls to battle over independence, behavior control, and autonomy with their families. They were motivated to separate from their parents earlier and further than were girls. Boys' vocational and sexual identities were seen as separate. In contrast, girls remained more compliant, continued dependency relationships with their parents, and did not express an intense internal need to break familial bonds. A decade later, however, another study described little difference between the sexes with respect to autonomy (Moriarty and Toussieng 1976).

Douvan suggested that the adolescent girl may be unable to correlate her hormonal changes with feeling states and that this periodicity may disrupt her development of self-concept. The cyclic, uninterpretable character of her internal cycles may make her more dependent on external information for self-direction.

Educational and occupational choices are significantly influenced by parents, peers, teachers, and counselors (Houser and Garvey 1985). Houser and Garvey found that students who were career oriented saw their parents as emphasizing and favoring that choice. Both traditional and nontraditional women selected careers that they felt were consistent with what they believed significant men in their lives favored, although a woman's career choices were influenced by the perception of her mother as a role model. Crawford (1978) noted that college seniors who were nontraditional pioneers had better-educated mothers than those who were traditional. Women who were raised by working mothers tended to be more career oriented than those who were not, particularly if their mothers had positive attitudes about employment. An individual's career choice is also influenced by locus of control, fear of success, and sex-role orientation. Those with an internal locus of control are more likely to be able to succeed in a nontraditional area. Likewise, sex-typed individuals are more motivated to keep their behavior consistent with cultural expectations, and androgynous individuals are less likely to regulate their behavior according to cultural prescriptions.

Hennig and Jardim (1977) pursued the issue of women's success as leaders from a developmental perspective. They studied a group of women managers and found that most often each was an only child or had no male siblings. They enjoyed a close relationship with an active father who did not emphasize sex roles, and both parents allowed them to develop their own interests and strengths without feeling denigrated or controlled. Although they viewed themselves as social deviants of some sort, they were successfully able to adapt to this sense of being different. As adolescents, they resented the so-called female role since it placed restrictions on them. Early in their lives, autonomous functioning without dependence on parental figures and making independent decisions became important.

Achievement-oriented girls have been reported to be less socially developed, less mature in their attitudes toward friendship, and less concerned with boys and popularity than were the more "feminine" girls (Douvan and Adelson 1966).

High-achieving women also demonstrate differences in their tolerance for being perceived as deviant. Chusmir (1985), comparing men and women managers with regard to the need for achievement and affiliation, found that executive women were higher in measures indicating need for achievement and lower in need for affiliation than men. While these data do not tell us about the origins of these traits or the behaviors they influence, they suggest that high-achieving women may be different from lower-achieving women and from men. The one longitudinal study in the literature containing a substantial number of women physicians indicated that academically achieving women reported poorer family relationships than less-achieving women, and they tended to give the worst ratings to the quality of the father-daughter relationship. This study also found that achievement was less influenced by marriage and family size than by motivational and personality factors shaped early in life. There was no connection reported between mother-daughter relationship and daughters' later career choice or development (Graves and Thomas 1985).

Rushing (1964) found that girls revealed a significant association between their aspirations and their perception of dissatisfaction with the father-daughter relationship, whereas boys did not. One interpretation is that women who perceive their fathers as distant may interpret this attitude as being a reaction to an imagined inadequacy. For such women, successful professional achievement would compensate for the personal inadequacy and help them gain paternal acceptance. Another view suggests that high-achieving women entering professional activity that is traditionally male would wish to establish closeness with their fathers through professional activity. Some of these data appear to contradict the Hennig and Jardim data and underscore the differences of opinion on the relationship between family influence and achievement.

Kanter, in her 1977 book on men and women in corporations, described the roles of women in corporations as mother, seductress, maiden aunt, or kid sister rather than colleague and peer. Milwid (1982) added a fifth category—the good daughter. Women in her study reported being deferential, and were careful to be nonthreatening and to see the men they worked with in family roles. She noted that "the psychological baggage women bring to masculine culture is packed with the need to be nice and to be liked." Those interviewed indicated that they needed to learn how to be more assertive, firm, and self-confident.

The so-called feminine characteristics of responsiveness, accommodation, and nurturance make it difficult for many women to assume and project authority. They often feel uncomfortable about relinquishing these traits or allowing the emergence of others which are characterized as "masculine." Conflict is generated between their needs for competence and success and the comfort of a socially sanctioned role. Relinquishing familiar postures, then, may be at the risk of reduction in self-esteem and loss of traditional affirmation.

As Moulton (1977) has indicated, women are accustomed to assuming a "good girl" role, often achieving success by maintaining a self-effacing facade, avoiding situations of possible disapproval, relying on authoritative directives, and not saying no. They are unaccustomed to open public rivalry or hard negotiation. Some research (Dunbar, Edwards, Gede, et al. 1979) suggests that women become anxious after asserting themselves, whereas men experience relief.

Transferential and sociocultural responses continue to be described as limiting career progress for women. Obviously, in academia as well as in corporations, new employees and faculty—male or female—may experience difficulty, particularly as they move up the ladder. Special conflicts, however, are often engendered in women when they are faced with the necessity of making unpopular decisions, defining priorities, and making choices—particularly when these represent compromises with previously held values and beliefs or when they expect to be isolated or disliked for them. This occurs in part because the internalized self-concept of most women does not include authority, assertiveness, and leadership, and it does include a great need for affiliation. Women's focus on relationships fosters increased sensitivity to criticism and a greater need for approval. This often determines their style of interacting and responding in leadership roles (Gilligan 1982).

Cultural expectations have a substantial impact on women's assumption of leadership roles. Sociologists suggest that women's opinions spark negative and resistant responses, and their credibility in positions of leadership is significantly less than men's, on the basis of their gender. Since women are socialized to achieve vicariously and to measure their success by the success of individuals to whom they are related, with whom they identify, and to whose success they have contributed, direct action on their own behalf is unfamiliar (Lipman-

Blumen 1983). In positions of authority, men predominantly lead men to whom they relate as peers and competitors; women lead men to whom they are socialized to be less assertive. These factors inevitably influence the expectations and success of women in leadership roles.

Hennig and Jardim indicate that as women evolve in their careers they develop competence associated with strict attention to their tasks. Their data show that the women desexualized relationships at work and their communications there centered on the job. A close fatherly relationship with their boss served to support and encourage them. He often became a mentor. Personal growth and satisfaction were more significant work-related goals than monetary rewards. In contrast to successful male executives, women managers tended to stay with one company through most of their careers.

The assumption of leadership roles by women is further complicated by the lack of peer support and of mentors or models functioning in similar roles or assuming equivalent responsibilities. Thus, women must cope with their own and others' resistance to their assumption of the attitudes and behaviors necessary for effective leadership, and they face conflict generated by contradictory self-perceptions and expectations.

The power of gender-role expectations is illustrated by a description of the analysis of a series of Tavistock-type group experiences held at a university undergoing major turmoil as the result of an initiative by women to gain greater access to positions of power and authority. Mayes (1979) found significant and pervasive differences in behavior depending on the gender of the group leader. In female-led groups, male members were either hostile and less cooperative or they were dependent. Men described feelings of loss of control because their ability to function "as males" was hampered, and they expressed relief and a sense of "return to normalcy" when they were able to join male-led groups. Initially, the women in female-led groups were assertive, instrumental, and task oriented. However, over time, they became "less assertive, less identified with the leader, and sought to keep male attention in a traditional manner." Women who refused to relinquish their assertive roles received the majority of male and female anger. Groups with male leaders reported traditional sex-role patterns of behavior in both men and women.

Another study emphasized that different attitudes toward male and female leaders have important implications for both perceptions and

37

actual performance (Yoder, Adams, Grove, and Priest 1985). The authors note that in order to be helpful a mentor should fill the "masculine" role of team player and possess needed information and expertise. This makes mentors powerful. Johnson (1976) found that women were perceived to be inferior to men in sources of power. It is possible, then, that potential female mentors may consider themselves to be inadequate to the role, and novices may avoid female mentors in favor of males whom they perceive to have more power. Both of these possibilities are inconsistent with the leadership qualities inherent in a mentoring relationship. Although women professionals do appear to have mentors, Roche (1979) indicated that they rarely have female mentors. Since in most fields there are few women leaders, women on either side of the relationship are in unique situations. This adds to pressures and the situation itself is anomalous.

A recent study of women leaders, including vice presidents and managers, in male-dominated fields such as banking, law, and architecture, reported that these "successful" women continued to feel excluded from office networks, increased resistance to them in higher echelons, and a sense of the intractability of male orientation and culture in their fields (Milwid 1982). Earlier in their lives, they had believed in a revolution that seemed to have been won and that gender was no longer a limitation to advancement. Few anticipated that it would be a factor that would so profoundly affect their professional development and lives.

Conclusions

These issues obviously suggest the need for ongoing investigation. It is sobering to note that a recent report issued by the National Research Council indicates that sex segregation in employment has not changed much since 1900 (Ilchman 1985). The authors suggest that 30 percent of workers would have to move into job categories dominated by the opposite sex to even things out. They conclude that women's occupational choices and preferences "play a limited role in explaining occupational segregation by sex," and they indicate that the barriers have to do with persistent effects of discriminatory laws, personnel practices, and beliefs about women's proper roles and traits. They also note that fear of sexual distraction and concern about women in supervisory and leadership positions are contributing factors. Their pessimistic conclusion is that the discrepancy in men's and women's career paths is reinforced by early rearing patterns, training programs, and even by tax structure. Thus, as I indicated earlier, change is likely to be slow.

The Red Queen's advice to Alice was that it would take "all the running you can do to keep in the same place. If you want to get somewhere else you must run at least twice as fast as that!" (Carroll 1977).

REFERENCES

American Medical Association. 1979. *AMA Council on Long-Range Planning and Development: Women Physicians in Organized Medicine* 43:729–731.

Association of American Medical Colleges. 1985. Kathleen Turner, personal communication, December.

Association of American Medical Colleges. 1986. Kathleen Turner, personal communication, August 8.

Block, J. H. 1982. Psychological development of female children and adolescents. In P. Berman and E. Rainey, eds. *Women: A Developmental Perspective*. Department of Health and Human Services, Public Health Service, National Institute of Health Publication no. 82–2298. Washington, D.C.

Braslow, J. B., and Heins, M. 1981. Women in medical education: a decade of change. *New England Journal of Medicine* 304(19): 1129–1135.

Bullough, B., and Voght, M. 1973. Women, menstruation, and nineteenth-century medicine. *Bulletin of the History of Medicine* 47:66–82.

Carroll, L. 1977. *Through the Looking Glass*. New York: St. Martin's.

Chusmir, L. H. 1985. Motivation of managers: is gender a factor? *Psychology of Women Quarterly* 9(1): 153–159.

Corner, G. W. 1937. *The Rise of Medicine at Salerno in the Twelfth Century*. Philadelphia: W. B. Saunders.

Crawford, J. D. 1978. Career development and career choice in pioneer and traditional women. *Journal of Vocational Behavior* 12:129–139.

Douvan, E., and Adelson, J. 1966. *The Adolescent Experience*. New York: Wiley.

Dube, W. F. 1973. Women students in U.S. medical schools: past and present trends. *Journal of Medical Education* 48:186–189.

Dube, W. F. 1977. Medical student enrollment 1972–1973 through 1976–1977. *Journal of Medical Education* 52:164–166.

Dunbar, C.; Edwards, V.; Gede, E.; et al. 1979. Successful coping styles in professional women. *Canadian Journal of Psychiatry* 24:43–46.

Epstein, C. 1975. Encountering the male establishment: sex-status limits on women's careers in the professions. *American Journal of Sociology* 15:6–9.

Flexner, A. 1910. *Medical Education in the United States and Canada: A Report to the Carnegie Foundation for the Advancement of Teaching*. New York: Carnegie Foundation.

Gilligan, C. 1982. *In a Different Voice*. Cambridge, Mass.: Harvard University Press.

Graves, P., and Thomas, C. 1985. Correlates of mid-life career achievement among women physicians. *Journal of the American Medical Association* 254(6): 781–787.

Hennig, M., and Jardim, A. 1977. *The Managerial Woman*. New York: Anchor/Doubleday.

Houser, B., and Garvey, C. 1985. Factors that affect non-traditional vocational enrollment among women. *Psychology of Women Quarterly* 9(1): 105–117.

Ilchman, A. 1985. *Women's Work, Men's Work: Sex Segregation on the Job*. Washington, D.C.: National Research Council.

Johnson, P. 1976. Women and power: toward a theory of effectiveness. *Journal of Social Issues* 32(3): 99–110.

Kagan, J., and Moss, H. A. 1962. *Birth to Maturity*. New York: Wiley.

Kanter, R. M. 1977. *Men and Women of the Corporation*. New York: Basic.

Kilson, M. 1976. The status of women in higher education. *Signs: Journal of Women in Culture and Society* 1:935–942.

Lipman-Blumen, J. 1983. Emerging patterns of female leadership in formal organizations: must the female leader go formal? In M. Horner, C. Nadelson, and M. Notman, eds. *The Challenge of Change*. New York: Plenum.

Ludmerer, K. 1985. *Learning to Heal*. New York: Basic.

Mayes, S. 1979. Women in positions of authority: a case study of changing sex roles. *Signs: Journals of Women in Culture and Society* 4(3): 556–568.

Milwid, M. E. 1982. Women in male-dominated professions: a study of bankers, architects, and lawyers. Ph.D. dissertation, Wright Institute, Berkeley, California.

Moriarty, A., and Toussieng, P. 1976. *Adolescent Coping*. New York: Grune & Stratton.

Moulton, R. 1977. Some effects of the new feminism. *American Journal of Psychiatry* 134:1–6.

Nadelson, C., and Notman, M. 1978. Women and biomedicine: women as health care professionals. *Encyclopedia of Bioethics*, Vol. 4. New York: MacMillan.

Rinke, C. 1981. The economic and academic status of women physicians. *Journal of the American Medical Association* 245(22): 2305–2306.

Roche, G. R. 1979. Much ado about mentors. *Harvard Business Review* 57:14–28.

Rushing, W. A. 1964. Adolescent-parent relationship and mobility aspirations. *Social Forces* 43:157–166.

Shryock, R. H. 1966. *Medicine in America: Historical Essays*. Baltimore: Johns Hopkins University Press.

Suter, L. E., and Miller, H. P. 1973. *Income Differences between Men and Career Women, Changing Women in a Changing Society*. Edited by J. Huber. Chicago: University of Chicago Press.

Turner, K. 1981. Memorandum no. 81–7 to the Women's Liaison Officers, Association of American Medical Colleges, Washington, D.C.

Yoder, J.; Adams, J.; Grove, S.; and Priest, R. 1985. To teach is to learn: overcoming tokenism with mentors. *Psychology of Women Quarterly* 9(1): 119–131.

3   DISCUSSION OF DR. CAROL NADELSON'S PRESENTATION: WOMEN IN LEADERSHIP ROLES

DOUGLAS B. HANSEN

Dr. Nadelson, as a psychiatric leader, is trying valiantly to keep up with and accommodate to the rapid cultural changes being thrust upon us. But in one of her other lives she is one of those who promote major cultural change. I was surprised that she does not sound more sanguine about the ultimate success of the women's movement. Perhaps she is pessimistic because she expected more and faster change; the statistics were not encouraging to her. Maybe she is tired from her multiple duties and ceaseless travel, or maybe she is a realist. Cultures do not readily change, and once they do they have a strong tendency to revert to original forms—a phenomenon we see around us in the world political arena. Whatever Dr. Nadelson's reasons are for pessimism, I am going to take her pessimism as the jumping-off point for my discussion.

Let me paraphrase and emphasize the highly cogent position taken by Dr. Nadelson. When women have had significant influence in medicine, and by extension I believe she would argue leadership in other areas, it has often been due to external factors. The factors she mentions are war, physician shortage, and major cultural reorganizations. These historical periods when women were prominent have not produced permanent attitudinal change in society. The flowering of woman's productivity and leadership has quickly evaporated when business as usual returns. The attitudinal changes favorable to women that occurred during these periods have faded rapidly, showing a remarkable impermanence. Dr. Nadelson's observations are that improvement in women's leadership positions has not come about evolutionarily or automatically and, therefore, there is little sense of permanent progress.

If her argument is accurate, I conclude that we must do something different than we have to maintain and further women's prominence and leadership. Dr. Nadelson is dedicated to this cause, and I am for the cause. I need to make this statement here because this is a highly charged political issue and what I say could easily be misconstrued. From a moral and ethical position I favor equality for women, and from a practical point of view our nation and the world need all the talent, brain power, and leadership we can get. It is apparent, however, that moral arguments and practical considerations have not been sufficient to advance this cause, as outlined by Dr. Nadelson.

As psychiatrists our specialty is to take a biopsychosocial point of view. We do not view persons or societies in fragmented terms. Let us apply this comprehensive psychiatric view to the problem we have posed. The causative argument for the poor position of women is often cast in social psychiatric terms. I start with the easy one because it is obvious there is prejudice against women. We all know about job and educational barriers, lack of peer supports, "old boy" networks, derisive jokes, the problems of expectations, and restrictive roles.

The psychological perspective emphasizes considerations mainly having to do with the internalization of early experiences, such as the roles played by parents, identifications, ego ideals, expectations, the responsiveness to or discouragement of emerging propensities in the child, and so forth. Considering just these aspects of the biopsychosocial spectrum, I believe that psychological programming is far more important than social in maintaining the historical problem we are discussing. I do not believe that social factors are nearly as important as we seem to suppose. Of course, I cannot prove this, but if you will bear with me I shall argue by analogy.

Waves of immigrants came to this country during the last century and all were subject to strong and open prejudice. I think it is an impressive statistical finding that many of these immigrant groups attained income levels comparable to white Anglo Saxon Protestants over a similar number of generations. They accomplished this through hard work, thrift, and emphasizing the education of their children. They did this within close-knit families with strong family values; single men and women have never done well.

There were exceptions, however. Irish immigrants, although they achieved income parity, did so at a slower rate than the other groups. Some believe this was because the Irish chose to depend on the political system for improvement of their lot and not as much on themselves with hard work, thrift, and education. Clearly, the Irish were not subject to more social prejudice and discrimination than the other groups.

Some groups, such as American blacks, have not yet achieved economic parity, and it is often said that this has to do with discrimination—a social psychiatry argument. However, other races with high visibility, such as the various oriental groups, have moved to economic parity with the same speed as the white immigrant groups despite their skin color and different culture. To crown my argument, black immigrants from the West Indies achieved economic parity rapidly and at the same rate as the Jews, Italians, Poles, and others despite their color, existing prejudice, and job discrimination. Since social psychiatric considerations in our society have not effectively impeded the success of immigrant groups, regardless of color, I would argue that psychological factors are the dominant ones in holding people back.

I believe this is an effective argument by analogy that the differences in men's and women's leadership and position are explained more by psychological variables than by social barriers and discrimination. Social barriers are obvious and unpleasant. Although not the most important within this context, they can be isolated and easily legislated against; this is not so for psychological aspects, which cannot so easily be isolated and proscribed and which occur in the heart of the family. From this you can gather that I have chosen the psychological as more important than the social in assessing the cause of Dr. Nadelson's lament that women have not maintained their leadership gains over the centuries—that there is an ebb and flow but no permanency to the attitudinal shifts favorable to women. Dr. Nadelson already discerns the ebb tide setting in.

We have yet to consider the biological dimension. I recently asked our group of third-year psychiatric residents what they could tell me about women as leaders. The majority of the group are women and include the most active participants. One attractive woman, who was embarrassed by what she said and who asked to remain nameless, responded that men make better leaders because they are more narcissistic than women. This caused a humorous reaction in the group. I was not sure why she was so embarrassed, because I agreed with her. I think that the same point is made by Gilligan (1982) in her book, *In a Different Voice,* and reiterated by Dr. Nadelson. Women specialize in relationships and keeping things together more than men. That leaves a different role for men—a less object related, less accommodating, more instrumental role that is consistent with leadership.

This leads me to the biological and psychobiological or, as Edward O. Wilson (Lumsden and Wilson 1981) would say, the sociobiological. I believe that we can find additional reasons in this discipline for the difficulty women experience in becoming and staying leaders in this and all societies, at this time and all other times.

Let me repeat, I am trying to explain Dr. Nadelson's facts; I am not trying to make a political statement. Biological explanations have historically been used and misused against women, but that is not my intent. I think we now have the outlines of new biological discoveries that can be of use to us in rational discourse.

The studies of Robert Stoller and others come to mind as differentiating males and females neurologically and thus, to an extent, psychologically. The infant psychiatrists and psychologists have opened our eyes to a vast range of phenomena of which we were ignorant until recently. The nervous system perceives selectively—prefers and attends to some things over others, and we have only begun to learn the dimensions of this discovery. It also learns some things with one or a few trials, while other things may take many repetitions or are actually unlearnable. We are programmed more than we have wanted to believe, and again man's narcissism is offended as it was successively by Galileo, Darwin, and Freud. In short, it is likely that our genes influence our perceptions, preferences, our yearnings and learning, wishes, interests, and so forth. If this is so, then our genes influence how we relate to the world and to each other, and they ultimately influence the culture we create. This is part of the hypotheses of Lumsden and Wilson (1981), which state that genes influence culture and conversely that culture influences our genes—that over the long pull culture and genes coevolve and are in many ways a package.

These authors show us it is statistically almost certain that any persistent social-psychological difference in a group will, after thirty to forty generations, become encoded in the genes as propensities and preferences. The sex-role differences in society have existed in primates and man for millions of years. The reasonable hypothesis is that the preferences, propensities, and traits that contribute to our sex roles are built into the nervous system and into our genetic code. I hasten to add that we do not know a lot about this or the practical implications such concepts hold for us. However, we do know that certain children have strong tendencies to prefer girl games and girl activities and other children prefer boy activities and objects. Occasionally this happens cross-gender, apparently driven by constitutional factors. Of course we know this can happen psychologically as well in compliant youngsters pressured in highly deviant mother-child relationships.

Using such biological and sociobiological concepts, I can argue that statistically women are biologically more prone to be interested in preserving relationships or have some precursor of this trait and conversely that in all societies girls are also socialized to preserve relationships—making biology confirm the culture and culture confirm the biology. That is, genes and culture support and stabilize each other in a conservative, slow-to-change matrix. In such a scenario, temporary cultural changes would tend gradually to revert to some basic historical norm. This is exactly the situation that Dr. Nadelson has described and chronicled in her discussion of the ebb and flow of women's position.

Conclusions

To state this again, it is highly possible that male and female differences in relatedness, dominance, and submissiveness, in preferred sexual fantasy, in preferences, subtle yearnings, and attractions are part of our evolutionary inheritance as well as early socializations. If this is so, it explains Dr. Nadelson's historical summary and answers her implied question concerning the low incidence of women leaders, our lack of success in altering the sex roles, and her discouragement that society continually reverts to old forms. It may be an old form indeed— an archtype that is encoded genetically in tastes, preferences, interests, wishes, and so forth. If so, equality defined as males and females having a similar proportion of leaders may not be a legitimate goal for us. I know that any such limitation on freedom to choose goals for ourselves is offensive to us. But we have Dr. Nadelson's facts and figures to deal with. If such gene-culture interactions prove to be a valid thesis, we may need to reevaluate our goals. In the meantime, the least we can strive for is to allow everyone's individual strivings for leadership an opportunity—a goal we can all embrace and which is perfectly consistent with my argument and the one presented by Dr. Nadelson.

REFERENCES

Gilligan, C. 1982. *In a Different Voice*. Cambridge, Mass.: Harvard University Press.

Lumsden, C. J., and Wilson, E. O. 1981. *Genes, Mind, and Culture: The Coevolutionary Process*. Cambridge, Mass.: Harvard University Press.

4   THE MYTHS AND NEEDS OF
CONTEMPORARY YOUTH

SAUL V. LEVINE

We in psychiatry and the other mental health professions have pro-pounded, propagated, and perpetuated various myths regarding normal and abnormal youth amid our patients, our media, and our public. We have adopted one major theory of normal behavior based largely on psychopathology, and, while this has had obvious advantages in en-abling us to study the behavior of people, there is little doubt that it has also constrained us in our efforts to both understand and evaluate youthful behavior.

Myths about Adolescents

1. CONTEMPORARY YOUTH ARE MORE AT RISK, MORE OUT OF CONTROL, AND WORSE OFF THAN BEFORE

While there are no doubt unique current problems, some of the comments by pundits and seers of today are no more accurate than similar comments made even centuries ago. Allow me to present some examples that will illustrate this point dramatically. In the third century B.C., Socrates said, "I see no hope for the future of our people if they are dependent on the frivolous youth of today, for certainly all youth are reckless beyond words."

In the eighth century B.C., Hesiod stated that, "Our adolescents now seem to love luxury. They have bad manners and contempt for au-thority. They show disrespect for adults and spend their time hanging around places gossiping with one another . . . they are ready to contradict their parents, monopolize the conversation in company, eat glutonously, and tyrannize their teachers."

In the second act of *A Winter's Tale,* William Shakespeare has one of his characters state, "I would there were no age between ten and three and twenty, or that youth would sleep out the rest for there is nothing in the between but getting wenches with child, wronging the ancientry, stealing and fighting."

My favorite above all, however, is a profoundly gloomy set of words carved in a 4,000-year-old tablet in the biblical city of Ur. It goes as follows: "Our civilization is doomed if the unheard of actions of our younger generations are allowed to continue."

Obviously, the more things change, the more they stay the same. In my opinion, we are not witnessing a recent deterioration in our youth, but some adult commentators have always seen youth as on the road to destruction.

2. THE GENERATION GAP IS EVER WIDENING

The generation gap was a phrase used widely during the 1960s and given its most forceful emphasis by anthropologist Margaret Mead (Mead 1970), who observed that adults were like immigrants to a new land, getting used to the novel dress, values, language, and behavior of their youth. In the 1960s, as now, this was grossly overstated. It is just not so that adolescents today are vastly different from their parents. There have been a variety of longitudinal and cross-sectional studies of youth and their parents in different cultures. Polls in the United States and Canada (Yankelovich 1974) and studies by social scientists and clinicians (Offer 1970) have shown just how remarkably convergent are the parental and adolescent generations. In religious values, political identification, mores, values, career aspirations, and economic goals—there is surprisingly close approximation in all of these areas between the adult and youth generations. Not only is this in contradistinction to commonly held beliefs; the truth is probably to the chagrin of many well-meaning adults, who secretly harbor hope that the ensuing generations will represent "better" values and goals. The 1960s saw many adults imbuing the "flower children" with just such enhanced and, as it turned out, invalid characteristics.

3. ADOLESCENCE IS A TIME OF INEVITABLE TROUBLE, TURBULENCE, AND TURMOIL

Ever since Anna Freud postulated the concept of *Sturm und Drang* as almost an inevitability of the adolescent stage, the storminess and turbulence of youth have constituted a veritable built-in expectation of adults about young people about to embark on that phase of life. We know from our clinical experience and from studies (e.g., Rosenthal and Jacobsen 1968) about the power of expectations in shaping behavior; the tail ends up wagging the dog. How many of us have had the experience of parents of wonderful prepubertal children agonizing with us over the forthcoming inevitability of disaster? A self-fulfilling prophecy is set up that bears no relation to fact. Turmoil is not only not inevitable; we have learned that most adolescents go through those memorable years fairly smoothly (Offer 1970). We should not base our conclusions about normal adolescents on those disturbed young people that we see in our offices and wards. This is not to say that there are no difficulties associated with these important formative years, but we should beware of applying the principle of universality in both our pronouncements and our prognostications without valid foundation.

4. THE 1980s CONSTITUTE THE WORST DECADE IN HISTORY FOR SOMEONE TO BE YOUNG

I have immense trouble with those doomsayers who wail a litany of woe about this age being the most oppressive to our youth. Is it worse for young people now than in World War II? Is it worse now than during the Dark Ages, or during the time of child labor, or at the turn of the century when the life expectancy in North America for adults was in the thirties? In some ways, this is the best time for our young people, especially in Western technological societies. There are more opportunities—yes, even for the adolescents we work with—than ever before. Rather than the commonly held notions of undue stressors of young people, what may make the 1980s particularly difficult for some young people is the rapidity of change and the unpredictability of the future. We live in an age now when there have been more scientific publications in the last five years than in all the preceding millennia. The technological and psychological effects of this creativity and productivity will begin to be felt only in the next decade. While we are preoccupied with the constraints offered by society on our youth, it is in fact the bewildering array of choices and ambiguities that are particularly oppressive to our young people—but not the commonly held and hackneyed oppressiveness of drugs, television, divorce, and annihilation, to name but a few common *bêtes noirs*.

5. YOUTH IS THE MOST DIFFICULT PERIOD OF LIFE

While there is no doubt that there are specific tasks of youth that must be at least addressed, if not resolved, to call this the most difficult period in the span of one's lifetime borders on the ludicrous. There are very few adults who would not gladly trade at least part of their existence for an opportunity to relive some of their adolescent years. Perhaps it is overstating it to define an adult as "an adolescent with a mortgage," but there is a point to be made—that adolescents have degrees of freedom unheard of before and perhaps never to be replicated again. It is fallacious to ascribe irresponsibility to them, but certainly, there are fewer responsibilities demanded from and owed to others. It is doubtlessly easier to be an adolescent than to be aged, or a disenfranchised, lonely, middle-aged individual, or an unemployed adult. While youth is particularly buffeted by dramatic internal changes along a variety of dimensions, we are all constantly reassessing and reevaluating ourselves in light of changing social and psychological conditions and circumstances.

6. THEY'LL GROW OUT OF IT

This particular myth is the other side of the coin of the inevitability of *Sturm und Drang;* that is, if adolescence is, in fact, merely a predictable stage that a young person will go through with difficulties, then we do not have to take their symptoms and signs seriously. We then have to simply tell parents and others that it is "just a stage," and "they'll grow out of it"; statements that I am sure most of you have heard from time to time. This contradicts longitudinal studies (Masterson 1967) and our own clinical experience. Furthermore, it is both disrespectful and invalid; we know that adolescents with problems become adults who are a population at risk. The specific symptomatic or clinical manifestations may differ depending on the age, but there is no doubt that a young person in significant trouble will not grow out of it without some kind of significant intervention. This need not take the form of psychotherapy, but the obstacles and hindrances to smooth growth and development have to be overcome via an injection of new or redirected energies.

7. IDENTITY IS RESOLVED DURING ADOLESCENCE

Eric Erikson (1968) did adolescents a favor when he postulated the concept of identity as the central task of their age. However, this is a task that adolescents only begin to grapple with during that period of life and never resolve completely. Further, identity is merely a rubric that subsumes important subtasks: impulse control (sexuality and aggression); intimacy (close friendships); independence—individuation (emotional, physical, economic); initiative—industry; ideology (values, beliefs).

Identity diffusion is not the inevitable alternative to not resolving one's identity in those years; nor is it an identity-related disorder (DSM-III 1980). Also, identity is not the sole domain of adolescents; they have not cornered the market on questions like: Who am I? Where am I going? How and why? Which adults among us, clinicians included, do not ask themselves regularly these same existential questions? We are constantly reassessing ourselves, and our self-purviews change with circumstances, our age, and the tenor of the times.

8. ADOLESCENT SUICIDE IS AT EPIDEMIC LEVELS

It is true that the suicide rate among adolescents has risen over the last three decades. It is also true that it is the number 2 or 3 cause of death in the fifteen- to twenty-four-year-old age group. We must remember, however, that there is very little, comparatively speaking, cardiovascular disease or carcinoma during that period of time; it is the most healthy period of all the years of one's life. There is also more honest and reliable reporting to account for at least some of the increase. We should bear in mind that the adolescent suicide rate has actually leveled out over the last few years, that the suicide rate is higher in the elderly and much higher among lonely middle-aged individuals. Each suicide is obviously a tragedy, especially among young people in whom promise is unfulfilled, and the pain and suffering engendered in surviving family and friends are never to be healed. But

52

all this is very different from saying that there is an "epidemic"—the word that is used in almost every newspaper headline having to do with adolescent suicide. There are specific subpopulations (like certain subsections of Native Canadian and Native American youth) among which a disproportionate number of young people do attempt and complete suicide each year. It is to these populations that extra resources should be directed. This is very different from, again, making global generalities about all adolescents as being on the verge of self-destruction. We should be wary about making alarmist statements to the media and others in order to further our cause for needed services or other resources. In the end we do ourselves a disservice, because our credibility is destroyed when the truth is revealed.

9. ADOLESCENT SUBSTANCE ABUSE AND DRUG USE ARE AT EPIDEMIC LEVELS

While the latest statistics have shown drug use and abuse to be ubiquitous among young people, the current data are, if anything, more optimistic than they were ten years ago in most American and Canadian urban centers. (The current "crack" abuse notwithstanding.) Furthermore, to pretend that drug abuse is a phenomenon of youth is surely to beg the question. Who are the diazepam and sedative casualities in our midst? Who are the alcohol users and abusers around us? Who are the cocaine users and abusers in our society? And who are the cigarette addicts? The answer to all of these questions, of course, is the adult generation. I submit to you that an adolescent who is stoned, or constantly on marijuana or hashish, has a major emotional problem but that the issue of drugs is almost an irrelevancy. Any self-respecting clinician can get them off those particular substances in very short order, but we are still left with an individual who is in dire emotional straits. Furthermore, the dealers and pushers of some of the most abused and destructive drugs throughout the world are in fact representatives of the medical profession. Once again, we have an example of parents, the media, and clinicians with vested interests in convincing the public of the seriousness of their cause, proclaiming disaster, and evoking panic. This is not to minimize an area of legitimate concern, but one should avoid responding to and spreading simplistic notions and pointing fingers at paper tigers. The use of mind-altering chemicals is now universal and necessitates worldwide concern, but cogent concentration on populations at risk as well as prevention and general education is preferable to media melodrama.

10. ADOLESCENT SEXUALITY IS RAMPAGING, RAVAGING, AND RAPACIOUS

Once again we have another example of media preoccupation doing more to alarm and effect change than to report accurately. While there is no doubt that there are now converging statistics between males and females, there are still many young people who do not feel comfortable with the pressure to perform—sometimes perpetrated by peers, parents, and publications. There is an old saying that boys use love to get sex and girls use sex to get love, and this is unfortunately still valid, especially among some younger adolescents and even young adults. But increasingly, many young people do not wish to engage in sexual intercourse before they are either married or involved in a meaningful relationship. *Playboy* magazine was talking about a "sexual revolution" in the mid-1960s, before any statistics gave credence to that as a fact: another example of expectations shaping behavior. In a review of the effects of sex education and family life education courses in English-speaking countries, we found that knowledge changed rather dramatically after the courses; attitudes—toward others—changed in a more liberal (tolerant) direction, while behavior changed almost not at all. We do have problems in some populations with early teenage pregnancies, venereal disease, and other kinds of sex-related issues like exploitation and destructiveness. But to raise red flags and state with certainty that these problems are ubiquitous or universal is to mislead and to misguide and, further, to deprive those individuals who are really at risk of needed services and resources.

11. YOUTH UNEMPLOYMENT IS THE ISSUE FOR ALL YOUNG PEOPLE

There is no doubt that we have a major unemployment problem, with double-digit figures of unemployment for young people between the ages of sixteen and twenty-five. However, to pronounce that we need universal make-work programs or occupational subsistance programs for all young people is ludicrous, expensive, and invalid. There is no doubt that, for an individual who wants to work and needs to work, to be unemployed is demoralizing and degrading. This is particularly true in a middle-aged individual who has dependents to support. When we are talking about young people, however, such notions do not always apply to the situation. The youth unemployment statistics are augmented by individuals who work for a while and then stop, who work and get unrecorded money, who work part-time, or who do not really want to work. It is obvious that we have too many people who are able-bodied, want to and need to work, who cannot get jobs and suffer the psychological and other consequences of that situation; however, most of these people are not youths.

To the extent that we do have a youth unemployment problem, more than 60 percent of our youth unemployment statistics are accounted for by less than 20 percent of our youth population. The young people who make up those double-digit unemployment statistics can be identified early in elementary school. These are potential school dropouts who have difficulties with literacy, structure, rules, and social relationships. These young people can be picked out as early as in grade 1 to grade 11 as being on a downward spiral. What we do not need are mass universal assistance programs for all young people. What we do need is nothing short of a Head Start program, taking the enormous resources (that are promised by all the political parties for all young people) and diverting them to those specific subpopulations who particularly require those resources of money and personal support. Failing that, we are using superficial tactics to approach deep wounds, which will do nothing to prepare our vulnerable young people for the future.

12. YOUTH ARE OVERWHELMED BY THE SPECTER OF NUCLEAR ANNIHILATION

Another area of intense concern to many of us is the psychological effects of the specter of nuclear war on our developing youth. Surveys are reported that appear to show large numbers of adolescents seemingly preoccupied with nuclear annihilation. Again, this is contrary to most clinical experience. In collating thousands of letters in our nationally syndicated column directed at Canadian young people, we found that not one writer ever discussed the arms race or related subjects as causal or contributory to their concern. Certainly if young people are asked questions directly about their concerns about nuclear war, they will, as they should, respond with fear and loathing. Many of us are members of organizations aimed at nonproliferation of nuclear armaments; we have to be especially careful about making critical pronouncements to our patients and youth in order to vent our own political persuasion. I am not suggesting that acne and girlfriends are the only concerns of young people; far from it; but it is a far cry from saying that many young people are overwhelmed or stunted in terms of their own emotional growth and goals because of the nuclear arms race. As a matter of fact, youthful involvement in antinuclear campaigns can serve as an ideological rallying cry and become an important growth and therapeutic vehicle for them.

13. TELEVISION IS DESTROYING OUR YOUTH

Television is blamed for illiteracy when our population is more literate than ever before. It is blamed for violence (it is estimated that most young people see 13,000 murders on television prior to reaching adulthood) at a time when the level of violent crimes in our society has, if anything, diminished on a per capita basis over the last few years. It is blamed for suicide, at a time when suicide rates seem to have leveled off and when there is little evidence to support the correlation between television watching and self-destructive tendencies. Television violence and sexually suggestive television have been blamed for many social problems, but the evidence is underwhelming. Even supportive laboratory experiments have not been generalizable to the community. There is no doubt that lowest-common-denominator content is served up to young people who sit like mindless blobs watching the stuff, which is probably written by upper-middle-class literates. What is most destructive about television, however, is not the behavior that it engenders but rather the passivity and vegetation it generates. But that is no reason to blame television for all the ills of youth and society.

14. YOUTH ARE VICTIMS OF SOCIAL OPPRESSION AND MUST BE PROTECTED

To blame society entirely for the ills of youth is to avoid teaching them responsibility and accountability. Youth are no more victims than are the rest of us. Youth are also the benefactors of society's advances. In fact, the majority of crimes of violence on the streets are perpetrated by young people. While hurting young people have to be helped, dangerous youth have to be controlled. Our own track record with out-of-control youth is abominable. I am a firm believer in discipline and consequences; justice must not only be done but must be seen as being done by the public at large. Society must have the sense that it is being protected from the young people who, for whatever reason, are destructive and dangerous. Just as society can be oppressive to youth, so too can some youth be oppressive to society.

15. MISCELLANEOUS MYTHS

There are many other myths that we propagate; we should be careful about ascertaining the facts rather than elaborating our fantasies. Is youth the age of narcissism? Are youth more narcissistic than we are? From what we have found in our syndicated column, there is a "paradox of narcissism" that makes for excrutiating personal gain. If individuals are so narcissistic as to feel that their preoccupations and conflicts are exquisite and unique, they never get the opportunity to share them with others or check whether they are shared by other people. In these instances, narcissism breeds inevitable suffering.

Another myth is that we have harried and hurried children as a result of our parental generation pressure to perform adult tasks too early. While a spate of recent books has appeared about this, there is very little factual evidence to support that theory.

Anyone shopping in the northeastern United States for dairy products will conclude from the milk cartons that we have an epidemic of missing children. The myth is that abduction abounds. When one looks at the statistics, it turns out that many of these are runaways who return home within a few weeks or months; very few are the victims of diabolical or degenerate psychopaths. The media preoccupation, however, and public proclamations give the impression of panic in the streets and an epidemic to be confronted. It is wise to warn our children about avoiding the seductive offers of strangers, but the obsession with street proofing turns ours into a paranoid culture.

Much has been written about the exploitation of young people by cults. While this culture has certainly contributed to those concerns, the fact is that we are talking about a minuscule proportion of the youthful population and one which, when all is said and done, comes back home. Again, reading media accounts and other public pronouncements, one gets the impression that our youth are there for the taking by the prevalent malevolents of the world.

And there are still other myths. Why do we provide a steady diet of destruction and demise? Why do we have to become alarmists in order to get desired changes, benefits, and legislation for our youth? We set up the expectations to fulfill our prophecies, and we engender panic in many cases. We end up losing our credibility when those who have the pursestrings in their control ask us to provide accurate data. We do not have to prophesy danger, degradation, and demise in order to achieve our aims and objectives. It is invalid and demeaning to us.

Needs

After this discussion of various myths about adolescents, let us go on to look at the needs of youth from a developmental and experiential perspective.

1. LOVE

Adolescents, like children, need an abundance of love. While this may sound like a cliché and even trite to some individuals, if child rearing is not performed in a context of caring, one might as well forget civilized behavior among our youth. It is no accident that Freud included the capacity to love (give and receive) as one of the mainstays of normality. Erikson postulated that love plays a major role in an infant's earliest experience of trust. The contention that love is not enough is, of course, valid. It is not sufficient, but it is absolutely necessary in the development of our youth. (In a context of love, paradoxically, parents can get away with terrible behavior; in love's absence, nothing can supplant love.)

2. SPACE

Youth need space, physical as well as emotional. They need room to develop, room to learn about oneself and one's limits, as well as one's potential, space to make mistakes, to experiment with one's life. This refers also to time to develop. We cannot, as parents, clinicians, and authority figures, constantly be exerting pressure and putting constraints and our expectations on young people. They need space to engage the world and themselves in order to take advantage of opportunities. Space, then, refers to physical, as well as emotional and temporal, dimension.

3. PEERS

Most adolescents need peers for development, to measure them-selves, to monitor their progress, to size themselves up, to test out their ideas and behaviors vis-à-vis others, and to experiment with new forms of ideas in relation to themselves and their parents (Douvan and Adelman 1977). These social experiences are vital in the development and maturation of youth. The friendships made through adolescence are clearly some of the best and most poignant intimacies ever expe-rienced. Individuals may be separated by many years and by many miles, yet, given the choice of an individual with whom they can com-mune almost immediately, many adults choose those precious friend-ships made during adolescence. The necessity for peers during adolescence has been used in both intervention and various forms of social therapies, including positive peer counseling and self-help groups. Intentional social systems and communal experiences are particularly effective with deviant young people.

4. TRADITION

We are so preoccupied in this day and age with the present and future that we often relegate the past to some forsaken role. The identity-related question, "Who am I?" also implies, "Whence do I emanate?" One's heritage is vital in defining one's present identity. In order to make a gestalt of one's life, his or her past, ethnic, religious, and familial roots become ever more important. Enriching rituals of childhood and adolescence are temporal and social milestones that enable people to savor memories of their past and come to grips with their rapidly chang-ing present. Even if the young person is going to rebel against the traditions that have been taught, at least he or she has something to come up against. The nebulousness and ambiguity of nothingness do not provide one with traditions to learn about one's past and, therefore, make it impossible to define the present.

5. LIMITS

Another need is limits. If one cannot envision child rearing in the absence of love, it is equally impossible to consider bringing up children without any degrees of limitations or constraints. After all is said and done, adolescents do need nonnegotiable noes; they need limits and "thou shalt not" bottom lines. I have them, you have them, why should they be different? This is part of their development, of learning about themselves and society. Behavior and misbehavior cannot always be rationalized, reduced to psychodynamics, explained away, or excused. At some point, responsibility has to be taken. To demand adapting to social rules is, in fact, doing young people a service. This goes for every society and every social system. To provide limitations is a prerequisite for civilizing our youth.

6. THE AVAILABILITY OF ADULTS

In our experience, one of the most common complaints of young people is that they perceive that adults are not interested, or not available, or that adolescents cannot talk to them. Whether this is real or imagined is probably less relevant than their perception of the validity of that feeling. It is true that adults are sometimes too busy, too preoccupied, too involved to have enough time for their adolescents. We are not discussing here only the availability of parents. We can all think of important adults like aunts and uncles, teachers, or others who played major roles, even if fleeting, in our own development and directions. A subsidiary need to available adults is models and mentors. Many of us can think of important adults who play a major role in defining our choices. This is equally true for young people who are in dire emotional straits or in conflict with society. I can think of no better example than the individual who sets the protagonist in new exciting, constructive, and prosocial directions (see Brown 1965). As clinicians and teachers, we often do not recognize the pivotal role we sometimes play for young impressionable individuals who may benefit from our enthusiasm, forward thinking, and dedication to a way of life.

Discussion

While I have decried the principle of universality in condemning young people to all be suffering from the same blights of maldevelopment and social oppression, there is a spectrum of needs and problems that disproportionately afflicts some young people. There is a role for the principle of universality, but not as patch-up, isolated, or ineffective generalized programs. The principle I am propounding is that it should be ensured that all young people benefit from the opportunities for education, vocation, and recreation, irrespective of socioeconomic class or background. As a wealthy society, it is incumbent on us to make resources available so that all our young people are imbued with a sense of optimism and enthusiasm regarding their country, their society, and, above all, themselves.

The need for belief and belonging are higher order needs for all young people (Levine 1979). This is an area that has been given little attention by clinicians and theoreticians. Adolescents are potentially highly motivated, with an enormous amount of energy that can be captivated and committed to creativity and productivity. We have seen numerous examples in recent past generations that, in times and regions of external conflagration, indices of social deviance and deterioration among young people (hospitalization, imprisonments, suicides, etc.) diminish when they get involved in outer-directed meaningful movements that give them a belief system. This ideological thrust, together with a powerful supportive group, has been exploited in institutions such as the Peace Corps, Vista, Cuso, and Katimivak. These serve prosocial and developmental needs, but belief and belonging can also be utilized in therapeutic communities for preventive, remedial, and rehabilitation purposes. To the extent that we can captivate and mobilize our young people in constructive directions, it will reflect not only on us as a society but also on them in their believing in themselves. To the extent that creativity becomes meaningless to us, in that our sole *raison d'être* remains acquisitiveness, competition, and materialism, then there will always be groups with overriding philosophies and ideology that will attract many young people who are not satisfied (Levine 1981).

Conclusions

As opposed to a litany of woe, there has to be a realistic view of difficulties, to be sure, but there has to be a light at the end of the tunnel, a payoff, if you will. A reward clinically is, certainly, that our patients will improve. From a broader perspective, we have to hope that our domestic and social interventions do, in fact, work and contribute not only to the growth of the individual but also to society as a whole. From the perspectives of society, it is obvious that we can afford to be optimistic about our young people in particular and about ourselves and our society in general. It is important to remember that our young people need us because we are their foundation; but we need them because they are our future.

REFERENCES

American Psychiatric Association. 1980. *Diagnostic and Statistical Manual of Mental Disorders. (DSM-III.)* 3d ed. Washington, D.C.: APA.

Brown, C. 1965. *Manchild in the Promised Land.* New York: Macmillan.

Douvan, E., and Adelson, I. 1977. Adolescent friendships. In J. J. Conger, ed. *Contemporary Issues in Adolescent Development.* New York: Harper & Row.

Erikson, E. 1968. *Identity: Youth and Crisis.* New York: Norton.

Levine, S. V. 1979. Adolescents, belief and belonging. *Adolescent Psychiatry* 7:41–53.

Levine, S. V. 1981. Cults and mental health: clinical conclusions. *Canadian Journal of Psychiatry* 26:534–539.

Masterson, J. 1967. *The Psychiatric Dilemma of Adolescence.* New York: Arm Hill.

Mead, M. 1970. *Culture and Commitment: A Study of the Generation Gap.* Garden City, N.Y.: Doubleday.

Offer, D. 1970. *The Psychological World of the Teenager.* New York: Basic.

Rosenthal, R., and Jacobsen, L. 1968. *Pygmalion in the Classroom.* New York: Holt, Rinehart & Winston.

Rutter, M.; Graham, P.; and Chadwick, O. 1976. Adolescent turmoil—fact or fiction. *Journal of Child Psychology and Psychiatry* 17:35–56.

Secretary of State. 1985. *Social Trends Analysis Directorate.* Ottawa: Government Printing Office.

Yankelovitch, D. 1974. *The New Morality: A Profile of American Youth.* New York: McGraw-Hill.

5 ARTHUR RIMBAUD: THE POET AS AN ADOLESCENT

DAVID A. HALPERIN

Arthur Rimbaud, the nineteenth-century French poet, early captured the literary imagination to assume a unique status within the literary pantheon. He has provided generations of literary-minded adolescents with a striking benchmark for achievement and creative fecundity. Withal, his total withdrawal from the world of letters at the age of nineteen—his total refusal to participate in creative literary activity after that age (Starkie 1947)—has presented continuing questions and abetted his elevation as a quasi cult figure.

Rimbaud is considered one of the greatest French poets of the nineteenth century. However, he was a poet whose work has been influential throughout our Western literary culture. He helped to create new paths in literature and foreshadowed the concerns and even the language of poets as diverse as Paul Claudel, Hart Crane, Andrei Mayakovsky, and Allen Ginsberg. Along with Baudelaire, Rimbaud introduced into the world of poetry the use of scientific and industrial metaphor and a willingness to consider the moral, social, and psychological issues created by the urban technological world that was being created in his contemporary France. Rimbaud's influence was to be reflected in artistic movements as diverse as Surrealism, Futurism, and Symbolism.

Yet he self-consciously renounced any artistic concerns at the age of nineteen and thereafter lived the life of an adventurer and explorer. This chapter will explore this monumental act of literary renunciation within its cultural context and as a reflection of the problems Rimbaud faced in his transition from adolescence to maturity within a tumultuous and rapidly changing environment.

As the psychoanalyst attempts to explore artistic creativity and the relationship between the artist and his creations, Freud's (1908) dictum that "analysis can do nothing towards elucidating the nature of the artistic gift, nor can it explain the means by which the artist works— artistic technique," seems particularly relevant. His recognition of the limits of the perceptions afforded by psychoanalysis—"he lays down arms before the problems of the creative [artist]"—seems particularly appropriate in attempting to explore the questions raised in the lives of those figures, such as Rimbaud, whose genius manifested itself at an early age. Moreover, the exploration of these issues is particularly difficult in the case of Rimbaud because he saw himself and was seen by his contemporaries and literary successors as a figure of archetypal importance.[1]

Verlaine considered Rimbaud to be *le poet maudit* (the accursed/ damned poet), and this aura of being a uniquely accursed individual helped to create an atmosphere in which every aspect of Rimbaud's life assumed larger-than-life proportions. This mythic quality has been enhanced by the very intensity of Rimbaud's poetry, which conveys a cogency and a relevance that is quite unexpected when we consider it as the creation of an adolescent boy who was born in the provincial, drab, industrial frontier town of Charleville in northern France on October 24, 1854. This quality is alluded to by Schmidt (Rimbaud 1975), who comments that, as he prepared the translations,

> Rimbaud seemed to me a kind of mirror, and my early translation of his poems were essays in narcissism. It was a childish preoc-cupation: I set myself the task of entering his strange world as I perceived it; to seek his path even where the wind at his heels had effaced it. I came at least to see his life as incidents in a life that we—he and I—somehow, somewhere shared. My own adoles-cence was swallowed up in the new one his poems revealed to me. [P. xiv]

Thus, like all great art, Rimbaud's poems enable the reader to reeval-uate and appreciate with renewed intensity significant aspects of his own life. But, as we examine the manner in which life was transmuted into art, we must not fall into a reductionist fallacy that robs the artist of his uniqueness.

Rimbaud's genius did not lie exclusively in his invention but in his ability to appropriate the intellectual and artistic currents that were reflected in the endeavors of lesser figures (Starkie 1947). He utilized popular intellectual currents such as mysticism and occultism in the service of his own artistic and personal needs. It is intriguing to examine the manner in which he selected otherwise eccentric and irrational elements of the popular culture of his day in the expression of his uniquely personal themes. While his work has been characterized as expressing "a limited and familiar core of themes—a child, a child as a poet, and the absence of a mother's love—love was denied by his own mother, and we find it denied by women again and again in his poems" (Schmidt, in Rimbaud 1975, p. 4). But it is important to recognize that the very absence of certain issues or themes from his work is also a matter of significance.

The Poet in His Family

Rimbaud's father was a remarkable man for his period. The son of peasants, he rose through the ranks of the French army to become the political officer and governor of a region in the then newly conquered Algeria. During his twenty years in Algeria, he was able to master Arabic, and he subsequently translated the Koran into French. In the aftermath of the Revolution of 1848, he was transferred back to metropolitan France. He met and married Vitalie Cuif, Rimbaud's mother, while posted to the barracks at Charleville. Aside from his translation of the Koran, later literary projects such as memoires of his military service never materialized.

Rimbaud's mother was the daughter of prosperous farmers. She was a pious, rigid, Catholic woman who appears to have been endowed with social aspirations and the peasant's traditional financial caution. She has not had a good press either in Rimbaud's poems or in the recollections of his friends. But it was to her farm that Rimbaud returned throughout his life. Its serenity is reflected in his beautiful nature poetry. And it was there (in the barn) that he wrote his major work, *A Season in Hell (Une Saison en Enfer)*.

Jean-Arthur Rimbaud was the second of four children. An older brother, Frederic, was born a year after his parents' marriage. Mrs. Rimbaud apparently identified him with her own wastrel brother, and

Frederic was later to become a day laborer. Arthur had two younger sisters, both of whom had literary interests. Vitalie's diaries are a major source of information about Rimbaud's life. Isabelle idealized Rimbaud and later nurtured him through his terminal illness. Her husband ultimately became one of Rimbaud's literary executors (although her refusal to record Rimbaud's final words, which she described as being "so beautiful but so strange," has always seemed to be a final victory of prudery over poetry).

Nineteenth-century France fostered a culture in which literary concerns and literary figures were given an importance that contrasts with the relatively peripheral position writers have always been given in American society.[2] The intensity and the depth of its literary culture are exemplified by the fact that Rimbaud's first poem, *Ver Erat* (*It Was Springtime*), was written as a classroom exercise in which students were expected to develop Latin verses on the theme presented by an ode of Horace. The Rimbaud family shared these literary concerns, particularly as the rewards and opportunities available then to a literary prodigy can be compared only to the status afforded in modern America to top athletes and rock stars.

Rimbaud's parents' marriage was unhappy. His earliest memory was of his mother and father struggling over a large silver urn that fell to the ground, emitting a frightening sound as it fell. This early memory dramatically presents the conflict between his parents. It also dramatizes the conflict within himself. In a sense, his adult life's erratic course may be seen as part of the process of resolution of his conflicting identifications between his father's life as man of action (albeit with literary pretensions) and his mother's literary expectations as a vehicle for her social aspirations.

Rimbaud's maternal grandfather died when he was five. His youngest sister, Isabelle, was born soon after. Then, when he was six, his father deserted the home. There is no record of any further contact between them. The only possible literary reference to him may occur in a composition that Rimbaud wrote when he was ten (Schmidt, in Rimbaud 1975, p. 5): "My father was an officer in the King's Army [the composition is set in sixteenth-century France] . . . His character was quick, fiery and he was often angry and would not stand for anything that displeased him. . . . Oh. How many times he promised money, toys, treats, once even five francs, if I could read something for him. . . ."

In this remarkable school composition, he notes his father's interest in his studying the classics and, prophetically (later in the essay), his resentment toward Rimbaud's studying "dead languages." Nonetheless, to be involved in literature is clearly presented as a means of obtaining his father's approval. As Esman (1984) has noted, the flowering of the adolescent artist is facilitated by an identification with an idealized father or father surrogate, a dynamic process that presents itself repeatedly during Rimbaud's creative evolution.

During this essay, Rimbaud describes his mother as "sweet, quiet, upset at very little yet maintaining perfect order in the house." He was later to view her control and her need for "perfect order" in a very different light as exemplified by the anger and rage rampant in his *The Poet at Seven* (*Poet à Sept Années*). But, during his prepubescent years, Rimbaud, superficially at least, appreciated his mother's investment in his literary abilities. In this regard, their relationship is quite consonant with Greenacre's (1957) formulation that: "Genius is a gift of the Gods, already laid down at birth . . . a sport development which finds especially favored soil for its evolution in families where there is good inheritance and favorable background for identification" (p. 9). But, in assessing the role psychodynamic factors play in encouraging the flowering of artistic factors, Ehrenpreis (1984) notes that:

> . . . it is one mark of genius that the work transcends the circumstances of the life. The most detailed familiarity with a poet as son, husband, and father need not equip one to judge his poems. When a poet endures a troubled life, is his talent part of the illness, or is it his spring of health?
>
> Reaching for themes and images, into his most intense and profound experience, does the poet reflect the sufferings that he peculiarly endures, or does he give body to intuitions shared by all suffering men?

This caveat is particularly applicable to the poetic work of Rimbaud.

Early Poems

His first poem in his *Collected Poems*, "The Orphan's New Year" (*Les Étrennes des Orphelins*), illustrates this problem. On first inspection, it is a rather sentimental poem. Written when he was thirteen,

67

Rimbaud exhibits in it one of the major themes that mark his later work—the absence of maternal love. But this poem should be considered in the context of other almost contemporaneous works such as "Feelings" (*Sensation*) or "The Blacksmith" (*Le Forgeron*). In "Feelings," his relationship with women has a more playful spirit: "And I will wander far, like a wild vagabond, throughout nature—happy as if I had a girl."

In "The Blacksmith," Rimbaud identifies with the new revolutionary egalitarian and more aggressively masculine world that was soon to express itself in the *Commune*. The appeal of Rimbaud lies, in part, in his ability to express the multiplicity of feelings that surface during adolescence. As these poems illustrate, Rimbaud feels the absence of maternal love and wishes that he could playfully wander with a young girl. He attempts to deny the impact and pain of separation from the past by discovering an independent and viable past of his own. The multiplicity of themes—of his trying out a variety of objects for identification—shows Rimbaud as an adolescent attempting to clarify his feelings and create a more cohesive sense of his own identity. What is remarkable even in these early poems is his directness of expression wherein his poetry becomes a vehicle in which to sort out his aspirations from his confusion.

Rimbaud's father was both a man of action and a man of letters. For Rimbaud, his poetry was an aspect of his identification with his vanished father. But it was also a vehicle for his being accepted within the world of adult men. The transition from the expression of tender feelings toward women expressed within his early poems and his later misogyny may reflect his search for acceptance from this male world. And, in this period of transition, he was influenced by a succession of ill-disguised surrogate fathers.

The first of these figures was Georges Izambard, a teacher at the *collège* (high school) in Charleville. Izambard was a radical for the period. He gave Rimbaud copies of the subversive writing of Victor Hugo (then in exile in England for his radicalism). The pious Mme. Rimbaud disapproved of this self-proclaimed anticlerical and freethinker. Rimbaud idealized Izambard and regarded him as a heroic representative of the counterculture. On his side, Izambard regarded Rimbaud as an intellectual equal. The intensity of their relationship and some measure of Rimbaud's hunger for masculine approval is indicated in his letter to Izambard that ends, "I love you like a brother,

I will love you like a father" (Schmidt, in Rimbaud 1975, p. 47). And, most curiously to a modern sensibility, despite the intensity of his letters to Izambard, there has never been any suggestion of a sexual liaison between Rimbaud and Izambard.

In the midst of this ferment, when he was fifteen, despite Izambard's advice (although with his implicit support), Rimbaud ran off to the Paris of his dreams. This episode marks the beginning of his fevered creative activity. His first stay in Paris lasted only a few weeks. In a subsequent letter to Izambard, he described how he was arrested as a vagrant and placed in jail. He was finally released in Izambard's custody and returned to live with him and his two maiden aunts in Douai for a few weeks. Needless to say, Rimbaud's mother was very unhappy over this entire incident (Schmidt, in Rimbaud 1975, p. 37).

He returned to live with his mother. But this return home was brief. He soon fled again to visit Izambard. This second elopement was a happy trip that he subsequently celebrates in poems in which Nature appears as a teasing but seductive country wench. It was during this trip that Izambard introduced him to a friend, Paul Démény—a poet who had already achieved recognition and whose modern importance appears to lie in his having been the recipient of many of Rimbaud's most important letters and poems. Démény regarded Rimbaud with a sense of equality for his obviously burgeoning intellectual gifts and poetic abilities. This second episode was finally terminated as Rimbaud was forced to return home at his mother's insistence, humiliatingly under police escort.

Early Creative Maturity

At fifteen, Rimbaud was on the threshold of his creative maturity. In attempting to appreciate the interaction between his personal growth and subsequent artistic development, the psychoanalyst is faced with the remarkable problem that while these issues are raised with other artists during a period of years or even decades, for Rimbaud, all of his development as a poet is telescoped into weeks or months and documented primarily in a few short letters. Nonetheless, despite the mythology that has grown up around Rimbaud, it is possible to see the youth beyond the poetic mask.

In July 1870, Napoleon III undertook the Franco-Prussian War. His decision was taken lightheartedly and without any apparent appreciation of the potential catastrophe that was to be realized. In October 1870, the Germans occupied Charleville (indeed, after the war Charleville lay just inside the French border). Rimbaud had just returned home from his second visit with Izambard. Throughout that winter, Rimbaud remained at home in enforced idleness—school had been suspended. In his poems of this period, for example, "Angry Caesar," he glorified the revolutionary French past and the heroic resistance of the French revolutionary armies in 1792 against the invaders. The spirit within these poems is strikingly contemporary and reminiscent of the work of Bob Dylan and other protest poets of the 1960s. The actual armistice was signed in January 1871, and in February, Rimbaud took advantage of this cease-fire to elope, again, to Paris.

Rimbaud wandered around a Paris that was ready to explode into the *Commune*. In the aftermath of the debacle, France was split between a revolutionary Paris and the provinces. There was a sharp cleavage between the representatives of radical change (Marx was to hail the *Commune* as a harbinger of worldwide revolution) and the representatives of the established orders under Thiers, at Versailles. During these chaotic weeks, Rimbaud wandered in a city without controls. And it was during these weeks that he underwent an experience that he never explicitly described but was presumably a homosexual rape. This experience formed the basis of his poem, "The Stolen Heart" (*Le Coeur Volé*), which he sent to Izambard in a letter dated May 13, 1871:

The Stolen Heart
My weeping heart on a deck drools spit;
They soil it with cigarette butts,
They spatter it with slop and shit;
My weeping heart on the deck drools spit.
The soldiers drink and laugh at it;
The sound of laughing hurts my guts . . .
Soldiers' cocks are a black burlesque;
They rape my heart with what they say. . . .

The poem is an extraordinary cry from the depths of a violated humanity. It was soon after this incident (March 1871) that he returned to Charleville.

Starkie (1947), in her definitive biography of Rimbaud, considers this incident to be "... the turning point of his development, and [one] would have traced to it the source of much of his later maladjustment and distress. It is only after this experience that we find in him a disgust of life, an inability to accept it as it is, coupled with a desire to escape reality. ..."

On his return to Charleville, Rimbaud began to neglect his personal hygiene—he wandered around the city and cried a great deal while distancing himself from his friends. He describes his sense of alienation in his letter of May 13, 1871 to Izambard: "I is an other . . . You are no teacher for me. I give you the following: is it satire, as you would say? Is it poetry? It's fantasy anyway. But I beg you, don't underline in pencil, nor too much in thought" (the poem "The Stolen Heart" follows). Rimbaud concludes with "That does not mean nothing" (Schmidt, in Rimbaud 1975, pp. 100–101). Izambard's response to this letter was to treat the poem as satire and parody it. He was obviously incapable of dealing with the intensity of Rimbaud's feelings.

Long-range diagnosis is always a risky business. Nonetheless, given the limitations of attempting to diagnose an illness at a distance in time, place, and person, it seems quite clear that after this incident in Paris, Rimbaud suffered a depression that appears to have been of psychotic proportions. A note of caution is in order, however, because Rimbaud was a youth of extraordinary articulateness and was acutely sensitive to the "normative" depressions that attend the process of separation and transition during adolescence. Indeed, Schmidt (Rimbaud 1975) notes that the characteristic word Rimbaud uses throughout his poetry is *saison* (season), a reflection of his and the adolescent's sense of the transitory. Rimbaud himself rationalizes his self-neglect and his lack of hygiene as an act of initiation into being a poet. Yet the acts speak eloquently for themselves even as they are consciously described in his letter of May 13, 1871, to Izambard:

Right now, I'm depraving myself as much as I can. Why? I want to be a poet, and I am working at making myself a visionary: you won't understand all, and I'm not even sure I can explain it to you. The problem is to attain the unknown by disorganizing all the senses. The suffering is immense, but you have to be strong, and to have been born a poet. And I have realized that I am a poet. It's not my doing at all. It's wrong to say I think. Better to say: I am thought. . . . [Rimbaud 1975, p. 100]

And in a letter to Paul Démény, he developed these ideas at greater length:

A poet makes himself a visionary through a long, boundless, and systematized disorganization of all senses. All forms of love, of suffering, of madness; he searches himself, he exhausts within himself all poisons, and preserves their quintessences. Unspeakable torment, where he will need the greatest faith, a superhuman strength, where he becomes among all men the great invalid, the great criminal, the great accursed—the Supreme Scientist for he attains the unknown. [Rimbaud 1975, p. 102]

In both letters, the poet is a figure of greatness, but he also is a figure who must undergo unspeakable degradation in order to realize his exalted vocation. Rimbaud rationalizes his "madness" and his "disorganization of the sense" as part of the price he must pay to successfully complete the mission he has undertaken. However, his joining the poet's vocation to his own very real suffering may also represent his attempt to find a redeeming value in the suffering he had experienced. Rimbaud's need for the "greatest faith, a superhuman strength" reflects his sense of himself as having become "among all men the great invalid." These letters describe in existential terms his profound depression and sense of worthlessness. Rimbaud sought the vocation of poet prior to these experiences, but this vocation was now transformed into the central part of a process of reconstruction.

After Izambard's parodying rejection, Rimbaud sought out a new surrogate father. He found one on August Bretagne—"the old priest"— a self-described mystic, student of the occult, and poet (his actual occupation was tax collector). Bretagne introduced Rimbaud to the works of Eléphas Lévy, whose *Histoire de la Magie, Les Clefs des Grands Mystères,* and *Dogma et Rituel de la Haute Magie* were widely read and influential popularizations of cabalistic ideas.

Interest in occultism was very strong in nineteenth-century France and America. And, as Zweig (1970) has noted, both Baudelaire and Rimbaud considered themselves to be "alchemists of the word." The redoubtable Enid Starkie feels that many of the obscurities of his verse and Rimbaud's poetic theories are cabalistic in origin. While Rimbaud's interest in these relatively esoteric ideas may simply reflect his participation in the intellectual concerns of his day, the resort to magic and occultism may also be an attempt to find a solution for personal problems. Rimbaud utilized cabalistic ideas to provide a structure for his poetry (much as did Yeats), but this should not blind us to the real possibility that his resort to magical ideas was an attempt to find magical solutions to his severe depression. Rimbaud's focus on the transitory and evanescent character of adolescence highlights his concern with the process of separation and individuation that forms so much of the burden of adolescents. And like modern adolescents, who sometimes deal with these issues by resorting to gnostic and similar species of "magic," Rimbaud embraced gnosticism to find a sense of continuity within a transitory world (Halperin 1983; Weber 1983).

Gnosticism is a complex phenomenon. An intriguing aspect of gnosticism is its emphasis on the androgynous nature of the divinity. This was in marked contrast to the authoritarian and patriarchal character of France during the Second Empire. Perhaps it was through gnosticism that Rimbaud was able to reach the following perception in a letter to Paul Démény dated May 15, 1871: "When the eternal slavery of Women is destroyed, when she lives for herself and through herself, when man—up till now abominable—will have set her free, she will be a poet as well" (Rimbaud 1975, p. 103).

The importance for Rimbaud of a woman's finding an independent vocation as opposed to being forced to realize her aspirations through man may be a veiled reference to his mother's overinvestment in his literary career as a means of realizing her social aspirations. Indeed, in gnosticism's emphasis on the androgynous nature of divinity, Rimbaud may have sensed the possibility of a pathway toward establishing more fulfilling relationships with women.

In poetry, Rimbaud found a vehicle for his entry into the adult world of men. Here, he was not unique. In late nineteenth-century France, there was a sense of the fraternity of artists—of artists being united against the Philistines. The famous painting by Fantin-Latour, *The Corner of the Table* (which hangs today in the Jeu de Paume of the Louvre), memorializes this spirit in its depicting a group of poets around a café table, including the "angelic" Rimbaud in the corner. A letter to Théophile de Bainville (whose memory is preserved primarily by a statue in the Luxembourg Gardens) expresses a similar spirit with its "Gentlemen of the Press, I will be upon action," that suggests that Rimbaud viewed the literary world as a select and esoteric social club. It was in this social context that Auguste Bretagne introduced Rimbaud to Paul Verlaine.

Auguste Bretagne suggested that Rimbaud send Verlaine copies of his poems. Verlaine was so impressed that he invited Rimbaud to visit him in Paris. Rimbaud met Verlaine in September 1871; he was sixteen. At their first meeting, Rimbaud presented Verlaine with his poem, "The Drunken Boat" (*Le Bateau Ivre*). It is an extraordinary work. Certain themes are notable:

> I drifted on a river I could not control
> No longer guided by the bargemen's ropes.

Within Rimbaud's world, he feels a profound inability to control himself or his direction. Nor are adults capable of providing direction because of their own vulnerability:

> They [the bargemen] were captured by howling Indians
> Who nailed them naked to colored stakes.

The presence of the Indians indicates a fascination with the primitive and uncivilized. It foreshadows his later journey to the "Heart of Darkness." But, characteristically, Rimbaud's response to this world without meaningful guidance and where rage may be expressed without control is to transmute his fears into a passivity that he hopes will enable him to reach some realm of transcendent beauty:

> Now I drift through the Poem of the Sea;
> This gruel of stars mirrors the milky sky,
> Devours green azures; ecstatic flotsam,
> Drowned men, pale and thoughtful, sometimes drift by.

As his identification with the thoughtful drowned men indicates, the fundamental affect of the poem is dysphoric. His depression is highlighted in the final stanza:

> Washed in your langors, Sea, I cannot trace
> The wake of tankers foaming through the cold,

74

> Nor assault the pride of pennants and flags,
> Nor endure the slave ship's stinking hold.

Given his turmoil in the aftermath of the events in Paris and his severe depression, it is hardly surprising that a relationship with Verlaine appeared to offer great opportunities. At its outset, Verlaine was involved in a superficially stable marriage with access to financial support and the possibility of providing Rimbaud with access to established literary circles and literary acceptance. Starkie (1947) has suggested that the homosexual affair was begun at Rimbaud's insistence. And, when his depression and need for support are considered (particularly after his humiliating rejection by Izambard), this is not surprising. However, given Verlaine's age (ten years older) and much greater experience of the world, the question of who initiated the relationship is more open.

What is certain is that the course of their relationship was extremely stormy. It lasted for two years. It was punctuated by numerous interruptions, followed by frequent reconciliations and subsequent desertions. They fled from Paris to Brussels, from Brussels to London, and back to Paris. Much of their time together was spent in drinking absinthe, smoking hashish, and arguing about Verlaine's expressed interest in returning to his wife, son, and wealthy in-laws. Separations and reconciliations were frequent. On one occasion, Rimbaud's mother met Verlaine's mother to discuss how to deal with their sons' peregrinations. During one of Rimbaud's separations from Verlaine, he returned home to his mother's farm. It was there, in the barn, that he wrote the only book he published during his lifetime—*A Season in Hell* (*Un Saison en Enfer*). He wrote this series of poems while sequestered in the barn, exempted from all family and farm chores by the woman he held in contempt—his mother.

Final Poems

A Season in Hell is an extraordinary work. It is an extended series of meditations on the poet's life and on the modern world. Formally, it is a series of prose poems, a poetic form that Rimbaud helped to originate in French. Emotionally, it is a cry from the depths—from the pit of depression. It is Rimbaud's celebration of his battle with/over himself during a period of severe depression—during the "dark night of the soul." In these poems, he forswears occultism, mysticism, and even the poetic life as a means of coping with his depression. It ends with:

> Yet this the watch by night. Let us all accept new
> strength and real tenderness. And at dawn, armed
> with glowing patience, we will enter the cities of glory.
> Why did I talk about a friendly hand! My great
> advantage is that I can laugh at old love affairs full of
> falsehood, and stamp with shame such deceitful couple—
> I went through women's Hell over there—and I
> will be able now to possess the truth within
> one body and soul.

Rimbaud saw this work as an essential expression of his innermost self. He had fantasies of the possibilities that might open to him if it received critical recognition (few copies actually sold). But, on another level, he seemed to regard this work of creation as being restitutive and integrative, in and of itself. Certainly, the final words speak to a process of integration that is the goal of the therapeutic process.

Despite the poems' brave words, Rimbaud could not fully separate from Verlaine, and he rejoined him in Brussels. This reconciliation, like the others, was short-lived. And, as Rimbaud was planning to leave him, Verlaine cried in a drunken rage, "If I can't have you no one will" and shot at Rimbaud. Fortunately for all concerned, Verlaine merely nicked Rimbaud with a bullet. He was subsequently arrested and jailed for two years. In the aftermath of Verlaine's attack, Rimbaud fled. Another father figure had betrayed him. Not surprisingly, the poems from this period show the influence of Rimbaud's increasing interest in folksong—it was as if he felt that the only parental figure that could not betray him was the unsophisticated and the untutored. The affect within these poems is lighter, as if the quasi-therapeutic work of *A Season* had been accomplished. In 1873, he stopped writing poetry; he was nineteen.

The Adolescent Becomes an Adult

After his final breakup with Verlaine, Rimbaud wandered throughout Europe, Asia, and Africa. His life sounds like the outline for a series of picaresque novels. He was briefly the manager of a circus in Scandinavia, a reader at the British Museum, then an art student in Munich. He is reported to have been a soldier in Java, deserted, and then shipped back to Europe on a tramp steamer. Once he walked over the Alps during the dead of winter to Italy. Throughout this time, he referred to poetry and to literary circles as "distasteful and disgusting." His sense of outrage reflected his intense sense of having been exploited by Verlaine and by the entire literary milieu. His frantic and manic-like activity seems to evidence, in part, a search for authority figures who would be more open about their agendas and who would accept him as an individual irrespective of his literary talents. The failure of poetry to provide either a constructive access to the adult world or magical solutions to his depression led him to explore other avenues. Withal, the possibility exists that Rimbaud's behavior does represent a bipolar affective disorder. And it is of interest that there has been considerable recent interest in the possible association of bipolar disorder and artistic creativity, particularly in poets.

Eventually, Rimbaud settled in Abyssinia. There is something extraordinarily disconsonant about the angelic young poet seeking to find fulfillment as a gunrunner to Menelik, emperor of Abyssinia, who was resisting the Italians who were even then attempting to conquer his kingdom. But, while this dissonance remains dramatic, it becomes comprehensible if Rimbaud's actions are examined within his historical context.

From 1880 onward, Europe was in the throes of expansion. The formation of the great colonial empires seized the imagination and captured the restless energy of the Continent. Rimbaud's activities were a part of this move toward imperial expansion. He was celebrated in the bulletin of the *Société Géographique* as one of France's great explorers in Africa. While his reports from Abyssinia may not have added to French literature, they reflect his continuing intellectual curiosity and a creativity of a different order. A comparison with his father, who spent twenty years in Algeria, is particularly cogent. Indeed, Rimbaud may have identified poetry with passivity because he associated it with his mother's investment in his literary career and with his own passive stance vis-à-vis male literary figures. Later, as he increasingly identified with his father, he sought the approval of men like his father who lived at the periphery of the French imperium.

The climax of Rimbaud's stay in Africa was his organizing an expedition from the coast to Menelik's headquarters in the highlands. The route Rimbaud traced was later used by the French when they constructed the railroad from Djibouti to Addis Abbaba. Rimbaud was the first European to blaze a trail over some of the most precipitous and hazardous country in the world. The organization of an expedition of 400 men through desert, across the Rift Valley, and onto the central Ethiopian plateau required skill of a high order. His financial rewards from this expedition were limited, but that should not obviate the courage, energy, and ability to lead men inherent in leading this expedition (and surviving it). Because of his extraordinary activity as a poet and the achievement of his brief literary career, there has been a tendency to overlook the achievements of his mature life. His actions after the age of nineteen belie the common view that his maturity was simply an aftermath. Rather, there was a redirection of creative energy towards an exploration of the outer world. As Edel (1975) noted: "It is a case of the artist moving from personal struggle and imagination into reality and then having no further need or impulse or material to go on shaping fantasies. The classic example, I suppose, is the French symbolist poet, Arthur Rimbaud."

Conclusions

Certain dynamic issues both dominated Rimbaud's life and appear as recurrent themes within his poetry. An examination of these issues makes his renunciation of poetry more understandable even if it is ultimately inexplicable. Certainly, his death, at thirty-nine, prevented him from realizing many of his plans.

The absence of a consistent father figure seems to have been of primary importance in his life. This absence is alluded to only once and in an early school composition. His literary career, however, was conducted under the aegis of a succession of paternal mentoring relationships: his letter to Izambard explicitly states, "I will love you like a father"; his relationship to Auguste Bretagne ("the old priest"); and finally with Verlaine (ten years his senior, an accomplished poet, husband, and father). The failure of these figures to provide consistent, nonexploitative support and their ultimate maliciousness (Izambard) or vengeful attack (Verlaine) led him far afield to find this support. His negotiations with Menelik were apparently shadowed with his desire to obtain Menelik's approval. Yet, because paternal figures were so inconsistent, it is not surprising that his actual relationship with Verlaine was conducted as a compulsive paradigm of desertion, separation, and reunion. Another aspect of Rimbaud's ambivalence toward Verlaine may lie in his adoption of the judgmental attitudes of mid-nineteenth-century France toward homosexuality. As his ultimate career choice demonstrates, Rimbaud both identified with and raged against La Belle France's indifference.

Rimbaud's relationship with his mother has deservedly drawn a great deal of attention. In *The Poet at Seven Years,* he describes his efforts to escape from the control of his rigid, puritanical, and hypocritical mother. Reality is more complex. During his early school years, Rimbaud was a notably docile and attentive child. His mother always expressed an interest in and fostered his development as a writer. She registered him in school at age seven particularly because she felt that she could not instruct him in the classics, which she felt would be necessary for his development as a writer. The rage expressed toward her in *The Poet* may have been stimulated by his anger at his separation from her occasioned by his entrance into school. Indeed, the development of a prodigy has been noted to be the product of a complex interweaving of parental support and/or parental overinvestment in which anger is a frequent by-product. Suffice it to say that *A Season* was written on the maternal farm. Rimbaud's later letters show a concern for her despite her rigidity and apparent inability to reciprocate. Some of the emphasis that has been placed on the poems, which express negative attitudes toward her (and other women), may reflect a certain politicization of Rimbaud's life that has tended to transform him into a homosexual martyr who fled France to escape the scandal attached to his affair with Verlaine.

A factor of primary importance in the development of his poetry and in the course of his personal life was Rimbaud's severe depression at age seventeen. On his return to Charleville, in March 1871, he began to neglect himself physically, distanced himself from his friends, and expressed his disgust with and disdain for life. The rationalization he used, that is, that a poet must deprave himself, should not conceal the presence of severe depressive symptomatology. Subsequently, he dealt with his heightened sense of vulnerability by developing his theory of the poet as seer. Presumably, in his guise of the poet as master scientist, Rimbaud hoped to restore his sense of integrity to himself as the great invalid.

The question arises of the degree, if any, that his poetry was directly therapeutic? This question takes on a peculiarly modern quality when some of the themes of his poetry are examined. Rimbaud was very interested in the experience of childhood and the particular intensity of the child's vision. Unlike his contemporaries, he did not see children either as small adults or as total innocents. His *Poet at Seven Years* explicitly discusses childhood sexuality:

> He passed, stuck out his tongue, then pressed two fists
> in his crotch, and shut his eyes to see spots.

This depiction was as unacceptable in 1871 Paris as it was to be in 1905 Vienna. Moreover, like Freud, he was interested in dreams and the evocative nature of words and sounds. Likewise, his interest in the occult and cabalistic was a part of the welter of popular concerns about the uncanny, which expressed itself in figures as disparate as Madame Blavatsky and Sigmund Freud. Rimbaud was hardly involved in developing an understanding of the psychodynamic development of the individual. But his concerns about childhood and its vicissitudes lend a certain poignant intensity to his poetry and may have enabled him to use his poetry in the resolution of his inner conflicts. That resolution allowed him to identify more fully with his father, who saw literature as the product of a life lived at the cutting edge of the French Empire.

Like other explorers, such as Henry Morton Stanley, Rimbaud's childhood was marked by conflict with an absent father figure. His quest for identity led him initially to seek approval from a series of literary mentors. His renunciation of poetry appears to have been the act of an individual who refused to pay, by his personal submission, the price for entry into the literary salon. He left Paris to describe his world, but only in reports to the *Société Géographique*.

NOTES

1. A. J. P. Taylor's recent characterization of Dylan Thomas as the Rimbaud of Cwmarvon Point confirms this, as does the recent play, *Dark of the Moon*, or James Ramsey Ullman's popular novel, *The World on Fire*, which provide modern illustrations of the continuing impact of his legend.
2. There is a Quai Arthur Rimbaud in Charleville and a Promenade Marcel Proust in Cabourg. One of the most fashionable boulevards in Paris is Avenue Victor Hugo. Compare this to the objections raised

against naming streets and bridges after figures such as Walt Whitman and Herman Melville.

REFERENCES

Edel, L. 1975. *The Stuff of Sleep and Dreams*. New York: Avon.

Ehrenpreis, I. 1984. Art, life, and T. S. Eliot. *New York Review* 31(11): 5–7.

Esman, A. 1984. Giftedness and creativity in children and adolescents. *Adolescent Psychiatry* 13:62–84.

Freud, S. 1908. Leonardo da Vinci and a memory of his childhood. *Standard Edition* 11:63–139. London: Hogarth, 1961.

Greenacre, P. 1957. The childhood of the artist. *Psychoanalytic Study of the Child* 12:47–72.

Halperin, D. 1983. Gnosticism in high tech: science fiction and cult formation. In D. Halperin, ed. *Psychodynamic Perspectives on Religion, Sect and Cult*. Littleton: John Wright-PSG.

Rimbaud, A. 1975. *Complete Poems*. Trans. P. Schmidt. New York: Harper Colophon.

Starkie, E. 1947. *Arthur Rimbaud*. New York: Norton.

Weber, V. 1983. Modern cults and gnosticism: some observations on religious and totalitarian movements. In D. Halperin, ed. *Psychodynamic Perspectives on Religion, Sect and Cult*. Littleton: John Wright-PSG.

Zweig, P. 1970. *The Heresy of Self-Love: A Study of Subversive Individualism*. New York: Harper Colophon.

6 WHEN ADOLESCENTS WRITE: SEMIOTIC AND SOCIAL DIMENSIONS OF ADOLESCENTS' PERSONAL WRITING

BONNIE E. LITOWITZ AND ROBERT A. GUNDLACH

While all adolescents write in school, many write outside of school as well. Some adolescents in therapy show their private writings to their therapists. In this chapter, we look at such writings (personal diaries, letters, and notes to therapists) and seek to understand through these examples the purposes writing serves for adolescents who choose to write. Our examples are drawn from four sources: an eighteen-year-old middle-class boy's journal written over four years; the letters of a seventeen-year-old middle-class boy from the same suburban school; the script of a thirteen-year-old inner-city black boy; and the diary written by a twelve-year-old middle-class, inner-city black girl over three years.

Writing in general and adolescents' writing in particular have received attention from psychoanalytic theorists and psychotherapeutic researchers. Jacobson (1964) describes the traditional, drive-discharge-model view of writing as an object onto which energy can be cathected:

> First of all, the intention normally arises from a previous interest in and concern with the issue about which the author wishes to write. The issue is the object which must become enduringly vested first with libidinal, aggressive, and neutralized psychic energy to the point where the plan to write about it turns into action. Of course, the writing will never proceed if the writer does not have sufficient self assurance at his disposal, self assurance which must

be based on an awareness and realistic evaluation of his abilities, and on a sufficient and sound cathexis of the function of writing. [P. 81]

In other words, both what is written about and the activity of writing per se must be invested with psychic energy. There is, in addition, narcissistic gratification as the writer enacts (or approaches enactment of) his ego ideal and ambitious fantasies, which may be further fed by recognition and acclaim, but these self-investments are seen as secondary to the primary investment in an object by means of writing or in writing itself. In a sociocultural context that values writing, this activity may entice the writer to narcissistic rather than libidinal gratifications. In general, however, as a cultural activity, writing is viewed as a sublimation (i.e., it is invested at a distance with neutralized drives).

Since it encourages the reactivation through the transference neurosis of personal object relations, writing has traditionally played no role in psychoanalytic therapeutic communication. In fact, Freud designated oral language as the privileged means of communication in the talking cure. Consequently, writing has come to be seen as a resistance to the real work of analysis or, alternatively, as an acting out of a need in regressive states to hold on to the analyst between sessions.

In contrast to the traditional psychoanalytic position, theorists whose view of object relations is rooted in social interaction rather than object cathexis (Greenberg and Mitchell 1983) might see writing as another form of symbolic communication between self and other through which a sense of self (true self, identity) develops. From this perspective, the presentation of self and the invocation of other(s) is as critical as the cathected topic and activity (as per Jacobson 1964). Therefore, the importance of writing to the individual is not necessarily solely one of secondary narcissism.

Perhaps due to this shift in theory—or simply because so many patients do write—some authors have reexamined the place of writing in psychotherapy, both as facilitating the therapeutic process and as reflecting therapeutic progress (e.g., Rampling 1980; Ryle 1983; Solow 1969; Widroe and Davidson 1961). Several authors have stressed the usefulness of writing in the treatment of particular patients such as borderlines (Domash 1976) or hospitalized patients (Hofmann and Lewis 1981; Schowalter and Lord 1972) or patients who are withdrawn and have difficulty communicating secrets (Oberkirch 1983).

Frequent topics of recent articles are the place of writing in adolescence and the use of writing to shed light on development during this period, especially as manifest in diary writing by adolescent girls. Blos (1962) has described this activity—typical for adolescent girls but less so for boys in America—"from middle-class families where literary efforts are valued," along traditional lines as follows: "The diary assumes an object-like quality" of a "female confidante, . . . stand[ing] between . . . make-believe and reality" and "filling the emotional void felt when the novel instinctual drives of puberty can no longer be articulated on old objects and cannot yet be articulated on new objects" (pp. 94–95). In affording the writer the opportunity to try out feelings and aspirations, the diary serves both as an arena for role playing (i.e., identificatory processes) and as an inhibition to premature action (e.g., sexual acting out).

Two recent articles elaborate on Blos's observations. Dalsimer (1982), in her review of Anne Frank's diary as a window to the inner world of female adolescence, underscores the functions of Anne's diary for the tasks of normal adolescence: to reveal herself safely to a nonjudgmental other, to create an other ("you," "Kitty") with standards and prohibitions who replaces the lost parents, and to recapture aspects of the earlier relationship with parents. (This last function, which Dalsimer connects to Winnicott's transitional phenomena, we will discuss in relation to Vygotsky's concept of egocentric speech.)

Sosin (1983) also uses the concept of transitional object (Winnicott 1953) to describe diary writing by seven adolescent girls (ages twelve to eighteen), who discuss this activity in later interviews (at ages eighteen to twenty-three) with the author. Sosin describes the self-mirroring and self-soothing functions of diary writing (e.g., "it was kind of like being my own mother in a way," p. 98) and also emphasizes the use of the diary to inhibit acting out and to contain volatile affects. She concludes, "These functional aspects of the diary become internalized into the evolving psychic structure just as the analogous functions of the therapist in the context of a positive transference are internalized" (p. 101).

In this paper, we extend this analysis of the functions or uses of writing in some adolescents' lives. By analyzing not only a diary written by an adolescent female but also a play, a journal, and letters to a therapist written by three adolescent males, we seek to broaden the range of written forms typically considered and to emphasize that adolescent males as well as females make use of personal writing. We have also recast the psychodynamic and psychoanalytic issues discussed in the professional literature from a psycholinguistic perspective. Our purpose here is to give more attention than is usually given to the properties of writing itself—the unique characteristics of written discourse as an expressive and communicative medium. Such an approach is important, we believe, in supplementing the more familiar approach that views writing simply as a transparent medium, a clear window on psychodynamic meanings that exist beyond the sentences in the text.

Our analysis is based on two assumptions. The first is semiotic. Writing is but one among many semiotic systems available to adolescents. It serves, along with other semiotic systems (such as gesture, facial and body expression, dress, and speech) as a means of representing who one is, how one feels, what one knows and wants, and so forth, in culturally appropriate ways. While writing is one system among other systems of semiotic exchange by means of which subjectivity is established, it nevertheless has unique properties. Writing creates an object by leaving a visual trace—the text—which, unlike the auditory trace, may endure over time and space. Thus, writing permits material expression yet suspends the consequences of utterance and therefore allows greater control over the nature and level of challenge from an interlocuter.

This last observation implies our second assumption: all writing is social, by which we mean that all writing arises out of and always embodies interpersonal relationships. In other words, every piece of writing presents a self and invokes an other or others, who may or may not be the consciously intended audience of the piece.

Drawing on these premises, we will explore three uses of writing by adolescents. First, writing may be used to externalize and objectify an inner feeling or content. Second, writing may be used to continue a process begun in speech by which social dialogues become part of an inner discourse. Last, writing may be used to experiment with various writer-audience or self-other relationships.

In the last section of the chapter, we will discuss examples of writing from several adolescents as illustrative of these various uses. In the end, it should be clear that writing affords some adolescents yet another semiotic means to address the particular developmental tasks they face—for example, sorting out past parental identifications and

85

forging an identity through new identifications, establishing relationships of varied closeness with others, finding roles to play and ways to meet the greater adaptive demands of society, and gaining increased psychological independence through greater control of semiotic systems.

Uses of Writing by Adolescents

In examining our first proposed use of writing—to externalize and objectify inner feelings or content—we find an exploitation by adolescents of the unique semiotic properties of writing. Writing makes thought corporeal, and many writers have echoed E. M. Forster's (Murray 1968) claim, "How can I tell what I think until I see what I say." Writing creates an external object to a greater degree than speech because writing remains; it leaves a trace, whereas speech quickly fades. Research shows, for example, that young children cease writing on pads ingeniously designed to leave no trace. Writing creates iconic images that have a reality (i.e., a material presence, beyond a mere recoding of or a coding alternative to their spoken equivalents).

The material product of writing, combined with its potential distance from the one who produces it, creates paradoxical reactions. On the one hand, people are often more fearful of committing themselves in writing than in speaking, as if the commitment were more real because it is enduring. (Note how legal evidence privileges the written over the oral.) Also, writing may wander away from one's possession and therefore one's control. On the other hand, the only way Luria's (1968) mnemonist could relieve his overloaded memory was to write unneeded information on a slip of paper and physically throw it away. Similarly, young children who are too ashamed of thoughts or actions to tell another may be willing to write these out to be read later or simply to be thrown away. In this way, one can externalize inner thoughts and feelings and rid oneself of them.

As there is a lessening of affect through mediation from experience to speech, there is a further weakening of affect in writing. Writing can therefore serve to tame and control emotions that threaten to overwhelm the subject. Writing, serving as a substitute action, can inhibit another action. For example, one abusive parent found that writing in her diary what she wanted to do to her child substituted for the abusive acts themselves.

In writing, one can create an objective reality—a possible world—with its own context and truth conditions. Even the youngest child understands that books create a play world in which animals can speak and cars can fly. In their personal writing, teenagers create possible worlds in which they can express and try out various feelings and ideas. Like Forster, they can see on paper what they think and, perhaps more important, feel. Sometimes, these feelings are destructive, suicidal, or alienated; often, as Inhelder and Piaget (1958) noted in describing the resurgence of egocentricism in adolescents, they are grandiose:

> To fully understand the adolescent's feelings, we have to go beyond simple observation and look at intimate documents such as essays not written for immediate public consumption, diaries, or simply the disclosures some adolescents may make of their personal fantasies. For example, in the recitations obtained by G. Dumas from a high-school class on their evening reveries, the most normal students—the most retiring, the most amiable—calmly confessed to fantasies and fabulations which several years later would have appeared in their own eyes as signs of pathological megalomania. [P. 344]

Inhelder and Piaget do not address the question, Why do adolescents so often prefer personal writing to express unacceptable feelings? We suggest that writing permits a presentation of the self and its inner world with greater distance from and control over the audience.

Writing is more an act—that is, a piece of volitional behavior, in the intuitive sense—than speaking, speech act theory not withstanding. As an act, writing indicates both its message and the writer—the one who performs the act. Writing as a presentation of self or as a performance is evident in the ubiquitous presence of the author's name on pieces of writing by children and adolescents. Even private writings such as personal diaries are identified by author's names or titles—for example, "writer in renaissance"—and seem to indicate, "This object equals me." Much adolescent writing seems to fluctuate, as do other adolescent behaviors—for example, dress, speech, and manner—between the same poles of flamboyant showing off and insecurity, between competence and incompetence. Comments, corrections, or criticisms of adolescent writing can generate the same narcissistic injury as in these other areas.

Yet, compared to speech, writing permits a distance of both discourse participants. One does not have to share writing with another person until one is ready, if ever. In this sense, writing is more private than speaking, which is immediately shared and open to reaction. The writer can control if and when (sometimes, where and how) he will expose himself and his thoughts to his audience. This aspect of writing may make it particularly useful when the reception by others of feelings or ideas is a concern. For this reason, adolescents who are extremely vulnerable and sensitive to reactions may find writing, especially personal writing, the best way to express certain feelings and ideas—for example, ambitious ideals, grandiose fantasies, and secret desires.

At the same time, the writer himself becomes more distanced from his expression in writing than in speaking. Drafting, editing, and revising materials are based both on control of audience and on the distance of self from text. One can treat even one's own text as if written by another person—that is, one's self at an earlier time. From this greater distance, a writer may repossess his now-material thoughts and feelings. Whereas inchoate thoughts and feelings may be disorganized and disconnected, they become fixed in written words and phrases. Articulating in writing one's inner world requires a selection of categories and points of view and establishment of relations between ideas (e.g., topic and comment and sequence of events). This more ordered reality can be reinternalized at a higher cognitive level, creating a new inner world. Adolescent writing is filled with examples of problem solving, decision making, question answering, and organization of arguments and positions. Adolescents gain control over their inner worlds by reinternalizing what they write.

In summary, one function of personal writing for adolescents is, we hypothesize, that it externalizes an inner world by creating an objective reality as a context into which inchoate thoughts and feelings can be given expression and meaning. Part of the possible world created is the writer himself. This new reality can be subsequently reinternalized at a higher level of consciousness, completely disowned, or merely kept at a safe distance.

Even in discussing, as we have above, the privacy of writing with its focus on the writer and his relationship to the text, we cannot escape the social nature of writing. The remaining two uses of writing in adolescence we shall examine address writing as a social enterprise: first, as a continuation of a process begun in speech by which social dialogues become part of an inner discourse; and, second, as experiments with various self-other relationships.

The privacy of writing creates the appearance that writing is a solitary activity. Many writers, for example, comment on the isolation and loneliness of their profession. A closer examination, however, shows dialogue buried in every written monologue. The dialogic nature of both speech and writing is succinctly stated by Vološinov (1973): "any utterance—the finished, written utterance not excepted—makes response to something and is calculated to be responded to in turn" (p. 72). Our examples of adolescent writing are filled with questions and responses: the titles and opening lines of pieces are stated as questions, and they set up what follows as a reply; whole pieces serve as a response to earlier, pretextual questions; and rhetorical questions are liberally used throughout texts—often to set up internal arguments between different parts of the writer's self.

Writing is dialogic in nature precisely because it is dialogic in its source. As Vygotsky (1978) notes, all speech originates in social, dialogic exchanges between persons, from which speech becomes interiorized as inner speech for oneself. "Every function in the child's cultural development appears twice on two levels. First, on the social and later on the psychological level; first between people as an *interpsychological* category, and then inside the child, as an *intrapsychological* category" (p. 128). The functions, by means of which the child is other-regulated, are interiorized with the speech and become "self-functions." Thus, children learn to use language for self-direction and self-regulation—that is, the child treats himself as others had treated him. Social speech in the process of becoming inner speech may erupt in egocentric speech, an external form of speech as the child attempts to perform functions for himself that had been performed by an adult. Writing for oneself can be compared to talking to oneself, as essentially egocentric.

Typically, egocentric speech would increase in the service of a difficult task where the help of an adult needs to be invoked (Vygotsky 1962). But it also may occur in practice mastery of the language system (Weir 1962). Self-conversations, modeled on conversations with others, are much in evidence in adolescent writing. We find examples where adolescents use writing to help themselves work through problems, allay anxieties, and soothe or comfort themselves.

As social speech becomes interiorized as inner speech, we are told that the structure changes (Vygotsky 1962). Inner speech is sense saturated, predicative, and subjectless, lacking the cohesion required in other-directed discourse. Some personal writings by adolescents seem to conform to this pattern. Yet, the sentence structure or poetic forms of even the most primary process/free association–like pieces show that these examples are consciously (sometimes self-consciously) constructed presentations of self for other echoing past self-other communications. Such pieces are not inner speech made visible, although they may try for that effect. Just as fantasy is not inner reality but the individual's effort to deal with inner reality, so these pieces are the writer's attempt to express an inner world or state, which is possible only via conventions and rules.

In summary, adolescent writing also provides evidence for the uses of writing to internalize functions of an other for one's self. These functions have their roots in self-other dialogues and in the processes by which these become internalized. In the progression from dialogue to inner speech and monologue, some examples of adolescent writing are closer to one end than to the other—that is, some are more overtly other addressed. Yet, all examples manifest an awareness of writing as a particular form of addressed communication—one of greater distances and control but always responsive.

The dialogic source and nature of writing mean that it can be viewed as variations on self-other relationships. Specifically, adolescent writing can be viewed as attempts to master the author-audience relation imposed on young adults in our culture by their schooling.

Much of adolescent writing seems to result from the trying on of different identities for different audiences. Writing like a journalist, a poet, or a scientist is similar to earlier role playing, in which a child, for example, may try on a hat and handbag and speak like the mother. Both Vygotsky and Piaget agree that, in school-age children, play becomes dominated by games and athletics whose other-generated rules differ from the child-generated rules of preschool play, where a "new relationship is created between the semantic and visible fields—that is, between situations in thought and real situations" (Vygotsky 1976).

Neither theorist, however, sees adolescence as anything other than a further step in the progression away from preschool play. Yet, play in adolescence, particularly language play, reveals many aspects of preschool play, except that it is now "voluntary" and "logical" and takes full advantage of the symbolic capacities of adolescent cognitive and linguistic development (Inhelder and Piaget 1958; Litowitz 1985;

Vygotsky 1976). In fact, Vygotsky's (1978) insight about preschool play is even more evident in adolescent writing: all play involves rules that give rise to new forms of desires and relates those desires to a fictitious "I" (p. 100). Adolescents can experiment with the expression of varied desires (wishes) in semiotic exchanges of all kinds (e.g., dress, speech) including writing. Through experimentation, adolescents learn how to manipulate rules, conventions, and roles and to regulate desires. A feature of this process, critical to identification, is the positioning of one's self in relation to an other in discursive practices. Certainly, adolescence is a period of serious play, but, whereas early play creates possible worlds in action, later play creates possible worlds with words.

There is a great deal of language play in adolescence when teens delight in confounding their elders with new words and new meanings to old words in slang and jargon (Litowitz 1985). Simultaneously, there is a lot of trying on of other semiotic expressions: makeup, clothes, speech style, attitude, behaviors. Writing permits another area for play, especially role play, through which adolescents can try various identities as voices.

The source of these roles with their attendant rules and conventions are multifarious. Writing is strewed with the remnants of past dialogues, both personal conversations and didactic discussions. The choice of words (e.g., "puerile") and of phrases (e.g., "Is there life after X?" "To live life to its fullest") as well as syntactic and textual forms (e.g., rhetorical questions, conventionalized frames)—all bear the traces of the writer's past interaction with others. In a literate culture, many self-other communications come from interacting with texts—from writing in a particular style to the wholesale importation of phrases. We find echoes not only of reading but of schooling in general—for example, time lines from history class, lessons on tenses from language classes, and disembodied words memorized from dictionaries and the-sauri. The culture outside of school also provides resources—rock songs, videos and films, graphic insignia, and nightly prayers. All these bits and pieces from past voices crowd adolescent writing even more than mature writing since teens either cannot or do not feel the need to maintain one consistent voice throughout a piece. Consequently, an adolescent's writing, for all the sincerity and power of its emotional appeal, can simultaneously sound pompous and strained, like a child dressed up in too-large adult clothing trying to speak in a deep voice or with mother's rouge on trying to play the vamp. We are reminded by Vygotsky (1976) that, in play, children act ahead of their developmental level and strive beyond their present capacities.

In a more general sense, adolescent writing as addressed communication between self and other is evident in the frequent use of "I" and "you," in spite of the vigilance of schoolteachers. These discourse-personal indices creep back into adolescent writing, especially personal writing, as adolescents cannot or simply do not want—or perhaps do not need—to control the use of writing as an overt appeal to another person. Adolescents use writing to maintain a connection to an other person, to keep the experience of the other present and close. We see this in their notes and letters but also in diary entries that call out to another person, though they are not specifically addressed to any one. Winnicott's (1958) remarks on the capacity to be alone are particularly applicable to writing; one can be alone only in the presence of an other. In fact, it is often difficult to keep track of the number of persons and voices inhabiting a given text. The crowd can include voices from the past, peers and family members, authority figures, and appeals to a general public or to a specific person, as well as multiple parts of the writer himself.

In these ways, adolescents not only practice articulating ideas and mastering literate forms but also use this particular semiotic medium to develop an ongoing sense of identity—that is, a sense of person as well as personal voice. Unlike speech-act theory, which focuses on learning how to "do things with words" (Austin 1962; Bruner 1978, 1983; Searle 1969), the functions of writing we have examined are a continuation of the general semiotic processes by which one learns how to be—using the voices and meanings of social and cultural life to compose a sense of who one is in relation to others. Writing's unique semiotic properties enable adolescents to control communication with all sorts of others, including themselves (and parts of themselves). Because adolescence is a period of active mastery of forms and establishing identities, teenage writers better provide us with evidence than do those at earlier or later ages of these developmental processes.

Examples of Personal Writing by Four Adolescents

From our previous discussion it is clear that the three uses of writing are not separate and distinct from one another but rather overlap. In presenting examples now, we must emphasize that every piece of writing is plurifunctional. In articulating an inner reality, a writer may also be experimenting with conventional forms and invoking other voices; he may be soothing himself at the same time he is solving a problem or trying on an identity. Every piece of examined writing demonstrates the impossibility of writing without invoking an other or others, without drawing on prior (re)sources, and without experimenting with a textual form (cf. Halliday's [1973, 1975] interpersonal, ideational, and textual metafunctions).

CASE EXAMPLE 1

Martin is a thirteen-year-old black boy, living in a predominantly black section of a large, northern city, who comes to a local hospital for therapy. He comes late to sessions and finds it difficult to talk. However, he comes to the hospital at other times and leaves written notes in his therapist's mailbox. One such communication is the following play (punctuation added):

Play

An XConvick

Cast:

L —— The wife of x con

P —— Daughter of x con

M —— no relation to x con

W —— X convick

Play picks up at two oclock and x con cruzing down the street doing 65mph. Cops pull him over to the side. Asks questions, runs him in on no sticker on license plate. Cost $150.00 to get him out. $50.00 to get the car back from pound. The cage is open. Jail bird flies out of cage.

One day later, happy on high one or the other. Two days later comes back to x-con family. Welcomes him with numbers and all. "How was work today?" Ex-con: "It was O.K." "Did you get you licence stright yet." "No not yet. I go to court next week to get the $50.00 back with my drivers licence." O.K. So. Ex cons wife to me. "Pick up that crumb." where ex con hits me. I should have hit him back but I caught myself. Then he hit me three or four more times. I was a crillimetter away from knocking teeth from him with a pot.

The End

Credits * * *

Martin's mother had recently remarried a man whose initial was W, so that the play's cast exactly replicates Martin's family. The plot concerns the revelation of W's criminal nature to Martin's family who blatantly ignore what is obvious to the writer. Martin's message is "You're so hard on me but you love an obvious criminal; you even allow him to punish me for 'a crumb.' " Echoes of past discourse are evident in both the dialogue and phrases like "the play picks up," "the cage is open," "jail bird flies out of cage." It is unclear what Martin's intent was—to redress a wrong now that he has control over the characters in his drama or to express emotions that he could not speak. Note that part of what is expressed is Martin's self-control over his own aggression toward W. Martin could have chosen stream-of-consciousness poetry, a letter or note, or a diary, but he chose a structured play, a time-honored genre (in both drama and psychodrama) for the direct expression of familial relationships. It is also not clear whether he could not finish the play because he did not know how or because he did not need to—that is, that the structure got him started and enabled him to accomplish what he needed. Evidence for the latter view is the shift in pronouns, signaling the writer's inability to suppress speaking directly (versus through his characters). Note, however, the final return to structure in "The End" and "Credits * * *."

CASE EXAMPLE 2

Paul is a seventeen-year-old boy in therapy. Recently, Paul moved from a more rural environment to a suburb in a big city. He is intelligent, articulate, and literate. Since beginning therapy, Paul has become greatly intrigued by Freudian psychology. The following piece, written by Paul for his therapist, shows the use of question answering to work through problems. The evocation of past dialogues is very clear in this self-conversation presented to his therapist:

Why must people be people? Ill-logic. To be an adult; to lose control. Suceptable to age; dissapation. Two attitudes merge into one highly-flawed monstrousity of a scheme: the way to live? Hardly. Personal freedom cannot be achieved. A simple relationship: Freedom vs. Nature. Nature always wins; an unbeatable competitor. Them. Why do they persist in life: Thrive on causing pain. Is there life after childhood? No, a shift in attitude, values, morals, standards, and every other radical, undefinable term occurs. I hope never to become an adult. Freedom becomes slavery. Life becomes death. Life is so simple, yet we make it complex. The point of no return. To live life to its fullest can and must be an illusion. Only in death can this illusion become reality. Only in death!

Although this piece may seem a free-association soliloquy (i.e., a form of self-addressed inner speech), closer examination reveals many stylistic devices, such as rhetorical questions, verbal ellipses, and parallel constructions, which the author uses to create the mood of a prose-poem and which differ radically from the structure of inner speech.

In another note, Paul represents the fact that every person has both unconscious and conscious desires and thoughts as a dialogue between the two voices of his unconscious ("I") and his conscious ("you")— a bivocality incorporated from the discourse with his therapist. He presents both parts of his psyche but, interestingly, takes the role of his unconscious for himself.

The Dream
. . . You can't escape me. I'm here; I'm always here. What's wrong? Do I remind you of Dr. Jekyl and Mister Hyde? I am. I confuse you driving the sleep which you think is so comfortable. You awaken; I disguise. I enter your memory, paging through your library, picking good events, bad events, symbolic of your conflicts. Bad deal, huh? Without me, you'll suffer. No release. With me, you'll suffer. Bad dreams, nightmares, utter confusion. . . . I'm a dragon beneath your surface, stirring about. You are conscious. I make the puzzle pieces fit. Make sense now? Of course! Try me later. I don't conform to the rules of logic or rational. I don't have to. I'm a dream.

In yet another note, Paul speaks directly to his therapist and in the process addresses his unconscious, the universe at large, and a special young lady.

95

I am so depressed, Happiness is a buried emotion. Fuck my un-conscious. I love her, so if you can hear me unconscious, leave me alone. My brain is a prick; the worst kind. Let me be. Can't anybody relate to my problem or am I alone in a dimension of the universe yet unexplored. If I lose her, therapy will be worthless; I'll just cry and withdraw until I'm a catatonic introvert. B——, save me. This is a plea not to instill guilt but to let you know the power you have over me.

With this one piece, the author speaks as patient to psychiatrist, as one part of himself to another part personified, and as lovesick romantic to the unattainable object of his desire. All these dialogues are presented in a communication to his therapist.

In yet another voice, this same depressed youth, at the mercy of his mind and brain and lady, begins a well-written, carefully researched school paper on children's dreams with the following flourishes:

The road to the completion of this paper was a long and difficult one. [Paul names and thanks the two men who have influenced him.] The hours which I have spent researching, compiling, and summarizing my topic have all paid off in what I feel is one of the most significant achievements of my life. . . .

One of the first attempts to explain dreaming was by Sigmund Freud, a bright German doctor. . . .

In this example, the reader can see the writer struggling with a particular voice—the research scientist—writing for a larger public audience. This author-audience relationship is a consequence of his identification with and idealization of the two men, a teacher of psychology and his therapist, whom he thanks in the preface, and connects the writer in a direct line to Dr. Freud. One can see Paul trying on the conventions and rules of a more publicly addressed communication—the prerequisite acknowledgment preface, conventionalized phrases, and identifying appositive clauses.

CASE EXAMPLE 3

Alan is an eighteen-year-old attending the same suburban school as Paul. Alan is a good student who has a close relationship to his parents and two older brothers. Alan has kept a diary throughout his high school years, but the history of the diary over the four years shows its varied uses. In the beginning the diary was personal. Then, in the summer of his sophomore year, Alan used the diary for daily assignments in a journal-writing course. For eight weeks, Alan would write something in his diary every night, prepared to convey his thoughts (though not necessarily the writing per se) in the next day's class meeting, where he would be expected to comment on his classmates' thoughts. After that summer, the diary once again became personal, until the beginning of his last year in high school. For a senior English course, Alan was asked to write in a diary every day. The entries were checked but not read by the teacher. By the middle of his senior year, Alan ceased writing in his diary (although he claims he will resume the diary in college).

Shortly after Alan began his diary, he filled in the first page with the following epigraph: "writer in renaissance" (*sic*). Some time later, he seems to have realized that he had misheard the expression, "writer in residence," perhaps collapsing it with "renaissance man," for he crossed out the above and retitled his diary: " 'Poetry and other written works' by Alan ———." Indeed, all of the first entries are short poems. Since each entry is dated, one can see the urgency of the early writing with two, three, and sometimes four poems bearing the same date.

The poems express either idealistic themes, for example, utopias—hoped for or failed—or cosmic concerns (e.g., why are we here; why do we have to die; man's place in the universe; the inexorable and swift passage of time). The poems bear such titles as "Mother," "Vivo," "Meaningless Child's Play," "The Human Bomb," "Aloft," and "The Ultimate Dream." Current political issues, such as the Vietnam War, nuclear destruction, and conflicts in El Salvador, are woven into many entries. For example, here is a poem about time that reworks the time line from history class and tense from language class:

Tense
Animals big and small,
Recorded history,
Jesus Christ? A.D.
Renaissance, presidents, transportation
World wars, one and two
Viet Nam, young men too

> Space zap, micro electronics
> The 5th dimension,
> New life, black holes
> Can't I stay to watch the end,
> I feel like Ive been here forever.

Often the poems seem to be an answer to a question, sometimes explicitly stated in the title—"A Utopia?" "The Perfect Machine?"—or, in the opening lines, "Is it so?" "What's this you say?" For example, the following poem, whose title is influenced by Alan's beginning Spanish and Pablo Neruda's *Memoirs* (confieso que he vivido), is filled with questions. The juxtaposition of positive and negative, good and bad, is a frequent strategy in Alan's writing, as if the writing permits him to list assets and debits and make a final accounting.

> Vivo
>
> Is this all?
> Fun, knowledge, yet sadness, pain and end
> Where's the rest?
> Here or not?
> Good times and bad times,
> Do we get our share?
> Is this all?

The last entry in this section is a prose piece titled, "Society," expressing familiar themes of nuclear destruction and World War III, stupidity of our leaders, pleas for change, and so forth, ending with "It's not a chess game !!!!!! It's life. It's the survival of humanity. We must change before it's too late. One more war, and the winner will be no one."

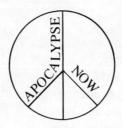

It is interesting to note in this last piece the use by Alan of other symbolic media: films (*Apocalypse Now*) and graphic symbols (the peace insignia worn by Alan on a silver necklace at this time). While writing is clearly a mixed medium for younger children, adolescents' personal writing retains this quality even though it disappears from school writing (Gundlach 1982).

In a later section, Alan's poetry becomes longer and more ambitious. One can see the influences of school, home, and the larger culture. In the following reworking of the time theme, for example, the reference to infinite and infinitesimal comes from a soliloquy in the movie, *The Incredible Shrinking Man*:

It's About Time

Time,
Where the infinite meets the
Infinitesimal, yes,
One and the same, It all depends on you
It can mend and bend—all to shape
   your mind,
I think, my years turn to seconds,
Or, do my seconds turn to years,
We ourselves are timelords,
However, the time we are allowed
   to be timelords is too short,
And nothing, nothing can be done.
"I," says the timelord, "will live forever"
"And I," says time, "Will not."

At one point, Alan's brother wrote him some "bedtime limericks, to be read before going off to sleep." Alan was delighted with the rhythmic force of the limerick form. Several entries thereafter were either directly in that form or influenced by it:

A mind full of complication
A life awaiting anticipation
Not knowing what to do
Is it coming closer to you
As an eternity has now become frustration.

99

Although based on fact
Was it ever really exact?
What I thought I knew
Might not have been quite true
And so it remains, and I know not how to act.

Along with rhyme and stanzas, Alan experimented with other literary touches such as the expression of affect through repeated phrases, exclamations (Oh!), and intensifiers (so, do). In the following example, one can see Alan trying out but not quite mastering these devices:

The sky is open and the sun is
Out, with each breeze my mind drifts
Today, like many other days, memories of
Yesteryears traverse my mind. And from
These, how much happiness I behold and
How much pain I do feel.

I can remember how I cried, how
I laughed, what I felt and what I saw.
And all the beaches I have seen,
And all the water I have swam,
And all the land beneath my feet,
Oh! my memories are so sweet.

I have as many as I can dream,
The more the merrier as it would seem.
And although my memories are incomplete,
Compared with those whose are replete,
I find I do not have to compete,
For myself, I have enough, and so replete.

During the times that the diary was used more as a journal for his classes, Alan's style becomes conventionalized and academic. He is careful to anchor his prose in the specific context of the text, to set up an argument and let the reader know where he is going.

Journal
At this part of my journal, being the first part, I guess I should write about something of first importance to me. I'm not sure this

is of first importance but what this boy had to say bothered me. He's a very nice boy, and I will develop what happened to be a very interesting yet disturbing incident. . . .

Or, the following example shows Alan, now taking his brother's role, trying to recast for the reader a previous discussion with his brother:

Is a bicycle the same bicycle if all of its parts have been replaced throughout its lifetime? This question, being as intriguing as it is, has to be given a lot of thought. This was a question brought up by my brother from his philosophy class at college. I will try to express my feeling about this question now. . . .

Some entries use this more elaborated textual style to refute those who have questioned his motives:

The decision as to what college I wish to go to and when I want my interviews, etc., is a tough choice. I am often told by people that my lack of resoluteness is due to my inhibitions about attending college. This is fallacious!

At other times, Alan seems to be justifying himself to himself against an internalized standard (e.g., superego):

Now that my team is 1-12-1, I think I can say that I have become accustomed to losing. Although at every game I give all I have to come out victorious, I do, and I will not lie, go into the game with a small, preconceived notion that we will lose. Is that so bad. I know one should not go into a game with a bad attitude but what could anyone expect.

Alan uses the diary to work through recurring themes (e.g., time, ambition) in the form of addressed communications ("I"/"you") that are really self-conversations:

Life is such a short part of time. Just a few minutes ago it was the bi-centenial. Why so fast. I'm in no hurry. If it is so short, can't I live forever. To die, you wouldn't even know it, would you? I don't want to. Life is fun, even with its bad times and bad people. I want to stay alive. Not die. Why do I have to die? I want to see what the future holds, in space, death from war, intelligence, everything could happen. Everything I see before me could change so much in the next few decades. A funny thing, though, is that I don't even notice many changes. . . . I guess the changes come about gradually. I want to see all the changes, meet the next Newton or Einstein. How smart they were. Incredible. As long as I leave this planet with something behind, not body or thoughts, just some of the nice things I've done for people.

It is clear that the mention of Newton and Einstein provoked an unreported grandiose fantasy about Alan's own future. The last sentence is a response to this silent fantasy as much as it is a resolution of the piece's stated theme—his necessary mortality.

The themes Alan addresses in his journal are the everyday concerns of adolescence: too much to do in school, not enough time with his girlfriend, waiting for his SAT scores, lamenting his soccer team's losses. Some entries itemize the day's activities; others are obsessive ruminations on one issue such as performance at soccer or on the SAT exam. Periodically, an entry will deal exclusively with the sad state of Chicago's sports teams or the national election for president. Several entries at the end of the journal are simply verbatim copies of popular song lyrics and one, of the poem "Casey at the Bat." In the following entry, Alan addresses a universal adolescent problem—acne—in a parody of academic discourse (note similarity to opening about college):

Have you ever thought about what factors affect your score on a test after you have finished it? Many people would argue that it is not possible to influence your score on a test already taken; however, I disagree.

In my view, there is but one way to have a factor in your score, the way is worrying. I feel the amount one worries is directly proportional to the possible increase in score. Thus, the more you worry, the better you do. Many people would probably think I'm crazy, but it has worked for me.

What is the only disadvantage to worrying? Well, I suppose it's not healthy for people, but for me, it has only one effect. The effect: an increase in the number of zits. Yes, the more I worry (and I do worry a lot), the more acne I get.

Overall, the diary has permitted Alan to express not just opinions but feelings and, through this externalization, to reflect on his experiences:

An experience that I had never known. She and I were there. I thought the feeling was mutual. As it turned out, it was only a one way street. I had heard it from her friends, I thought I knew it all. I really knew so little, it got me into a predicament. She was foreign, dark, and many of the things I wanted. She told me I reminded her of someone she had known. She said she liked my eyes and they melted her like butter. With all these hints what did I have to lose. I went ahead and asked, she said it couldn't be. She had someone and at the moment she could not get free. I shown very happily, although not inside. I think she has lied, I didn't know why. It hurts me now to feel this way, I know I can overcome it. I'm not sure how to act with her, ignore her or be nice, I guess I'll do whats natural. I am sure this experience will help me, like others I have had. I'm not sure how this will help me, but I shall pay attention.

CASE EXAMPLE 4

Doris is a twelve-year-old black girl, a good student, who lives in a middle-class black neighborhood of a large northern city. Three years ago, while Doris was at summer camp, her older half-brother (eleven years older, from her mother's first marriage) murdered her mother, her father, and her older (by two years) brother. Doris has been adopted by her aunt (the mother's sister) and husband, who have a daughter. For about a year, Doris has been in therapy that focuses on her suppressed grief reaction. Doris began her diary at summer camp three years ago; she wrote periodically over the next two years; and she continues to write at present. Doris does not write specifically to her therapist. She recently gave her diary to the therapist to look at for a short while and then asked for it back so she could continue to write.

Two major themes alternate throughout Doris's diary: her relationships to her new ''mother'' and ''sister'' and her relationships to boys. The diary allows Doris to objectify feelings for which there may be no other audience available or desired. Sometimes the result is to distance herself from situations and thereby to gain control through this media-

103

tion. Other times, the result is to keep feelings and experiences present through their written *re*-presentation. The range of feelings talked about in the diary is impressive: rage at others and herself; jealousy and loneliness; loss and mourning; and sexual excitement and love.

In many ways Doris's diary is a typical example of the genre so often mentioned in relation to adolescent girls. Its tone is gossipy and chatty; its themes are focused on romantic attachments: "Terry has been cool this year and now he goes with Jeannie. Oh, and guess what, Mia likes Chris. My God. What has the world come to?"

As mentioned in the literature, the diary seems often to be a trusted confidante who listens to secrets and gives advice: "Today I got back from Carbedale. We had a surprise party for Jackie. Oh and Joey isn't nothing. He lied to me. I was going to have a party but mom said no and I'm very angry. I don't know if I should tell her. What should I do?" A closer examination, however, shows more voices than simply those of a writer and her fictive confidante. Traces of past oral discourse are present everywhere, accounting for the difference in tone (more vernacular than literary) between this diary and Alan's (above). Many entries include expressions from speech to set up topics, such as "see," "oh," "guess what?" Often, words that would be stressed in speaking are written larger, darker, underlined and with exclamations, giving the text more of the affective expression of talking. In one entry, the "test of love," a ritual speech finds its way into her writing, not making any sense without the usually accompanying daisy (whose petals are plucked with each phrase):

Test of Love
loves, not, loves, not
loves, not, loves, not, loves
not, loves, not, loves,
not, loves, not, loves,
not, loves, not, loves,
not, loves, not, loves,
not, loves, not, loves,
not, loves, not, loves,
loves, loves, loves, LOVER

Both the typically adolescent theme of romance and the more particular theme of Doris's changed familial circumstances are really variations of the questions, who loves her; whom does she love; how will she know when she is loved; what's the difference between "like" and "love"; and what about hate? The following long outburst covering many pages of the diary was written in her mother's presence. The enraged Doris uses writing as an aggressive act expressing her anger at the mother but not risking the mother's response. It is interesting to note in this piece that the writer attacks the mother, who is physically present but deaf to the abuse, and appeals to an unnamed ally and to God, who are physically absent but responsive.

I HATE MY MOTHER. She is really pissing me off. I mean she get's mad very easily. I know my real mother wouldn't have said anything but everything is going wrong with us. I'm not sure if I can stay here much longer. All of this is affecting my school work. I mean it I really don't like her. I just can't stay here any more Maybe I will run away, or kill myself. I don't think all this is happening because of me. I just think that she should have more patience. I'm really getting sick of this. I mean it, I hate her. Sometimes I wish some one else adopted me or I should go to the adoption agency. Oh God please help me in this time of need. My mother is standing right in front of me now but I don't give a care. I hope she doesn't say anything to me or else I think I will go off. —— [the "sister"] is mad at me too. She's mad because I gave her my cold and I glad I gave it to her. I just don't know why everything is going wrong. I just don't understand. . . . I am so mad I'm going to curse. FUCK them. all of them. I mean it. Forgive me God for saying that. I just don't care anymore. Please God if you go any where else tonight come home. Please? I just can't stand it any longer. Please get me out of this mad house. . . . Just forget her. Try putting yourself in my position. You really wouldn't like it. . . . I feel like crying now but I couldn't do that in front of her . . . embarass me in front of all my friends. I really am not going to forgive her for that. . . . Well, now that I have calmed down maybe I can go to sleep. Dear God, Bless our Family in a very, very, very special way.

Note that God is appealed to for his powers of intervention—to rescue her and to help straighten out her "very unloving, confused" family—but also for his forgiveness for her outburst. God is part of a ritual closing for early entries, for example, "So God help me," "Thank you God good night." Here one sees a parallel between diary writing for some writers and other activities, such as nighttime prayers and confessions. God is absent from later entries that close with "good night" or "I'm tired."

The beginning of the diary is composed of short entries wherein a procession of names of young men appear as characters in Doris' narrative. They enter on one page only to disappear on the next. Even Doris, it seems, has difficulty keeping track, since the diary's frontpiece contains a list to which she continually adds names and past tense markers (d):

1. I love d Willie
2. I love d Martin
3. I love d Tony
4. I love d Eric
5. I love d Jackie
6. I love d Terry
7. I love d or like d Howard
8. I love d Robert
9. I love d Glenn
10. I love d Ethan
11. I love d Richard
12. I love Joe

Love blossoms daily, or so it seems, and disappears just as quickly. Occasionally, a sexual fantasy will emerge in the diary, seemingly motivated more by the writer than by the strength of her attachment to the particular boy.

Now I go with a boy named Willie. I love him. he loves me. I like him so much that I had a dream that we were married and I fucked him. When I woke up I was all sweatie. I even play games like we have a little girl and he is a basketball player and I am a lawyer. Well we are suppose to have sex again and have another girl. This is a story.

That last sentence indicates a need to keep the record straight for someone, but whom—the imaginary diary-confidante? the writer? an internalized adult voice? It is also interesting to note the shift in verb tenses from past to present: the dream was past, but the fantasy and written representation keep it present.

The later diary entries more often deal directly with the loss of her natural family:

> Today I feel lonely. I feel real lonely. I want and almost need a sister. I have been crying and talking to myself. Now that's terrible. I miss my brother [named] so that it is hard to have two older sisters. . . . Why did the fuck did my parents and [brother] have to die? I'm sorry for all of the good things I said about my family cause I hate them ALL!!!! Well, ever since [sister] introduced me to Howard, over the phone, he and I have been good friends. Yesterday we talked for a long time. we talked about sex and boyfriends and girlfriends. He is a really nice person. He helps me out with my personal problems and everything. He seems like my big brother. You know, he reminds me of my older brother who died as a baby. He's just like Family to me.

Although Doris only mentions in passing that she has begun to see a psychiatrist, there is increasing evidence in the diary of a self-regulatory voice.

> Happy New Year Diary. Sorry I'm late but I've been busy. My mother and I go to a physychiartrist (whatever) now. He's nice but expensive. I really don't think it's working but then again we've only gone one time. I go back tomorrow at 11:45. [Sister] and I consider ourselves real blood sisters now. I call her parents mom and dad and the same for her. We've had a few arguments this year but not as many as last year. . . . I'm going to wait for the right boy to come along. Besides boys don't really interest me as they used to. I really don't like parties and stuff anymore, either. Even if there is a good looking boy that likes me I won't rush into anything. If you've noticed I haven't had or said anything about a problem with my mother but I better not speak too soon because before you know it I'm going to be righting about how much I hate her and how I'm going to run away or kill myself. Good night!

A capacity for self-observation and self-reflection becomes more apparent. The parade of boys continues—but more slowly—and is seen from a different perspective of self-direction and control:

I have also decided already who I was going to give up my virginity to. Isn't that wild? well, I've given this lots of thought. A month to be exact. I based it on responsibility, personality, and how I really felt about them. . . . Oh, I can't forget I also based them on how good they are at making love. . . . I really don't know about the love making yet but I just know Tony is (good). . . . I don't even think I will lose my virginity until I'm 17 or maybe 16 or 18 but I don't know!

The expressions of frustration with her mother are still present, though less frequent. They are more focused on such typical adolescent conflicts as rebellion against constraints and reflect more typical adolescent solutions. In this final example, one can see a new awareness of variation in language style in her metacomments ("My slang, of course") and in her schoollike use of "example."

I went for a walk today. It was so exciting being alone, by myself. I thought about a lot of things. I think my parents and sister need a vacation. That means I could stay home by myself. All by myself. With my sister's BMW. Or they need to send me somewhere where I can be alone, all alone, by myself. Although whereever I go it would hve to have a phone and a black BMW with tinted windows. Get down! My slang, of course. Anyway, like I said, I enjoyed being alone. Not lonely but alone. While I was walking it felt free. Example: a bird flying through the air, not really knowing where he is going, but just the fresh feeling of being free and alone. I loved it! Good Night! (I'm tired!)

Conclusions

Taken together, Martin's script, Paul's letters, Alan's journal, and Doris's diary demonstrate how some adolescents use written language as a semiotic system—how they use written language, that is, to represent their ideas and feelings to others and to themselves. Moreover, as we read these texts, it becomes clear that, although the act of writing may be private, this physical solitude does not reduce the social character of written discourse. Everywhere in the examples we have discussed are echoes of the voices of family members, friends, and other people who inhabit the internalized social world of the adolescent writer.

These semiotic and social properties of writing offer adolescents important resources for undertaking developmental tasks such as sorting out familial and other identifications, exploring levels of intimacy and self-revelation in interpersonal relationships, and finding roles and voices suitable for meeting the demands made by family, school, and the larger society.

We do not mean to suggest that adolescents should be required to use writing for these purposes. Many adolescents find semiotic systems other than writing more powerful or more accessible and so represent themselves more fully in gesture, facial or body expression, dress, or habits of speech. Nonetheless, one conclusion to be drawn from our analysis is that adults who work with adolescents should be alert and sensitive readers of the writing adolescents do produce. A second conclusion is that developmental theories meant to illuminate the lives of adolescents in literate cultures need to account for written language as one semiotic system among many that an adolescent may use in forming a sense of self, in establishing relationships with others, and in contending with the expectations communicated both by people and by institutions.

NOTE

Earlier versions of this paper were presented at the Annual Fall Seminar, the Irene Josselyn Clinic, Northfield, Illinois, and at the International Society for Adolescent Psychiatry, Paris. The authors wish to thank Drs. William Bradbury and W. Thomas Love for their assistance with the data and Dr. Norman Litowitz for his helpful comments on earlier drafts.

REFERENCES

Austin, J. 1962. *How to Do Things with Words*. Oxford: Oxford University Press.

Blos, P. 1962. *On Adolescence*. Glencoe, Ill.: Free Press.

Bruner, J. 1978. Learning how to do things with words. In J. Bruner and A. Garton, eds. *Human Growth and Development*. Oxford: Oxford University Press.

Bruner, J. 1983. *Child's Talk: Learning How to Use Language*. New York: Horton.

Dalsimer, K. 1982. Female adolescent development: a study of *The Diary of Anne Frank*. *Psychoanalytic Study of the Child* 37:487–522.

Domash, L. 1976. The therapeutic use of writing in the service of the ego. *Journal of the American Academy of Psychoanalysis* 4(2): 261–269.

Greenberg, J. R., and Mitchell, S. A. 1983. *Object Relations in Psychoanalytic Theory*. Cambridge, Mass.: Harvard University Press.

Gundlach, R. 1982. Children as writers: the beginnings of learning to write. In M. N. Nystrand, ed. *What Writers Know: The Structure, Language, and Process of Written Discourse*. New York: Academic Press.

Halliday, M. A. K. 1973. *Explorations in the Functions of Language*. London: Arnold.

Halliday, M. A. K. 1975. *Learning How to Mean*. London: Arnold.

Hofmann, A. D., and Lewis, N. R. 1981. The needle of caring, the thread of love: creative writing on an adolescent medical ward. *Adolescent Psychiatry* 9:88–116.

Inhelder, B., and Piaget, J. 1958. *The Growth of Logical Thinking: From Childhood to Adolescence*. New York: Basic.

Jacobson, E. 1964. *The Self and the Object World*. New York: International Universities Press.

Litowitz, B. E. 1985. The speaking subject in adolescence. *Adolescent Psychiatry* 12:312–326.

Luria, A. R. 1968. *The Mind of the Mnemonist*. New York: Basic.

Murray, D. M. 1968. *A Writer Teaches Writing*. Boston: Houghton Mifflin.

Oberkirch, A. 1983. Personal writings in psychotherapy. *American Journal of Psychotherapy* 37(2): 265–272.

Rampling, D. 1980. Written communications in psychotherapy. *British Journal of Medical Psychology* 53(1): 11–18.

Ryle, A. 1983. The value of written communications in dynamic psychotherapy. *British Journal of Medical Psychology* 56(4): 361–366.

Schowalter, J. E., and Lord, R. D. 1972. On the writings of adolescents in a general hospital ward. *Psychoanalytic Study of the Child* 27:181–200.

Searle, J. 1969. *Speech Acts: An Essay in the Philosophy of Language*. Cambridge: Cambridge University Press.

Solow, R. 1969. Written communication as a reflection of the treatment process. *Reiss-Davis Clinical Bulletin* 6(2): 142–150.

Sosin, D. A. 1983. The diary as a transitional object in female adolescent development. *Adolescent Psychiatry* 11:92–103.

Vološinov, V. N. 1973. *Marxism and the Philosophy of Language*. New York: Seminar.

Vygotsky, L. S. 1962. *Thought and Language*. Cambridge, Mass.: MIT Press.

Vygotsky, L. S. 1976. Play and its role in the mental development of the child. In J. S. Bruner, A. Jolly, and K. Sylva, eds. *Play: Its Role in Development and Evolution*. New York: Basic.

Vygotsky, L. S. 1978. *Mind in Society*. Cambridge, Mass.: Harvard University Press.

Weir, R. 1962. *Language in the Crib*. The Hague: Mouton.

Widroe, H., and Davidson, J. 1961. The use of directed writing in psychotherapy. *Bulletin of the Menninger Clinic* 25:110–119.

Winnicott, D. W. 1953. Transitional objects and transitional phenomena. *International Journal of Psycho-Analysis* 34:89–97.

Winnicott, D. W. 1958. The capacity to be alone. *The Maturational Processes and the Facilitating Environment*. London: Hogarth, 1965.

7 SOCIOCULTURAL MATRIX OF ADOLESCENT PSYCHOPATHOLOGY

SADI BAYRAKAL

Adolescence does not occur in a vacuum. Basically, the developmental task involves a psychological disengagement from the family and a simultaneous engagement with society. The psychic structure of adolescence is, therefore, critically affected by the current sociocultural atmosphere (Blos 1979). The new communication technology, which carries the message of prevailing cultural values to each new generation at a much earlier age than ever before, consequently is playing a crucial role in the formation of adolescent personality, emotional health, and behavioral difficulties (Nichtern 1980).

One finds an unmistakable correlation between the deterioration of the social atmosphere in Western countries and the increase in emotional difficulties and behavior problems in the young people of these countries (Flacks 1974). As Lasch (1978) points out, "social questions inevitably present themselves as personal ones." An analysis of the interplay between the adolescent and his society is useful, since, regardless of the socioeconomic and ethnic background of individual adolescents, common features of intrapsychic organization, defensive maneuvers, psychopathology, and interpersonal problems and difficulties can be found. What are the fundamental characteristics of the current occidental culture and sociohistorical context of the common life experience of youth that shape their psychic structure? More specifically, what is the individual phenomenology of this process and its impact on the universal developmental task of adolescence?

Despite the gradual loss of strength and influence, the family as a basic institution with its intricate internal and external relationship still remains a crucial force in the formation of the disturbed adolescent (Rutter and Nicola 1977). In some cases, poor nutrition and intellectual stimulation, physical and sexual abuse, lack of space, and general deprivation of peace and security impair youths' physical and psychic growth (MacLeod 1973). There is an increasing polarity in the stereotypical view of adolescents held by adults in all social classes. Youth are seen as irresponsible, hedonistic, self-centered, and victimizing. Yet, at the same time, they are considered an endangered species—victims, confused people with an unenviable lack of future. In general, adolescents engender anxiety and hostility in the adult world. Adults deal with these uncomfortable feelings by shaming, reproaching, and provoking youth—reactions which are sadistic and destructive in nature (Anthony 1975). Jealousy in adults and a resurgence of their own unresolved adolescent conflicts can find solution in the projection of the negative aspects of the current culture onto youth.

The ensuing "confusion and ambivalence reflect the general crises of American culture" (Flacks 1974). Given this pressing need to defend themselves against such accusations and to deal with constantly changing moral and ethical values, adolescents tend to view adults as "obsolete," the past as "irrelevant," and the future as "unpredictable." To forge a sense of permanency and to blend the past, present, and the future into a coherent whole becomes an insurmountable task. Social discontinuity and alienation from familial and social roots take place insidiously. "Many feel forced into detachment and premature cynicism because society seems to offer them so little that is relevant, stable and meaningful" (Erikson 1965). Ego identity, which develops out of a gradual integration of all the adolescent's identifications, is transformed into "identity diffusion" (Erikson 1959). In allying and identifying with adults in his family, the adolescent may feel obliged to live out the anxieties and fears of these adults (Palframan 1982). When emotional civil war is raging furiously within the family, the adolescent cannot escape from becoming the scapegoat or from assuming a variety of "irrational roles" at the expense of his mental health (Ackerman 1980; Framo 1982; Rollins 1973).

The adolescent who is desperate to complete the separation-individuation process turns outside family—most naturally to his peers. The cutthroat competition that permeates from the wider society to peer culture makes meaningful peer relationships difficult. The adolescent cannot escape from competitive individualism in a society where "success at any cost" is the ultimate virtue. Every relationship becomes a show for one-upmanship. The cult of individualism gradually frustrates the adolescent's need for bonding with his peers. The culture of consumerism creates perpetually artificial needs and dissatisfactions. The more the adolescent turns to the outside world, the more he is caught in the web of competitive acquisitiveness. In fact, what he wears, owns, and uses form his image (identity); this forces the adolescent's search for authentic self-identity into the background, creating an inner vacuum. The illusions and fantasies fostered by "commodities" fill the vacuum. The result is an insidious shift from an emotional investment in human beings to an emotional investment in material objects. In this process, other people gradually become "objects" to use and exploit for self-satisfaction.

The compartmentalization of sexuality into attraction, performance, and orgasm is stripping sex of its interpersonal context and reducing it to just another market commodity. In addition, double messages and standards (such as, it is the in thing to do—no you have to wait until you mature; or every form of sex is acceptable—no it is not) create confusion for adolescents who are struggling with the issue of clarifying a psychosexual identity that is linked to a cultural frame of references (Woods 1979). The redefined role of the male, according to the new sexual mores, is not completely incorporated into an accepted repertoire of behavior, for example, being kind and caring. For the female, the projected role dichotomy—on the one hand a professional and working woman and on the other hand a mother and housewife—is still an unsettled issue. While female adolescents are still denied sexual freedom, male adolescents are confused about the boundaries of their relationship to the opposite sex, and "A painful identity crisis is thereby imposed on them" (Millet 1970).

As the denigration and eventual abdication of authority in the home, in the community, and in society continues, the adolescents' superego formation remains unfinished. Under these conditions, the adolescent has to fall back on the infantile, primitive superego based on archaic images of the parents. This is not a normal process of identification with ego ideals, as it should be; rather it is a regression to a much earlier level of functioning. As a result, the permissive society paradoxically reinforces the harsh, punitive forms of superego that thwart the ego's maturational process and force it to regress. Under the impact of the regressive state, the ego resorts to some unhealthy defensive maneuvers—grandiosity, self-contempt, splitting, and projection. The adolescent's identification with authority and eventually with socio-cultural values remains incomplete. Youth perceive themselves as perpetual children who have to deal with a primitive and revengeful authority (Rogow 1975).

As part of this culture, schools are far from being a milieu in which an adolescent's curiosity about himself, others, and a better understanding of his world is stimulated. He is not taught to interrelate all his knowledge and experience into a cohesive, meaningful world outlook. Neither is he encouraged to initiate or take an active part in areas concerning his own life or his community. He gradually becomes aware that he is "educated" to be a passive technician or employee fitting into a certain job. Work is envisaged as merely a necessary evil to earn a living; it does not foster self-esteem or a realization of a creative self. The adolescent is on the way to becoming a "one-dimensional man" who has no power over what he produces or why he performs a certain task (Marcus 1964). Despite all the information and experience he accumulates, he is not learning to integrate these into an understanding of himself, his work, or the society in which he lives. Thus, the adolescent finds it extremely difficult to make a closure of his developmental task to a vocation, work, or life philosophy (Keniston 1971).

Adolescents have to come to terms with disappointing and confusing local and global realities—the puzzling contradiction of wealth and poor quality of life, the level of available knowledge and prevailing degree of ignorance, being on the verge of an era of science fiction, and teetering on the brink of global destruction. In view of these startling paradoxes, the quest for a belief becomes an excruciating endeavor. Where does my personal future meet the future of the world I live in? Is there any meaningful belief I can trust and to which I can commit myself? The necessary dialogues and cross-fertilization of ideas in the educational system, community, or in the mass media are missing. The young remain hungry for a belief. The best spokesman for today's youth may be rock music—the frightening gloom of rock-video scenes, the pessimism, the aura of violence, and the nihilism of the lyrics. The music itself is screaming anguish and rage.

The total impact of all the sociocultural factors I have mentioned engenders a basic core of anxiety. "Anxiety is a feeling of loneliness, helplessness toward a potentially hostile world" (Horney 1950) with ". . . frightening images of the world as being devoid of food and love

115

and his self-concept of the hungry wolf out to kill, eat and survive" (Kernberg 1975). Despair and anger toward a perplexing world alternate with the basic anxiety that stems from a poorly formed ego identity and sense of helplessness. Anxiety is dealt with by using some unadaptive defenses that manifest themselves as emotional difficulties and behavior problems—drug abuse, compulsive sex, withdrawal, or aggressive acting out toward others and the self.

Psychic survival gains prime importance for youth. In order to protect the good image of self, a sense of hostility felt toward the world is projected outside. A false-self is established especially to protect the real-self from a fantasied retaliation (Laing 1971). The real-self is prevented from any meaningful contact with the outside world and gradually becomes detached from it. "The immediate sense of realness of the world cannot be sustained by a false-system" (Laing 1965). The experience of depersonalization seriously threatens the ego. One is then compulsively driven to seek company. Because the adolescent is still functioning on the infantile level of object relationship, he tends to be possessive and exploitative. His interpersonal relationships never become stable and give very little satisfaction. The adolescent may develop a fantasized relationship with an idealized magical figure (false hero) that he hopes will fulfill the need for relationship and will also protect him from the hostility of the world. Idealization of the self with dreams of omnipotence and unusual abilities may imbue this identification with a false hero. In fact, underneath, "It is the image of a hungry, enraged, empty self full of impotent anger at being frustrated and fearful of a world which seems as hateful and revengeful as a patient himself" (Kernberg 1975).

The body becomes a part of the false-self—some sort of appliance that must "turn on" and "tune in" (Slater 1975). The dissociation of the body from the self reaches a point where the adolescent starts to feel that his body belongs to others and he has no control over it. He feels anything but real and alive. Self-inflicted pain or pain inflicted by others becomes one way to feel real. The resultant, apparently senseless, violence also serves the purpose of taking revenge on a world full of bad images and persecutory intentions. This violence only augments existing persecutory anxieties. A lack of interest in feedback or objective assessment of reality increases the solipsistic character of the fantasies, which causes a gradual blurring of the boundary between the inner world and outer reality. Interestingly, some adolescents are aware of this psychotic process, but this awareness only intensifies the emotional terror.

Conclusions

The emotionally disturbed adolescent of today is caught in a vicious cycle of varying degrees of anxiety and aggression as a result of the interplay between the intrapsychic life and the outside world. The nature of the intrapsychic and interpersonal problems fosters borderline and narcissistic personalities. Their psychic energy is consumed mostly with the preoccupation of psychic survival. The spectrum of emotional difficulties they present ranges from apathy and free-floating anxiety to depression and psychosis.

Every era and culture develops its own peculiar form of personality structure and psychopathology, which is more discernible in the most disturbed members of society. In Freud's time, guilt and various forms of neurosis represented the characteristics of basic personality traits that were caused by excessive repression of basic instinctual needs. In the second half of the twentieth century, there has been a significant change in the underlying organization of personality from inner direction to narcissism and alienation from the authentic self. Although the result is individual psychic disturbance, the determinants of the shift in the personality organization are sociocultural evolution and existing norms in society. The sociocultural reality is first reflected on the malleable psyche of the child and adolescent. Gradually, this simple reflection becomes a well-entrenched inner reality and forms an independent existence. The most vulnerable member of society is "the adolescent who in due process is becoming psychologically and socially homeless" (Keniston 1965). Although the existing turmoil of the emotionally suffering adolescent is a serious challenge to mental health professionals, the ultimate factor is the culture, which should adapt to the emotional needs of its offspring. "The young really need a more worthwhile world in order to grow up at all" (Goodman 1960).

NOTE

This paper was presented before the panel on "Behavioral Disorders" at the organizing conference of the International Society for Adolescent Psychiatry, Paris, July 22, 1985.

REFERENCES

Ackerman, N. 1980. The family with adolescents. In E. A. Carter and A. McGoldrick, eds. *The Family Life Cycle*. New York: Gardner.

Anthony, E. J. 1975. The reaction of adults to adolescents and their behavior. In A. H. Esman, ed. *Psychology of Adolescence*. New York: International Universities Press.

Blos, P. 1979. *Adolescent Passage*. New York: International Universities Press.

Erikson, E. 1959. *Identity and the Life Cycle*. New York: International Universities Press.

Erikson, E. 1965. *Challenge of Youth*. New York: Anchor.

Flacks, R. 1974. Growing up confused: cultural crisis and individual character. In A. Skolnick and J. H. Skolnick, eds. *Intimacy, Family and Society*. Boston: Little Brown.

Framo, J. 1982. *Exploration in Marital and Family Therapy*. New York: Springer.

Goodman, P. 1960. *Growing up Absurd*. New York: Vintage.

Horney, K. 1950. *The Neurosis and Human Growth*. New York: Norton.

Keniston, K. 1965. *Uncommitted*. New York: Dell.

Keniston, K. 1971. Youth as a stage of life. *Adolescent Psychiatry* 1:161–175.

Kernberg, O. 1975. *Borderline Conditions and Pathological Narcissism*. New York: Aronson.

Laing, R. D. 1971. *The Divided Self*. Baltimore: Penguin.

Lasch, C. 1978. *Culture of Narcissism*. New York: Norton.

MacLeod, A. 1973. *Growing up in America*. Chevy Chase, Md.: U.S. Department of Health, Education and Welfare.

Marcus, H. 1964. *One Dimensional Man*. Boston: Beacon.

Millet, K. 1970. *Sexual Politics*. Garden City, N.Y.: Doubleday.

Nichtern, S. 1980. The missing adolescent. *Adolescent Psychiatry* 8:54–64.

Palframan, D. S. 1982. The discarded adolescent. *Psychiatric Journal of the University of Ottawa* 7:226–230.

Rogow, A. A. 1975. *The Dying Light*. New York: Putnam.

Rollins, N. 1973. Some roles children play in their families. *Journal of the American Academy of Child Psychiatry* 12:511–530.

Rutter, M., and Nicola, M. 1977. *Cycles of Disadvantage*. London: Heinemann.

Slater, P. 1975. *Pursuit of Loneliness: American Culture at the Breaking Point*. Middlesex: Penguin.

Woods, N. F. 1979. *Human Sexuality in Health and Disease*. New York: Mosby.

8   ADOLESCENT FILM PREFERENCES: THE WORLD OF *PURPLE RAIN;* A PSYCHODYNAMIC INTERPRETATION

LUCIA VILLELA AND RICHARD MARKIN

This study of film preferences in adolescence is based on the assumption that myths, fairy tales, and narratives in general are metaphorical attempts to understand and explain the perceived realities of our own selves—our origins, our future, our world. This is not a falsifiable assumption. It can only be granted as reasonable or rejected—the list of those who have granted it is impressive. As early as in 1725, Giambattista Vico (Bergin and Fisch 1984) was claiming that myths were civil histories in poetical form. Since Freud (1906), Lévi-Strauss (1958), and Lacan (1966), this list has been growing at an exponential rate.

We are also assuming that movies are modern forms of mythmaking and that, like myths, they provide clues to the conscious and unconscious shared wishes, conflicts, and fears of different groups and different stages of development in our society. If adolescents as a group share certain specific developmental characteristics, and if these characteristics differ from those of other age groups, then these differences are likely to be reflected in the adolescents' narrative preferences. This last proposition is falsifiable, and, in order to check its legitimacy, we distributed questionnaires on media preferences and collected responses from 296 adolescents—from ages fourteen through eighteen—and 160 adults—from ages twenty-six through sixty-five.

While we had not aimed at any systematic statistical controls or matched groups, the settings where our questionnaires were distributed tapped three different socioeconomic groups at the adolescent level

119

and three roughly similar groups of adults. We collected responses from students at a suburban high school, where the population was mostly white and middle class, and from adults at different suburban settings (schools, hospitals, business offices, and homes), where the population was also mostly white and middle class. We collected responses from students at a private, university-sponsored, urban high school, where the population was racially mixed, middle class, and intellectually sophisticated, and from staff and graduate students at the same university, where continuing-education classes attract a fair number of older, returning professionals and of part-time students. Finally, we collected responses from students at a public school located in a segregated neighborhood, where the population was exclusively black and below the poverty level or little above it, and from adult students at an open-admissions university, where the population was mostly black and economically mixed (from poverty level to middle class).

While we must warn against the generalization of results to other groups, within our sample, the existence of equivalences enables us to compare each group of adolescents to its equivalent reference group as well as to other adolescents.

Results were more complex than expected. Adolescents do share with each other preferences that they do not share with adults, but they also share with their group of origin (or similar groups) preferences that are not shared with other adolescents. For instance, students at the university-sponsored high school list *Purple Rain* as one of their favorite movies, as do adolescents from all socioeconomic groups. However, they also list *Amadeus* (about the tempestuous life of Mozart), a preference they share with adults at the same university and in the suburbs but not with other adolescents. Certain themes (such as physical danger, separation and individuation, self-cohesion and identity, commitment, and success) and interests (such as dance, physical strength, and physical skills in general) reliably distinguish adolescent from adult preferences. However, the prevalence of each theme, and the way themes and interests are combined and coded, seems to be the result of an interaction between age and group of origin. As shown in table 1, most adolescents are "turned on" by movies dealing with dancing, especially break dancing, but, in the suburbs, the movie *Foot-loose* (portraying conflict and reconciliation between dance-loving youngsters and dance-fearing adults) is a big favorite; while among students in the black public school and, to some extent, among students

TABLE 1
CONTRASTING AND SHARED PREFERENCES OF ADOLESCENTS AND ADULTS:
A COMPARISON OF THE TEN TOP CHOICES IN EACH GROUP

	Adolescents	Adults	Shared Preferences
Suburban middle class...........	Purple Rain	Amadeus	The Karate Kid
	Sixteen Candles	Terms of	Ghostbusters
	Footloose	Endearment	Romancing the
	Red Dawn	Places in the	Stone
	Indiana Jones	Heart	Gremlins
	The Terminator	Star Trek	
		The Return of the	
		Jedi	
		Entre Nous	
Urban middle class...........	Ghostbusters	Rear Window	Amadeus
	Purple Rain	Terms of	The Karate Kid
	Sixteen Candles	Endearment	Indiana Jones
	The Natural	Places in the	
	Gremlins	Heart	
	The Terminator	All of Me	
	Night of the	An Officer and a	
	Comet	Gentleman	
		Brother from	
		Another Planet	
		Beverly Hills Cop	
Urban poor.......	Nightmare on Elm	A Soldier's Story	Purple Rain
	Street	Beverly Hills Cop	The Terminator
	Beat Street	Indiana Jones	Gremlins
	Breakin'	Star Trek	
	Scarface	Trading Places	
	Teachers	Raiders of the	
	Silent Night	Lost Ark	
	Alone in the Dark	An Officer and a	
		Gentleman	

in the private urban school *Beat Street* and *Breakin* (in which poor but talented youngsters "make it" in the world of dance and music) are the winners. Table 1 lists shared and contrasting preferences for each group of adolescents and its equivalent group of adults.

The only movie listed as a favorite by all adolescent groups—and by few adults, except a small group of black females between ages of twenty-six and thirty—is *Purple Rain*, as can be seen in table 2, which lists the top twenty adolescent preferences and their comparative rat-

121

TABLE 2
MOVIE PREFERENCE OF ADOLESCENTS

	ADOLESCENTS					ADULTS				
	Sub (N=103)	UM (N=90)	UP (N=103)	Total (N=296)	Total % (N=296)	Sub (N=58)	UM (N=60)	UP (N=42)	Total (N=160)	Total % (N=160)
Purple Rain	29	23	71	123	42	1	2	10	13	8
Ghostbusters	26	46	4	76	26	10	2	1	13	8
Gremlins	12	6	36	54	18	4	1	2	7	4
Karate Kid	29	19	4	52	18	11	3	1	14	10
Indiana Jones	23	19	3	45	15	1	3	4	8	5
Sixteen Candles	17	15	...	32	11	1	...	...	...	...
The Terminator	9	6	13	28	9	...	2	4	6	4
Nightmare on Elm Street	6	...	15	21	7	...	...	...	...	...
Breakin'	6	...	12	18	6	...	...	...	...	...
Beat Street	2	2	13	17	6	...	...	...	...	...
Footloose	16	1	...	17	6	...	...	...	...	...
Friday the 13th	4	...	9	13	4	...	...	...	...	...
Teachers	1	1	10	12	4	...	...	...	...	...
Scarface	...	...	11	11	4	...	...	...	...	...
Missing in Action	7	...	4	11	4	...	...	...	...	...
The Natural	3	7	...	10	3	...	...	...	...	...
Red Dawn	9	...	1	10	3	...	...	...	...	...
Amadeus	...	9	...	9	3	7	13	...	20	13
Romancing the Stone	9	...	...	9	3	5	3	1	9	6
Silent Night, Deadly Night	...	...	9	9	3	...	...	...	...	...

NOTE.—Sub = suburban; UM = urban middle class; UP = urban poor.

ings by adults. Therefore, *Purple Rain* is the film we shall examine in some detail in this chapter.

In our analysis of *Purple Rain,* we are following a somewhat modified structuralist technique. We intend to identify a number of mythemes or binary oppositions around which the story can be organized, as Lévi-Strauss (1958) did in his analysis of the Oedipus myth. However, we agree with Turner (1969, 1977) and with Brooks (1984) that linguistic-based techniques often jeopardize their own goals by concentrating on the synchronic (i.e., the timeless) dimension and ignoring the dia-chronic (i.e., ignoring changes over time). Therefore, our analysis of themes will focus on their transformations over time and their rules of occurrence. We shall examine both plot and story and the tension between the two; this tension will then be interpreted in developmental and psychodynamic terms.

We are defining story and plot very much as the Russian formalists defined *fabula* and *sjuzét* and as the French structuralists defined *histoire* and *récit.* Story is the time-bound sequence of events referred to in a narrative in the order they are supposed to have taken place. Plot is the way and sequence in which the events of the story are presented to the viewer (or reader).

In contrast to most straightforward, so-called realistic American movies, in *Purple Rain,* plot and story are far from identical. *Purple Rain* has its own brand of punk-rock American surrealism, which forces the viewer to recognize that any retelling of a story, such as the one that follows, is already an act of interpretation.

Purple Rain is the story of a young and struggling musician who is both a composer and a performer and of his quest for love, success, and knowledge of self. The roads and streets traveled in this quest are full of torments as well as ecstasies; there is nothing bland or muted in the world of purple rain. The young musician, simply called the Kid throughout the movie, lives in a modest residential area in Minneapolis. He lives in the home owned by his black father and white mother, both onetime musicians who did not succeed in their chosen careers, who blame each other for their failures, and who are now locked in the bonds of an intense and violent love-hate marriage. The Kid ineffec-tually attempts to mediate their relationship and stop the violence. When he fails, as he usually does, he takes refuge in his basement apartment, which is full of unusual lamps and lights, masks, rotating statuettes, musical instruments, cassette players, and larger-than-life pictures and posters. Or, he escapes to an idyllic countryside on his motorbike, alone or with his newly found love, Apollonia,[1] an aspiring young singer who has just arrived in town. At work, in a club where rock fans congregate, the Kid has had a fair measure of success as a promising musician and the leader of a group called The Revolution. But the club owner is not pleased with his choice of songs—they are too controversial, too blatantly sexual, too full of anger and pain. The Kid is also having problems with members of his band, for he demands a lot and does not share the spotlight. And now a special cause of discord has arisen: Lisa and Wendy, the two girls in the band, have composed a song that he likes but refuses to use in their act. This discord is being manipulated by Morris Day, the Kid's main rival and the leader of a group called The Time, who wants to get the Kid fired. Apollonia's arrival in town further complicates the matter and intensifies the rivalry between Morris Day and the Kid. She falls in love with the Kid, but he finds himself treating her the same way he sees his father treat his mother. He is jealous, mistrustful, suspicious of her motives, and unwilling both to share his dreams with her and to help her with her own aspirations for a career. When she accepts help from Morris Day, the Kid hits her, and they break up. The Kid is getting himself deeper and deeper in trouble in his work and in his love life. At home, the violence is escalating. One night, as he comes home enraged, ready for a fight, he finds his father in the basement, playing a haunting tune—not too unlike the one the girls have composed—on the piano. It is a moment of few words and many shared feelings for father and son—the uncovering of an empathic bond that had seemed dramatically absent. A few days later, the father shoots himself in the head in a suicide attempt. He miraculously survives, and his tragic action shocks the mother out of her alcoholic haze and into the role of a concerned wife. Alone at home, in the room where it took place, the Kid relives the suicide attempt, which he had heard but not seen. The sound of the shot is reexperienced over and over again as the Kid looks at a coil of rope on the floor and paces back and forth in increasing agitation. A picture of himself hanging from the ceiling flashes on the screen. The Kid screams, grabs a stick hanging from the wall, and starts knocking down jars of preserves, dishes, shelves—whatever he can hit in the room—until he pulls down a cardboard box that comes apart revealing stacks and stacks of annotated music. As he picks up a page and recognizes it as the song he heard his father play, his rage

STAGE OF SHOCK AND DENIAL

Initially there is a stage of shock and denial regarding their child's homosexuality. All of the fears and prejudices of the parent regarding homosexuality are suddenly brought to the surface. During this time, the gay adolescent is in particular danger of being physically assaulted by the parent and, not rarely, of being physically ejected from the home. The adolescent may be overwhelmed by the magnitude of emotions expressed, and fear or humiliation may cause him or her to leave the home or run away. Within hours to a few days, the shock and disbelief usually organize into a more orderly system of denial. Parents may entreat their child to put these ideas out of his or her head, to pray, or refuse to discuss it further, insisting that it is merely a normal phase of adolescence that will pass or believing that it is a temporary effect of associating with an undesirable peer group. Parents, even those who may have suspected that their child was homosexual for a long time, may refuse to hear the child state that his or her homoerotic feelings antedate their discovery by the parent. The various methods of denial used by family members serve to externalize the issue from the adolescent and family, thus protecting the individuals from the painful feelings that recognition of a family member's homosexuality will cause. Not infrequently, especially if the adolescent recants his or her homosexuality, family members may remain in a prolonged state of denial.

CASE EXAMPLE 1

A seventeen-year-old boy's homosexuality was discovered by his parents near the end of his last school year. This boy, an exemplary student in an accelerated program of a private school, had been accepted to a prestigious university, entering in the fall. His father sequentially had him evaluated by two psychiatrists who found the boy to be without any disorder. The father then sent his son to see a priest, who also felt that family conflicts were more the issue than the boy's homosexuality. The father then specifically sought consultation with a psychiatrist who offered to attempt to change the boy's sexual orientation, but the boy refused to return after the initial session. One evening the boy's mother asked her son to recant his homosexuality. The boy refused, and in her frustration she struck him just as the father entered the room. Believing the boy to be assaulting his wife, he ordered his son out of the house. The boy found shelter with some friends for

167

about a month, continued in school, and then returned home when his parents threatened to withdraw all financial support for college. The boy's homosexuality was not further discussed by family members for the next three months, even though the boy continued to be involved in a homosexual relationship.

Some parents have continued for years to attempt to interest their sons or daughters in opposite-sex partners—despite overwhelming evidence that the child indeed has exclusively homosexual interests.

STAGE OF ANGER AND GUILT

Unless the parents have extremely rigid personality structures, the stage of denial usually gives way to a stage characterized by anger and guilt. The homosexual adolescent, if the fantasies of disaster are not realized, will often persistently continue to provide evidence that forces parents to move beyond their unrealistic state of denial. Not uncommonly, parental anger is focused on attempts to discover a proximate cause for their child's homosexuality. Without our group, the adolescent's parents often found out about their child's homosexuality at the same time they learned of the rap group and sometimes directed their anger at the group's leadership or sponsorship. Teachers, the school, the media, the adolescent's friends or intimates, or the other parent may be attacked. This behavior of parents is caused partly by the attempt to defend against the painful emotions aroused by the realization that a son or daughter has experienced homosexual feelings or behavior for a very long time. Parents feel guilty that they did not recognize their child's homosexuality or that they did not take any action to change the outcome. Of course, many societal myths regarding the etiology of homosexuality (the seduction of youth by homosexual adults; the presentation of sex education that includes information about homosexuality; the exposure to popular music; or the association with peers who are homosexual) support the notion that homosexuality is a condition acquired during adolescence. A parent often projects blame onto the other parent for not being a good enough mother or father, creating additional strain on the marital relationship at a time when clear communication is so important. Rigid or compulsive parents may look for external solutions, such as litigation, as a means of remaining detached from the drama that is unfolding in their own home. Almost universally, however, whether under the guise of taking over

168

where the other parent has failed or to correct what is believed to be one's own failure, the parent or parents of the gay adolescent make frantic and at times ludicrous attempts to alter their parenting practices, as though they hope to reverse events. Parents frequently revert to using disciplinary practices and having expectations that are inappropriate for the age of their child. In their attempt to turn back the clock, these parents almost invariably establish an unreasonable curfew, attempt to restrict access of the adolescent to friends, open the adolescent's mail, or search his or her room.

It is during this period that parents most often coerce the child into treatment, demanding a change to a heterosexual orientation. If the child resists the parents' prescriptions, residential treatment may be pursued. Parents seeking treatment for their adolescent often refuse to accept a therapist unless the therapist shares their belief that homosexuality is pathological. The adolescent is understandably unlikely to accept a therapist who holds such values. The exception is the younger adolescent whose homosexuality is discovered during the period of intense anxiety that typically occurs when the adolescent first acknowledges his or her homosexuality. He or she may be overwhelmed by the intensity of the family's negative reactions and, fearing punishment or wholesale rejection, may submit almost penitently to whatever the family requests.

A carefully chosen therapist who does not consider the adolescent's homosexuality as pathological, and who does not trivialize the adolescent's homoerotic feelings or behavior as a mere phase of normal development that will pass, but who is able to recognize the complexity of the family dynamics, can be invaluable in assisting the family to reach a new homeostasis that promotes rather than stifles the continued psychosocial development of the adolescent in an atmosphere of enhanced intrafamilial relationships. The perceptions of family members and the resulting dynamics are often distorted by years of misinformation that have been provided by the adolescent who has misrepresented and attempted to hide his or her homosexuality. The endorsement of prejudices against homosexuality, the reliance on stereotypes, and the family members' personal experiences will affect the dynamics at this time of family crisis. It is important to realize that both the adolescent and other family members often exaggerate each other's behavior, when talking to a third party, as a way of justifying their actions.

169

During this phase, parents, professing a concern for their loved one, may enumerate a dismal series of future events that the adolescent can expect, such as: narrowed career choices; no family life; or legal problems—most of which arc largely unrealistic and based on inaccurate stereotypes of gay people. Most of these responses, even those of apparent genuine concern, are displacements of anger, guilt, or loss by the parent, and the therapist must assist the family members in acknowledging these feelings. Unless family members are able to do this, they will be relatively inaccessible to new information and insights from others that will enable them to gain a realistic understanding of the issues so that they can be genuinely understanding of the experience of their adolescent.

STAGE OF ACKNOWLEDGMENT

After the stage of intense anger and guilt, a stage characterized by acceptance of the facts that their adolescent is sexually attracted to persons of his or her own sex and that this is likely to continue to be so follows. Parents with inaccurate information about homosexuality and gay life-styles, especially those with fundamentalist religious beliefs that condemn homosexuality, may resign themselves to believing that their child is immoral, pathological, or will forever be unhappy. In these families, various barriers may be placed before the adolescent, from emotional neglect to ostracism or expulsion from the family. Reestablishment of family support sometimes does not occur. One case in particular exemplifies most of these parental reactions:

CASE EXAMPLE 2

A fifteen-year-old female honor student, member of two school bands and of the school soccer team, chose to confide her homosexuality to a teacher. The teacher related this information to another teacher, who took it upon himself to disclose the information to the girl's parents. Her parents immediately forbade her to see any of her friends, screened all of her phone calls, drove her to and from school, and discouraged her from having any contact with her younger brother and nephews and nieces, and forbade her to leave the house after school. Within a week, she ran away from home and stayed with the family of another member of the group, refusing to disclose her whereabouts to her

170

parents. The group leader facilitated the parents' and child's entrance into counseling with a local agency in an attempt to resolve the family crisis. Both the child and her parents made exaggerated claims about the recent activities of the other: the child said she had been physically abused by her parents; her mother insisted her daughter had been attending a gay bar with live sex shows (actually a reference to a lesbian coffeehouse with poetry readings); and that the rap group was a cult of homosexuals using sophisticated brainwashing techniques. After several sessions the child returned home, but only after insisting that she be allowed to attend the rap group as a condition of her return. Her parents brought her to the group regularly, and the entire family entered family therapy with a mutually acceptable therapist.

Parents who have a broader knowledge of homosexuality in our society, who seek or are provided with accurate information, and who trust their own understanding of their child, begin to move toward the reestablishment of intimate family relationships. These families may not approve of homosexuality but recognize that their child is the same child as before revealing his or her sexual orientation. Fortunately, most families eventually reach this point, but not without much struggle, and the stress on individuals can take its emotional toll.

The Adolescents' Process of Disclosure

The group rarely pressured members to "come out" to their parents. The fears of the anticipated specter were so potentially threatening that telling one's parents was felt to be a most individual decision. Nevertheless, the group held telling one's parents to be a courageous, positive step. As the beneficial effects on the gay adolescents and the eventual improvements of family relations were observed by members, the group became a potent force in encouraging its members to come out to their parents.

Parental rejection was found to be temporary, and the support of the group made this potential for temporary parental rejection more tolerable. Most of the adolescents who did come out to their parents did not do so directly but rather began to eliminate their hiding maneuvers and prior vigilant caution until their parents confronted them. The predictions of the likely responses of parents were comforting to members involved in the process of disclosing their homosexuality. Only a small minority of the adolescents had disclosed their sexual orientation

171

to their parents prior to attending this group, but the proportion increased to over one-half for members who had attended at least ten times. Initially the leaders were alarmed at this powerful group influence and believed that the group was lending a sense of security that would not be obtained outside of the group. Fortunately, our initial fears about premature disclosure were generally unfounded, and most parents were able to move beyond their initial anger and rejection and reestablish a relationship with their child that was as good as or better than before.

These adolescents persistently and intensively examined parental motives and behavior, allowing them to develop a more empathic understanding of their parents and to have a deeper understanding of a variety of parent-child conflict areas, including those not directly related to issues of sexuality.

Before my experience with this group, I believed that the potential hazards of coming out to parents were too great for any gay adolescent who still lived at home. I no longer believe this to be the case for the adolescent who has a supportive network that includes peers and accepts his or her homosexuality. Each adolescent must carefully examine his or her particular situation, realizing that there is indeed a potential for extreme family reactions. The issues of personal safety and shelter, should parents react violently or expel the child from the home, should not be ignored, and provisions for temporary safe housing should be made before the adolescent embarks on this course.

The Peer Group and the Gay Adolescent

ACKNOWLEDGMENT OF HOMOEROTIC FEELING

During adolescence the peer group becomes increasingly important as the field where new ideas and roles are observed and experienced. Being accepted by a group of age-mates with whom one can share existence and establish intimate relationships is paramount to the early adolescent. These adolescents reported that between twelve and fourteen years of age they discovered that they were much more profoundly sexually attracted to persons of their own sex than were most of their age-mates. They almost immediately realized that "gay," "homosexual," or other, derogatory, terms were applied to persons who have such feelings. Most also stated that this was about the age when they first realized that they had felt sexually different for many years but may not have related these feelings to their image of homosexuality or homosexually oriented persons. It is understandable that this realization should occur at this stage of psychological development, for it is at about this time that the adolescent develops the capacity for abstract thought. The adolescent is now able to simultaneously recall the past, recognize present feelings and behavior, observe the expectations, rules, and reactions of society, all while imagining oneself in the future. Most gay adolescents can vividly recall the intense anxiety they experienced when they first discovered that they suddenly belonged to this group of people that is so vehemently despised by most others. The industriousness they mastered in childhood, the positive self-regard they may have developed, and the dreams for a happy and productive future seem to be dashed almost as soon as they enter the awareness of the gay adolescent. An ego crisis occurs that can be understood as the conflict produced by the juxtaposition of the negative views of homosexuality, which have been learned over their lifetime, with the incipient ego identity that is developing. Erikson (1963) defines ego identity as: ". . . the accrued self-confidence that the inner sameness and continuity prepared in the past are matched by the sameness and continuity of one's meaning for others, as evidenced in the tangible promise of a 'career.' " The normal developmental egocentrism of this age further compounds the anxiety and self-doubt of the adolescent who is recognizing his or her homosexuality. The young adolescent behaves as though he or she is at the center of others' attention and often feels as though others are observing him or her, almost with the capability of reading his or her thoughts (Elkind 1982). Perhaps this combination of developmental events is related to the high incidence of reported suicidal ideation in this group; slightly more than one-third of these adolescents mentioned having had suicidal ideation, most often occurring during early adolescence and relating to their sexuality.

Younger gay adolescents make one of three choices in dealing with their newly acknowledged sexual feelings: (1) try to change them; (2) continue to hide them; or (3) accept them (Martin 1982). These three strategies often follow one another over time, but this is not invariably the case. Very few younger or mid adolescents adopt the last strategy initially, but some persons who successfully suppress their thoughts about their homosexuality until later in life may come out at this stage seeming to have never adopted the other strategies. In using the term "strategy," I am implying a conscious awareness of the thoughts and feelings that lead to the conscious choice to engage in or avoid certain behaviors. I am not using this term to apply to those persons who have truly repressed their thoughts and feelings about their homosexuality. It is not that uncommon for some persons to experience many years of consistent or even exclusive homosexual experiences and homo-erotic feelings without ever acknowledging that this is an important part of themselves. The distinction between the conscious strategies that I am referring to and the unconscious mechanisms that one uses to ward off painful realizations is not always distinct. Well-learned and practiced strategies may become so habitual that one is no longer conscious of them. My impressions are based on observations of adolescents who are and have been aware of their homosexuality and were attempting to understand its meaning for them and for others in contemporary society.

From the time they first acknowledged their homosexuality, most of these gay adolescents went through a period when they attempted to change their sexual orientation—or at the very least hoped these feelings would go away. Few entered treatment for this purpose unless the family demanded this during the crisis period when the adolescent's homosexuality was discovered and the adolescent was experiencing intense anxiety, depression, or shame. Most attempts to change involve self-remedies, some of which may appear comical. Others that may be quite destructive are premised on the idea that homosexuality is antimasculine: wrists may be taped at night; efforts are made to walk with a swagger, bodybuilding may be entered into in a compulsive way; heterosexual dating and sexual activity may be frantically pursued; but, most commonly, attempts are made to use sheer will and self-recrimination to suppress homoerotic thoughts and feelings. Masturbation may induce increased guilt because it is associated with homosexual fantasies. Associations with same-sex peers may be terminated because of the erotic feelings that are aroused. At some time most of the gay adolescents made trips to a library where they sought information that might assist them in understanding their homosexual feelings. Unfortunately, most of the material available is inaccurate and biased against homosexuality and further assaults the adolescents' self-esteem. Depending on the support of the environment, the access to information, and the age and ego strength of the individual, the period of wanting to change one's sexual orientation may last from a few weeks to several decades. Usually within a few months to a year the adolescent has little desire to change sexual orientation but still remains extremely fearful of anyone's finding out.

HIDING HOMOEROTIC FEELINGS

Most adolescents ruminated about their homosexuality, usually the fear of being discovered and methods to avoid this. More than a few said that they thought about it every minute of every day, a fact that is not so surprising when one considers how often the average adolescent has thoughts relating to sexual or sociosexual activities. Exhibitionistic efforts to appear before their families and peers as undoubtedly heterosexual were made and included: heterosexual dating, involvement in contact sports, or rowdy or mildly antisocial activities. Other endeavors for which the individual may have had considerable interest or talent were sometimes purposefully avoided, such as dramatics, singing, dance, or the creative arts. Especially for boys, the self-conscious internal dialogue that accompanies the aforementioned behaviors may have marked deleterious effects on interpersonal relationships, particularly on the development of intimacy and friendship with other boys. Gay adolescents are forever monitoring themselves: "Am I standing too close?" "Is my voice too high?" "Do I appear too happy to see him (her)?" What should be spontaneous expressions of affection or happiness become moments of agonizing fear and uncertainty. Gay girls appear to suffer somewhat less in this regard, for girls are allowed a greater range of behavior in our society before they are considered to have crossed traditional sex-role boundaries. Some of the most painful moments occur when homophobic sentiments are expressed in a social setting, such as when an antigay joke is told, or when another individual, perhaps a boy with some traditionally feminine characteristics, is harassed or ridiculed or called some epithet that is commonly applied to gay persons. It is not unusual for a gay adolescent to join in these homophobic activities in order to maintain his or her own "cover." For similar reasons, gay boys and lesbian girls, often because of a fear of drawing attention to themselves, will not associate in their schools with other students whom they believe to be gay.

SOCIAL EXPERIENCE OF GAY ADOLESCENTS

The experience of the gay adolescent whose homosexuality becomes known or highly suspected varies. Verbal harassment, name calling,

175

baiting, and practical jokes are the rule, but physical assault does sometimes occur, not to mention the more subtle but important forms of social ostracism. Exceptionally popular individuals or those who were successful in high-status activities did not seem to suffer so much harassment. But these adolescents who enjoyed relatively high status among their peers often guarded the secret of their homosexuality zealously and appeared the most anxious about the prospect of disclosure.

Gay adolescents, whether they have come out or continue to hide, experience much of the heterosocial and explicitly or implicitly homophobic aspects of adolescent life as extremely isolating. Low self-esteem, academic inhibition, truancy, substance abuse, social withdrawal, depressed mood, and suicidal ideation are frequent but fortunately most often transient problems. Adolescence is a period of heightened awareness of sexual matters, and gay adolescents are apt to become frustrated by the variety of heterosexual and heterosocial outlets that are available to others while there are so few for them. Gay adolescents, wanting involvement in a peer group that accepts them and offers the possibility of establishing intimate relationships, often begin to search for other gay persons. They may call gay hot lines, search for gay newspapers, contact agencies that serve the gay and lesbian community, or frequent areas where they believe gay people are to be found. In most large cities there are a variety of gay and lesbian services, but most of these activities are directed to gay and lesbian adults, and many actively discriminate against gay youth because they fear reprisals if they serve young people. These and other barriers make it tremendously difficult for gay adolescents to succeed in meeting other adolescents in a positive and supportive environment.

Gay adolescents who attend a rap group may benefit from the experience in many ways, some of which have been discussed in earlier sections. But first, they must muster the courage to actually enter the group; the average time between finding out about this group and actually attending was about six weeks. The initial experience of coming to the group often had a profound impact on the adolescents' mood, particularly on that of adolescents who were extremely isolated or thought that teenagers experiencing similar feelings were extremely rare. Over a few sessions the adolescents' affect brightened considerably as they saw other normal boys and girls who were gay, shared common family and school experiences, and received concept validation of their feelings, fantasies, and behavior. Many of the adolescents from this group, including some who had been in therapy, reported that they had never shared any of this material with another person. One seventeen-year-old boy, attending the group for the first time, was quite obviously attempting to delay the close of the group. When confronted about this he matter-of-factly replied, "Now I have to go back for a week where I won't be with anyone gay. I have to think about how I talk and walk and what I say every minute of every day until I come back here."

Conclusions

This adolescent group exerted a powerful influence on members' willingness to disclose their homosexuality to their parents and friends. As myths and stereotypes about homosexuality were discovered not to be true, the shame about their homosexuality and the fear of disclosure were diminished. Through the sharing of past and current experiences concerning disclosure, anticipated reactions of others could be compared with actual reactions—allowing the development of realistic expectations regarding disclosure of their homosexuality.

Group members often socialized with each other outside of the group, and many close friendships, as well as a social network of peers, developed. Most of these adolescents had been quite socially isolated, and this was the first time for many that they had participated in extensive social activities with peers outside a classroom. Some of the members began to meet regularly outside the group to organize social activities for themselves and other gay teenagers.

Certain subgroups of homosexually oriented children, for example, juvenile male prostitutes and extremely feminine boys, do experience with high frequency important conflicts with their social environment regarding their sexuality. The nonclinical population of gay adolescents also experiences significant conflicts with their social milieu, particularly in the areas of family and peer interactions. Certainly, this group of adolescents may not be representative of the total population of gay adolescents, but I do believe that this group is much more representative than those on which other reports of gay adolescents have been based. Most gay persons appear to become aware of their sexual orientation during early adolescence. This awareness and its concomitant social, behavioral, and psychological ramifications interact with the

177

ongoing processes of social development and identity formation. Having the support of a gay peer group can be an important factor in promoting the gay adolescent to meet interpersonal challenges that are important for his or her uninterrupted development.

REFERENCES

Bell, A. P.; Weinberg, M. S.; and Hammersmith, S. K. 1981. *Sexual Preference: Its Development in Men and Women.* Bloomington: Indiana University Press.
Deisher, R. W. 1982. Variations in sexual behavior of adolescents. In V. C. Kelley, ed. *Practice of Pediatrics.* Philadelphia: Harper & Row.
Elkind, D. 1982. Piagetian psychology and the practice of child psychiatry. *Journal of the American Academy of Child Psychiatry* 21:435–445.
Erikson, E. 1950. *Childhood and Society.* New York: Basic, 1963.
Green, R. 1977. Atypical sexual development. In M. Rutter and L. Hersov, eds. *Child Psychiatry: Modern Approaches.* Oxford: Blackwell Scientific.
Green, R. 1985. Gender identity in childhood and later sexual orientation: follow-up of 78 males. *American Journal of Psychiatry* 142:339–341.
Martin, A. D. 1982. Learning to hide: the socialization of the gay adolescent. *Adolescent Psychiatry* 10:52–65.
Roesler, T., and Deisher, R. W. 1972. Youthful male homosexuality. *Journal of the American Medical Association* 219:1018–1023.
Saghir, M. T., and Robins, E. 1975. *Male and Female Homosexuality: A Comprehensive Investigation.* Baltimore: Williams & Wilkins.
Yalom, I. D. 1975. *The Theory and Practice of Group Psychotherapy.* New York: Basic.

12   THE BODY AS A TRANSITIONAL OBJECT IN BULIMIA: A CRITIQUE OF THE CONCEPT

CAMAY WOODALL

In recent years, explanations for eating disorders have been sought in the mother-infant relationship (Charone 1982). Problems with separation-individuation also have been implicated in the genesis of anorexia nervosa and bulimia (Selvini-Palazzoli 1978), as have Kleinian tenets (Chernin 1985; Woodall 1983). And Winnicott's (1953) construct of transitional objects has been invoked to explain the bulimic's attitude toward her body (Sugarman and Kurash 1982). But is there empirical evidence for these assertions? Do the statements of eating-disorder patients reflect a subjective experience that would support these assertions, especially in the case of transitional objects?

Winnicott (1953) proposed that infants are helped in the separation process by their ability to invest an object (e.g., a blanket or a teddy bear) with the soothing and comforting aspects of the early mother. The infant can then provide for herself or himself the comfort of the mother by holding onto this substitute object. Further, the infant can invoke this comforting at will and thus can begin to tolerate the mother's occasional absence without object loss.

Self-statements of bulimic and anorectic adolescent and older women (fourteen to twenty-six years old) were collected using a 100-item Sentence Completion Test devised by this writer for a larger study (Woodall 1983). Spontaneous metaphors referring to the body and self (e.g., "My self is nonexistent" or "My body is my enemy") were examined for their relevance to separation issues and to the concept of transitional objects. The same data were elicited from an age-matched group of obese females and normal females (i.e., those exhibiting no eating disorders). These self- and body statements are contrasted with the contention that, in bulimia, the body is a transitional object.

Sugarman and Kurash (1982) consider bulimia a problem of the Separation-Individuation stage, as do I. They disagree with Selvini-Palazzoli (1978), who concluded that the body in bulimia is a persecutory object produced by the internalization of the mother. Sugarman and Kurash state that, for them, bulimia represents "a more developmentally primitive ego boundary disturbance." They sum up their position in the following:

> Our working thesis is that bulimia reflects an arrest at the earliest stages of transitional object development. Specifically, the failure to adequately separate both physically and cognitively from the maternal object during the practicing subphase leads to a narcissistic fixation on one's own body at the expense of reaching out to other objects in the wider world, through the use of external transitional objects. This arrest in the area of transitional objects has profound consequences as regards self-other boundary differentiation, individuation, and capacity for symbolization. [Sugarman and Kurash, 1982, p. 58]

What at first seems to be a plausible conceptualization of the body in bulimia in fact can be argued on the basis of Winnicott's exegesis. Winnicott (1953) defines the transitional object as the first "not me" object that embodies the soothing, comforting qualities of the mother. This is precisely what the body is not in bulimia (and anorexia). The body is not experienced as a source of comfort—that is the bulimic's (or anorectic's) complaint. Data from the Sentence Completion Test indicate that the body is hated and rejected as the possession of the parent, who is experienced as frightening and rejecting.

More specifically, the body in bulimia is—as Sugarman and Kurash have said—a "not me," but this is not experienced as the bulimic's own decision. (This alone disqualifies the bulimic's body as a transitional object, since Winnicott stressed that the transitional object must be chosen by the child.) The bulimic does not choose to give up her body; it—specifically its surface—is claimed by the parent. This experience was reported by bulimic subjects (e.g., "I always saw her [mother] as needing me for a—gimmick. I never thought I could be like a help"). Bulimics and anorectics also reported that they were dressed up, placed in given situations, and expected to perform in prescribed ways.

Further, for the bulimic, there is no joy expressed in the exercise of bodily functions as Sugarman and Kurash contend. Their exercises and other compulsions seem instead a joyless wresting-away-from-the-other control of their bodies. It is done with a vengeance, not with exhilaration (e.g., "My body is the victim of my anger").

Thus, the problem seems a different one, that is, that food cannot be used as a transitional object. Food does not gratify the bulimic; it teases, frustrates, even feels good briefly in the mouth (the surface), but once inside it feels threatening. For the obese and the normal (no eating disorder) subjects, this was not the case. They reported that food does gratify them, does embody the soothing, comforting qualities of the mother. It feels "good" while being eaten and after. It nurtures like the mother it came from. And—as required by Winnicott—it is enough "me" to support the infant's feeling of omnipotence, that is, the mother's power is now within the self.

At this point, one could argue that food cannot be used as a transitional object by the bulimic because it is not separate from the mother. Food may be experienced as combining with the mother herself rather than being used symbolically. And it may be that food has never been separated from the mother because food's function of need gratification has not been fully accomplished. Need—organismic need in infancy— had not been met by "good enough mothering" (Winnicott 1953). There is no progression from need to gratification to state of no tension. The child does not rest between need states, does not develop trust of an "expectable environment." There is a split between safety and gratification, wherein safety feels ungratifying and gratification feels unsafe. Statements by bulimic women support this: "My food is scary yet safe—my hug" and "I can't enjoy food without feeling guilty." Evidence that food has not been separated from the mother was provided also by the following: "To me, food is a person" and "Food is an enchantress, a frustrating goddess." Food, for bulimics, seems to be a noun—"person," "enchantress." For the obese and the normals, food was an adjective: "My food is well-prepared," "My food is good for me." For bulimics, there would thus be no "dread of fusion" (Sugarman and Kurash 1982) if fusion were not already occurring for them when they binge. For then binging would not frighten them so much that they need to vomit (to undo the fusion).

181

Sugarman and Kurash specifically write that "Food is not the issue; rather it is the bodily act of eating which is essential in regaining a fleeting experience of the mother." This also can be contested. The second part of their statement points to the problem: food is indeed the issue because it supplies only a fleeting experience of the mother. Food gratifies the mouth—the surface, but not the stomach and gut, the inner body (e.g., "My gut is just a hole").

The bulimic subjects' narcissism—far from being an experience of exhilarating competence—seems instead a frenetic preoccupation with the display and adornment of the body surface (e.g., "My aggravation is . . . my preoccupation with my looks"). This preoccupation alternates—thus betraying its structure—with an aggressive giving up of the struggle altogether. One bulimic reported twice gaining thirty pounds and then losing it. This had to happen before her mother's eyes, she explained, in order to show her mother how miserable she was. Another bulimic saw her periodic obesity, about ninety pounds overweight, as a total giving up, which included not bathing or grooming. This woman began to examine her behavior in therapy, and she reported feeling alarmed as she approached normal weight, alarmed that she would become irresistible to men. She seemed to feel vulnerable to impingement and invasion by a powerful other. Thus, the bulimics' alleged narcissism may be instead a more complex experience. They seem to love and hate the body surface—love it as the only part the world responds to and hate its frequently oppressive upkeep. What is worse, they experience their emergent, inner selfhood as unacceptable to the other: "Why can't they accept my truth?"

Even the experience of being the same person as the mother seems not—as Sugarman and Kurash have said—an effect of the body as a transitional object. Rather it seems to be the result of the bulimic's main defense—identification with the aggressor. The bulimic becomes like the mother in an effort to reclaim her body surface. She herself now rejects and subjugates her body. Again, if the bulimic could experience her body as a transitional object—that is, as a source of pleasure—there would be no need to vomit. Vomiting is the evidence that food is experienced as frightening and "not me" rather than gratifying and "not me," which is Winnicott's requirement. Vomiting is also evidence that the inner body is incapable of gratification (e.g., "just a hole"). It may be that gratification of the mouth in bulimia (exemplified by comments such as "My mouth wants more" and "I eat so much my jaw hurts") is all the gratification there is, and this is quickly lost once food moves to the stomach.

The final question I address is why food cannot be used as a transitional object in bulimia. According to Tolpin (1971), the formation of transitional objects depends on prior "good enough" mothering. This goodness, which for Winnicott comprises the mother's reliability, nurtures the infant such that she or he is able then to invest the quality of reliable nurturing in an object that was originally provided by the mother and doubtless feels and smells like her (Blatt 1974). The object (e.g., a blanket) is reached for precisely at the moment of need for comforting, is ignored or even abused (stepped on, thrown around) in between, and is attacked when the infant is otherwise frustrated. Thus, it is used as the maternal object herself. The transitional object provides the experience of the infant-mother pair as a "way station or mental detour to the internalization of soothing structure for the infant who is 'hatched' from symbiotic merger while still vulnerable to disequilibrium" (Tolpin 1971, p. 328).

Conclusions

The usual and normal use of food reflects these descriptions. It is urgently sought when needed, ignored upon satiation, sometimes wasted and left around, and rejected during depression. Thus, food seems for most of us a reliable transitional object. It is suggested here that bulimics, by their use and abuse of food, are attempting to make of food a reliable transitional object, as a way to undo the mother's frightening unreliability. Two features of transitional objects are important to this contention: (1) the transitional object provides the sensory experience of the mother, that is, warmth, softness, and smell; and (2) it is a sensory experience the person can provide for herself whenever she needs it. Both of these are features of the bulimic syndrome.

Winnicott (1953) has written that the transitional object is not given up or mourned; it loses meaning. Tolpin disagrees and stresses that the object loses meaning—is decathected—between uses. This exposes its structure: the child has created it and the child decathects it. According to Winnicott, the child can only progress when the object survives this treatment, survives the use and abuse and remains "good." As applied to bulimia, progress from food as a transitional object would thus involve removing from it the added task of serving as parent equivalent, once internalization of its goodness had occurred. One bulimic, who was clearly outgrowing her binge and vomiting episodes, said of her regressions, "It's like a teddy bear I hang on to."

REFERENCES

Blatt, S. 1974. Levels of object representation in anaclitic and introjective depression. *Psychoanalytic Study of the Child* 29:107–157.

Charone, J. K. 1982. Eating disorders: their genesis in the mother-infant relationship. *International Journal of Eating Disorders* 1(4): 15–42.

Chernin, K. 1985. *The Hungry Self*. New York: Times Books.

Selvini-Palazzoli, M. 1978. *Self-Starvation*. New York: Aronson.

Sugarman, A., and Kurash, C. 1982. The body as a transitional object in bulimia. *International Journal of Eating Disorders* 1(4): 57–67.

Tolpin, M. 1971. On the beginnings of a cohesive self: an application of the concept of the transmuting internalizations to the study of the transitional object and signal anxiety. *Psychoanalytic Study of the Child* 26:316–352.

Winnicott, D. W. 1953. Transitional objects and transitional phenomena. *International Journal of Psycho-Analysis* 34:89–97.

Woodall, C. 1983. Eating disorders, body image and self-hate. Ph.D. dissertation, Rutgers University.

PART III

PSYCHOPATHOLOGICAL ISSUES IN ADOLESCENT PSYCHIATRY

EDITORS' INTRODUCTION

As emphasized in these volumes, the casualties of adolescence must be seen against the panoply of the kaleidoscopic social changes of recent decades. In particular, the recent focus on the family in its interactive patterns (competent vs. dysfunctional) has enriched our grasp of disturbances of self-organization, affect, identity formation, and value consolidation in contemporary youth. The depressed and suicidal adolescent continues to represent a large amount of psychopathology in adolescence. The manifestations of depression are protean, illustrating themselves in borderline and narcissistic states, eating disorders, as well as with sequelae of parental and sibling loss. A variant of depression may be viewed as a depressive affect or orientation in some adolescents. Whether the latter requires treatment is dependent on the depth and severity of depression. The following chapters deal with some of these issues.

Edward R. Shapiro and Judith Freedman focus on the relation of dynamic issues in families to the impulsive suicidal behavior of their narcissistic and borderline adolescents. They discuss their observations of a shared regression in these families during the adolescence of the symptomatic child in which there was an externalization and reenactment by family members of traumatic, early object relations. The adolescent contributes a statement about the "poison" in the family environment. The authors conclude that the suicidal act is presented as a solution to a dilemma and discuss various treatment approaches to the individual and family.

James R. McCartney writes that increasing numbers of adolescent patients are suffering from depression. It is the author's thesis that the task of adolescence is more difficult today since society does not support firm, consistent formation of object relations. This creates difficulty in developing a maturing sense of self, a functional autonomy. The depressed adolescent does not reflect this difficulty by developing the clinical disease depression; rather, by attempting to suspend maturation, he develops a depressed state, a predominant affect of depression. Treatment is determined by understanding adolescent depression from this growth and development perspective and providing a consistent, corrective psychotherapeutic relationship that stimulates growth toward autonomy.

Helen A. Widen explores the effects of sibling loss during adolescence. She notes that developmental tasks, normative crises, and preexisting pathology are affected and reports some specificity in the symptom response of late adolescent males. Widen recounts her therapeutic experiences with three college-age males in homosexual panic. Two cases, described in detail, had lost an older brother. The author focuses on the sibling loss, observing the gross defensive reaction to the event, connecting the event and its sequelae with the presenting complaint and interpreting character resistance to mourning and to integrating that event into an emerging adult identity.

Ruthellen Josselson considers the long-term influences of identity diffusion on late adolescent resolution. She found the literature confusing as to the degree of relative pathology subsumed under the heading "identity diffusion." Erikson and Kernberg differ on how transient or traversable such states may be. Her research studies the forms of personality fragmentation that underlie identity diffusion. For those who had been diffuse in identity and later resolved these conflicts, identity formation occurs in a characteristically totalistic fashion. The author concludes that symptoms of identity diffusion in late adolescence are to be regarded seriously.

Allen Z. Schwartzberg writes about the problems engendered by the remarriage family. He reviews the adolescent developmental tasks in this reconstituted group and notes that the young person faces a double termination process: loss of the role and status as a child and loss of the nuclear family while attempting to assume a role in the new remarriage family system. Schwartzberg believes that a key to the achievement of family cohesiveness is the development of strong couple bonding. He describes treatment of the adolescent and the family utilizing a family-systems perspective.

188

Richard C. Marohn combines his interest in the American western hero and villain and developmental aspects of self psychology in a study of John Wesley Hardin, an adolescent murderer, and his emerging psychopathology. Marohn explores available historical materials and the writings of Hardin to trace his growing difficulties with self-regulation, the temporary improvement derived from incarceration, and the final decompensation following release. The author concludes that Hardin's narcissistic behavior disorder was a failed attempt at self-regulation.

13 FAMILY DYNAMICS OF ADOLESCENT SUICIDE

EDWARD R. SHAPIRO AND JUDITH FREEDMAN

Two fifteen-year-old girls: one hanged herself in her mother's art studio; one was barely saved from going over the edge of a bridge. The first girl wrote, "I . . . told myself that I just couldn't handle all of Mummy's problems (which she invariably brings to me now), Daddy's problems, Laurel's problems, and most of all, my problems. I said, damn the family. I've carried them long enough, now I'll do something for myself. Then I went to the bathroom (to kill myself)" (Mack and Hickler 1981, p. 92).

The second girl remembered, "I pleaded with my father to get my mother a doctor because she was so upset. He said she needed to ask for one herself. Later, I called my aunt to help me get a doctor for myself. I thought of standing on the bridge to show my family I needed help and imagined my parents at the bottom of the bridge yelling up through a megaphone: 'Don't jump! We'll help you!' "

The first quotation is from a letter written by the girl who hanged herself. Her suicide was an act consciously aimed at rescuing herself from her family and from her experience of their overwhelming needs of her. The girl's writings and her family were studied after her death by Mack and Hickler (1981). The authors, who never saw the whole family in interaction or worked with the girl, concluded that her vulnerability to suicide lay in her "constitutional predisposition, her early childhood injuries, the patterns of her identifications and the structure of her personality" (p. 186). Though they recognized the parents' difficulty in responding to their daughter's physical and sexual anxieties, their focus was on her intrapsychic difficulties.

The second girl, a borderline adolescent saved from suicide, made her attempt with a fantasy of rejoining her family and getting them to respond to her needs. She was hospitalized and worked with intensively—both individually and with her family. The story that emerged helped both to clarify the relationship of the suicidal act to the family dynamics and to provide clues to the relationship between this adolescent's intrapsychic difficulties and the family turmoil.

Suicide is a complex, multidetermined symptom. In this chapter, we will focus on one aspect—the relationship of certain dynamic issues in families to the impulsive suicidal behavior of narcissistic and borderline adolescents. The conscious suicidal fantasies highlighted in these two cases—rescue of the self from the needs of the family (the narcissistic focus) and getting the family to respond to the needs of the self (the borderline focus)—will serve to underscore these issues.

We will illustrate how the suicidal outcome, for many of these patients, is not only a consequence of ego deficits or faulty internalization (Maltzberger and Buie 1980) but also a response to current repetitions of early experiences of psychological abandonment in the family. We will describe how unconscious ambivalence and narcissistic vulnerabilities in the parents may affect their early care of the child's body. With case examples, we will elaborate how, in early adolescence, when the child's body changes and his or her dependency needs increase, a shared family regression may be precipitated. In vulnerable families, the child's internal experience of not being cared for sensitizes him to the actualities of parental care in adolescence. Parental regression and lack of responsiveness in interaction with the child's fantasies and ego deficits may evoke unbearable rage or feelings of abandonment, which may eventuate in suicide.

Ambivalence, Narcissism, and the Care of the Child's Body

Feder (1980) suggests that the management of parental ambivalence prior to conception has an impact on the life of the developing child. Repression of negative aspects of parental ambivalence is readily seen when the reality of the newborn child's position as "displacer, interrupter of a supposedly idyllic [marriage], demanding narcissistic rival and destroyer of the mother's beauty, calmness and freedom" is denied and presented as the opposite: ". . . the idealization of the child and

192

the exaltation of maternity and paternity'' (p. 172). The intensity of the reproductive instinct and the undeniable love of parents for their children contribute to the repression of antireproductive wishes that are often expressed through unconscious fantasy and symptoms of open or silent rejection, hatred, incestuous activity, and neglect.

If parental ambivalence is unacknowledged and if aggressive infanticidal wishes and their derivatives are repressed, they may manifest themselves covertly in the parents' care of the child's body. The earliest source of the child's own investment in his body is through an identification with the mother's care of that body (Laufer 1981a). The nature of actual parental responses to the child and the conflicts manifested by them in their care of his body may have a direct effect on the child's capacity to take over the function of self-preservation and self-care as his cognitive and emotional capacities mature (Frankl 1963).

Normally, as the child's search for pleasure accommodates to reality, he gradually takes over the function of self-preservation in the late preoedipal and oedipal phases. Khantzian and Mack (1983) suggest that the capacity for self-preservation requires an internalization of parental communications that the child is someone of value who is worth protecting. The child's capacity for loving investment in himself may be limited by relative deprivation of love.

In early infancy, the child is totally dependent on his parental environment. The wish to be completely taken care of is linked to an unconscious infantile fantasy of merger with a gratifying mother. This fantasy is the context within which actual physical experiences, both those provided by contact with caretakers and those provided by self-stimulation, continue to be integrated throughout childhood (Laufer 1981a). In response to excessive frustration, this unconscious fantasy may serve as both comfort and retreat.

For the child to preserve this central dependency fantasy in the context of his increasing maturation and autonomy, parents must manage their own aggression so that they can provide adequate care (Galdston 1981). This management allows them both to respond to the child's body and to tolerate the child's use of aggression in the service of separation without reacting with retaliation or withdrawal.

Trauma during the childhood of the parents may, however, leave residues of heightened aggression or narcissistic vulnerability, limiting their capacities to respond. Consequent inability to tolerate the child's aggressive expression during weaning, toilet training, and later stages of separation may interfere with their provision of actual or symbolic holding of aggressive outbursts. In the absence of this containment, the child neither experiences the limits of his aggression and the boundaries of his body nor develops the security that goes with the increasing sense that his body will be cared for and his wastes managed and that neither he nor his parents will be destroyed by his aggression. Unmastered aggression cannot effectively be utilized by the child either in the service of need gratification or, ultimately, for self-protection.

Many of these parents secure their fragile self-esteem by requiring their children to experience them as appreciated, loved, strong, and nonaggressive. Since all children intermittently view their parents with more ambivalence, vulnerable parents may protect themselves by turning away from and, in a sense, by abandoning those aggressive aspects of the child. This withdrawal further contributes to the child's diminished sense of safety and to his increased vulnerability to traumatic and unmanageable feelings of helplessness.

In effect, such vulnerable parents cannot take care of the child and his body at times when the child's aggressive expression triggers anxiety about their own unacknowledged aggression or when the child fails to fulfill their narcissistic needs to be mirrored, loved, and admired. At such times, the child is forced prematurely to rely on his own ego resources, which may not be adequate to the task, to turn to alternative caretakers, or to regress to more adequately managed stages—possibly to some form of the central fantasy of reunion with the comfort-giving mother.

In adolescence, there is an alteration and realignment in instinctual drives, in the organization of the ego, and in relationships to objects, to ideals, and social relations, as well as a cognitive shift from the concrete to the abstract, the future and the hypothetical (Inhelder and Piaget 1958; Shapiro 1963). These developments, in conjunction with physical changes, provide the adolescent with a new experience of separateness (Erlich 1978).

The toddler's dependent needs include the need for nurturance, for negotiated management of urine and feces, and for help in the management of his separation anxiety. In adolescence, if the capacity for bodily care has not adequately been internalized, metaphorical requests may be presented anew for parental nurturance and for management responses to new forms of the adolescent's "messes" (i.e., drug use and unmanaged sexual and aggressive behaviors). With his revived

dependency and his capacity for representational and symbolic understanding, the adolescent is newly sensitive to unconscious messages
communicated by parents in response to his needs for limit setting and
for help in the management of his sexuality.

Narcissistic and Borderline Adolescents

Laufer (1981b) states that the adolescent's increasing sexual differentiation is experienced unconsciously as a loss of the fantasized union
with the mother, leaving the adolescent alone with his body for the first
time. This sense of aloneness is managed differently by narcissistic and
borderline adolescents.

Narcissistic adolescents have not had a gratifying early experience
of their mothers' loving investment in their bodies. The potential reex-
perience of this early frustration of bodily needs in adolescence results
in an unconscious sense of hopelessness, which the adolescent wards
off by an illusion of self-sufficiency (Modell 1975). The fantasized reunion for these patients is not with a gratifying mother but with a
powerful and narcissistically intrusive mother to whom the child must
submit in order to survive. In Laufer's words, "Making the body feel
dead and without needs is [their] only defense against experiencing the
[dangerous] wish to be intruded on by [the] mother."

In adolescence, because of their sense of never having had a "special" experience with their mothers, narcissistic patients are easily
overwhelmed by intense hatred and envy of those who they feel have
received what they have been denied. They protect themselves by
denying their needs, by projecting them onto others, and by controlling
them through "caring" behaviors.

When these mechanisms fail, narcissistic patients may turn to suicide
as a desperate attempt to control themselves. Suicide may then represent a statement that the body, even if dead, belongs only to them.
Unconsciously, the suicidal act both angrily removes the body from
the demanding and unresponsive mother and controls the terrifying
dependent wish to surrender to her. This notion is similar to the conscious fantasy of our first patient, who wished through her death to
remove herself from the draining needs of her family.

Borderline adolescents become engaged in passionate attempts to
repeat an earlier satisfying physical relationship to the mother that was
traumatically interrupted by the vicissitudes of separation-individua-

tion (Laufer 1981b). The repetition of this dynamic in adolescence, accompanied by excessive amounts of aggression, renders these patients continually vulnerable to losing control over their anger when they are frustrated by those who do not gratify their intense longings (Shapiro 1978). In response to such frustration, borderline adolescents may turn to suicide in a regressive attempt to reunite the body with the gratifying mother of infancy and to remain a part of her. This idea is similar to the fantasy of our second patient, who imagined that her suicide would correspond to her family's decision to respond to her needs.

FAMILY OBSERVATIONS

Laufer's studies of the fantasies and transferences of these patients are consistent with our group's observations of families with narcissistic and borderline adolescents (Berkowitz, Shapiro, Zinner, and Shapiro 1974a; Shapiro, Zinner, Shapiro, and Berkowitz 1975). We observed a shared regression in these families during the adolescence of the symptomatic child in which there was an externalization and reenactment by family members of traumatic early object relationships.

In families with symptomatic narcissistic adolescents, family interactions are characterized by failures to recognize, confirm, and respond to each others' actual attributes (a derivative of early difficulties in responding to bodily needs). In these families, members respond only to aspects of each other that support and stabilize their self-esteem. In an effort to stabilize a tenuous narcissistic equilibrium, parents may relate to their child with what has been called "pathological certainty" (Shapiro 1982b). This quality of relatedness is coercive in that the parents are certain, for their own defensive needs, that they "know" who their child is—who he "must be." In order to protect the parent from anxiety and to preserve the relationship, a vulnerable adolescent may attempt to become the person the parent requires. The cost of such compliance is a denial of the child's own needs, with consequent inner emptiness and loss of spontaneity and initiative.

The adolescent's unconscious awareness of his power to determine parental self-esteem may lead to an unrealistic grandiosity, which may interfere with the reality testing necessary for self-preservation. Our group has previously described (Berkowitz, Shapiro, Zinner, and Shapiro 1974b) narcissistic adolescents who regularly risk their lives in dangerous attempts to relieve their inner deadness and to aggressively take charge of their own bodies with the conviction that nothing serious can happen to them.

In families of borderline adolescents, we observed excessive anxiety and anger around the management of dependency needs during times of separation. Parents of these adolescents appear to have had adequate early symbiotic experiences, with subsequent difficulties in negotiating the anger experienced around separation. Aggressive meanings of autonomy and dependency are revived in their relationship with the adolescent, and they react with heightened ambivalence and denial and projection of aggression. The child's aggression is then experienced by them as something alien.

The borderline adolescent's own ego weakness, excessive aggression, and identity diffusion, with consequent sensitivity to parental views of him, contribute to his vulnerability to aggressive projections (Shapiro 1978; Zinner and Shapiro 1975). Shared family fantasies and projections result in an alienation of the "bad" adolescent from the "all-good" family group (Zinner and Shapiro 1975). The adolescent's dependent fantasies about a reunion with a nurturant mother become equated with a return to a purified family that will respond to his needs—at the cost of his differentiation.

For female adolescents, both narcissistic and borderline, these conflicted interactions and the derivatives of bodily care which they represent are often acted out around sexual issues, particularly in relation to the need for parental protection from sexual abuse and misuse. The two adolescent girls described at the beginning of this chapter are illustrative of both the internal deficits characteristic of these adolescents and the family dynamics that surround them.

Vivienne, the narcissistic adolescent, is well described by Mack and Hickler (1981) in terms of the vicissitudes of her narcissistic vulnerabilities. Both the authors and the family were committed to making the facts of this tragedy available for study, including the painful details of the family's experience. Our ideas about the relationship of Vivienne's family interaction to her vulnerabilities are, of necessity, speculations, since no objective scrutiny exists. Nevertheless, there are certain elements in Vivienne's writings as well as in the historical data produced

197

by the family that suggest the presence of the familiar family dynamics of narcissism.

In his clinical review, Mack points out the disturbance in mother-child bonding that characterized Vivienne's early years. Her birth itself was a performance for a crowded room of hospital staff present to observe the substitution of music for anesthesia. Mack writes, "[The mother] seemed as much to be launching the creation of a work of art as giving birth to an infant" (p. 129). In her own history of Vivienne's infancy, the mother describes her sense of an early mutual and reciprocal "tuning out" and alienation that resulted in the child's spending much time alone. The mother recalls her gratitude at having such a quiet baby since her earlier children were so active and exhausting.

When Vivienne was two, at the height of separation-individuation, the parents left her for a ten-week vacation. On their return, the child did not recognize her mother and would have nothing to do with her for several days. The Robertsons' (1967, 1971) studies of maternal absence during this period provide documentation of the powerful, long-lasting effects of such a prolonged separation at this vulnerable period. The historical data in Vivienne's case suggest the presence of early parental self-preoccupation and a relative insensitivity in terms of both understanding and meeting her needs for nurturance. There is documentation of Vivienne's subsequent tendency toward depression, of her sensitivity to the emotional pain of others, and of her controlled and aggressive isolation, which was manifest in her "biting and devastating humor."

When Vivienne was in grade school, her mother's interest in making unusual dresses for her—one manifestation of bodily care—was not affected by an awareness either of Vivienne's wishes or of community styles of dress. Vivienne's sister remembers the effect of being "different from everybody else" and the degree to which Vivienne was ostracized. She remembers how her mother "would make it seem that we were doing things to hurt her" and remembers her mother's constant intrusions, in which "she wanted us to share everything, and we did."

While her siblings moved outside to other relationships, Vivienne stayed close to home, becoming a "confidante and mediator" of family disputes. While her older and sexually more sophisticated sister could handle herself with boys, Vivienne's response to sexual passes was to frighten boys away by dramatically pretending to drop dead. This behavior is reminiscent of Laufer's notion of "making the body dead and without needs" in response to the intrusive narcissistic needs of others.

Our speculation is that Vivienne's emergence into adolescence with its alterations in her body heightened the stress on her fragile mechanisms for self-esteem maintenance and on her vulnerability to depression. These events deepened her dependency on her family and increased her separation anxiety and aloneness. The family's insensitivity to these needs and her own difficulties in acknowledging them may have supported her own sense of valuelessness. Though the authors state that Vivienne gave her family "few clues about the depth of her depression," the facts suggest otherwise.

Four months before her death, Vivienne took an overdose of pills. Though her mother then observed, "I don't see how anyone could stay sane with everyone's pouring out their problems to you—you have no outlet," she still, according to Vivienne's letters, continued "to bring me all her problems and load me down and I try to help her." Six weeks before her death, family counseling sessions were initiated because of father's business difficulties, and Vivienne wept silently and unreachably, telling her mother, "You wouldn't like it if you did know me."

During her last month, as her letters revealed, she practiced strangling herself, studying in a dissociated and scientific manner the effects, including looking at her bloated and disfigured face in the mirror and anticipating how her corpse would look. This study, not available at the time to the parents, was revealed later in all its gruesome detail. Again, the link to the narcissistic fantasy of taking control of the body, even in death, is apparent.

In the end, with her mother's rope, she hanged herself in her mother's art studio, almost certainly knowing from her experiments the horrifying image that would confront her mother at her discovery. It is our impression that this tragic suicide can be understood as a metaphorical statement by an adolescent who experienced herself as a narcissistically exploited "work of art"—with that representation being confirmed in actual family interaction. Her hanging was, in part, a desperate and aggressive effort to take control of her body, to turn passive into active, and to present her body to her family as a portrait of the underside of such human works of art—a body disfigured and alone.

199

Our second patient, Susan, a borderline adolescent, presents a different picture. Born to older parents who had been barren for twelve years and had prayed daily for a child, she was greeted with unambivalent joy. Despite the fact that the mother had a complicated pregnancy and delivery, requiring an extended postpartum hospitalization and a disruption of the marital life, both parents idealized the child.

The idealization persisted despite a gradual deterioration in the marriage. Her father's drinking worsened, and arguments between the parents increased. Susan's childhood was marked by a series of traumatic events that had never been discussed in the family and emerged only in the hospital after many months of treatment.

When Susan was eight, she was sexually molested by a married cousin. When she reported this to her mother, both parents told her she had had a bad dream. When they later learned of this man's molestation of other children, they said nothing to him or to Susan but decreased the frequency of their visits to his home.

When Susan was twelve, one of her father's friends made a degrading sexual pass at her mother. Her mother told the father, who never spoke to the man about it but continued the friendship. One day, when Susan was thirteen, this man invited her to go on an outing with him, with her mother's agreement. While they were away, he and Susan had sexual intercourse, which she reported to her mother. Again, neither parent confronted the man, though their friendship with him declined. Susan was warned not to spend time alone with older men.

The parents reported this history with blandness. Their denial and rationalizations ("we didn't want to make a scene," etc.) made evident their inability to recognize the kind of protection their daughter needed from them.

As she moved into her adolescence, Susan became promiscuously involved with boys. The father, who spent increasing amounts of time away from home, never talked to her about these relationships—he hoped that his wife "was managing things." When Susan thought she was pregnant at age thirteen, the mother scolded her and advised her about birth control but, not wanting to "upset him," did not discuss it with the father. Despite her disapproval of Susan's involvements with a disreputable group of friends, the mother continued to chauffeur her and to provide her with spending money.

200

While Susan's own aggressive outbursts, impulsivity, and lack of affect tolerance contributed to the chaotic nature of her relationships, the shared parental difficulty in managing their relationship to her bodily care was evident. Their manifest need was to remain in a positive "loving" relationship to her; they could not tolerate her anger, much less their own.

The nature of the family relationship with Susan was captured in her relationship with her horse. The loss of this horse, one year prior to her suicide attempt, was reviewed in the family therapy, with resultant clarification of central family themes. The following excerpt from that therapy illustrates the shared family understanding of the relationship of "love" to bodily care:

SUSAN: You don't believe I cared about Sandy that much.

MOTHER: I do believe it—it's fun to have him around, but not to take care of him. You love him, but who feeds and takes care of him?

SUSAN: I know—but it's different. It doesn't mean I love him less or that he didn't mean anything to me!

FATHER: Let's stick to the facts. How many times did you feed him?

DOCTOR: It's as though the two of you can't conceive of the possibility of loving somebody or something that you don't take such good care of.

MOTHER: Ouch! You're talking about us!

FATHER: If it was a car, I could see it. Something alive has to be taken care of.

SUSAN: (weeps)

FATHER: I think I did take good care of Susan—I—think I did! I don't have any kind of complex or guilt about that.

MOTHER: I think you're using the horse to cry about.

SUSAN: You don't understand what the doctor said!

MOTHER: Why are you crying?

SUSAN: I wasn't thinking of my relationship with Sandy as a person and a horse. I was thinking of it as mother and daughter, or mother and father and daughter. I'm your responsibility! The thing that was supposed to be taken care of was me! (weeps) I was supposed to take care of Sandy and I lost that right. You guys were supposed to take care of me and lost that right when I went to kill myself.

FATHER: I don't get this, Susan.

SUSAN: I couldn't kill myself when I had Sandy—I knew he'd be really hurt if I died. He needed me.

MOTHER: You don't think we need you?

The discussion reveals the ambivalent quality of relationships in the family, where aggressive and libidinal investments are intrapsychically separated but acted out in the relationship. In this family, the experience is that the object is loved openly and deeply, while, at the same time, it is starved and left in its own filth. Susan sees that she treated her horse with the same kind of "love" that her family gave her and begins to make the connection that such treatment kept her from her own self-hatred (she says, "I couldn't kill myself when I had Sandy.") The manifest love and covert aggression constitute the quality of "care" that each member of the triad provides for one another.

In the discussion, mother can recognize briefly her projection onto her daughter and begin to acknowledge an aspect of her own aggression. Unfortunately, what she does not recognize in her final comment is that her daughter needs her. Father's denial remains complete. The dissociation in this family underlines both the seductive pull of a purified, "all-loving" relationship that is overt and the total avoidance and acting out of their oral and anal aggression, the mastery of which is required for preoedipal bodily care and the development of the capacity for self-preservation.

This separation of manifest love from the requirements of bodily care was evident in father's repeated statement, "You've got to take care of yourself!" In the six months before her suicide attempt, Susan became increasingly involved in drug taking and in promiscuous relationships as her parents' fights escalated. On one occasion, the mother, who had stoically endured the increasing tension in the family, broke down in hysterical sobbing and screaming for a period of several days. Susan begged her father to get her a doctor. His response was, "She needs to ask for herself!" In a panic, Susan called her aunt to get a doctor for herself and had the fantasy of threatening to jump from the bridge and seeing her parents calling out to her from the bottom with a promise of care.

On the night before her suicide attempt, Susan had serial sexual intercourse with two of her boyfriends. Her behavior (as revealed later

202

in her therapy) was determined in part by her wishes to get a man to nurture her (as her father would not), to be in oral control of these males, to determine their erections, and to keep them in a position of interest in and attachment to her. The following morning, overwhelmed by shame, rage, and feelings of rejection, she ran to the bridge, stumbled over the divider, and stood poised over the water. A passerby grabbed her by the belt as she fell—falling, as she imagined, into the waters that represented a merger with the fantasy of a parental promise of care.

Discussion

Understanding the dynamics of adolescent suicide requires attention to the actuality of family experience. In our two case examples, which capture dynamic themes regularly seen in families with disturbed adolescents, the data confirm both Vivienne's fantasy that her family had narcissistic needs of her and Susan's fantasy that her family could accept her only if she gave up her differentiation from them (a differentiation which was manifest in the continuing existence of her unmet needs, including her need for limit setting). There was, in fact, sufficient evidence to support the psychological accuracy of the following statements from these adolescents: "My parents aren't interested in me" and "My parents hate me."

Our studies have indicated that, for many of these families, at the level of unconscious communication, such statements are true—though incomplete. It is also true that the adolescents have these same responses to themselves and that the parents have other, more complex responses, often including a profound degree of unconscious self-hatred. Nonetheless, it is likely that, were the parents able to acknowledge the truth of these statements, their children might experience a degree of liberation from the kind of dependent enmeshment so characteristic of these family relationships and be able to more freely examine their own difficulties.

Each of the suicidal adolescents had serious ego deficits: Vivienne, in her inadequate structures for self-esteem maintenance, and Susan, in her meager resources for impulse control and the management of aggression. In each of the families, the siblings appeared less dependent and had found other ways to manage family and internal tensions, though none was symptom free.

Each of these adolescents, if the difficulties were recognized, might have been approached individually—but probably not by their parents without help. In both families, parental blind spots in conjunction with the child's vulnerabilities made self-correction impossible. Vivienne's mother could not find out from her daughter what the difficulties were, both because of her unconscious wish to make herself feel better and because Vivienne could experience her questions only as intrusions. Susan's parents could not limit her dangerous behavior, both because of their unconscious anxiety and guilt about their aggression and because Susan's impulsivity and aggressiveness obscured her overt requests for intervention.

This complexity underlines the fact that the suicide of a child also represents the death of a family group, a group that is larger than the sum of the individuals who constitute it. The shared unconscious conflicts and fantasies of members of this group constitute an important aspect of the "holding environment" within which the child develops (Shapiro 1982a). Whatever the contributions of his own instinctual processes or the elements of his or her own ego functioning, his suicide is also a statement about the poison in this environment. A realistic reworking and detoxification of the covert hatreds and devaluations that constitute this poison would, at the very least, require an open acknowledgment of them in family discussions.

Unfortunately, such acknowledgment is usually not possible in these families because these truths are unconscious and particularly inaccessible when the adolescent is suicidal. At the level of unconscious fantasy, these parents feel that acknowledgment of their hatred would kill and that recognition of their lack of interest would starve. Consequently, their effort is to deny the accuracy of their child's perceptions and to present an unambivalent facade of love and involvement. The resultant enmeshment and mutual regression may then require combined individual and family work to help strengthen family members' capacities to observe and take responsibility for their own experiences.

The suicidal adolescent's recognition of his ultimate responsibility for his own aggression, envy, and wishes for revenge is essential for his treatment. The resultant improvement in reality testing helps the adolescent recognize that his hatred is ultimately not directed at his actual parents but at his projected representations of them derived from his childhood experiences. It is this tentative recognition that allows for the beginning of individual treatment.

204

During the adolescence of primitive patients, initiating individual psychotherapy may be difficult as a result of these externalizations and of the shared family regression that actualizes many of these conflicts. The adolescent may not be able to free himself enough from family ties to engage in a deepening therapy.

In a combined individual and family treatment, however, the adolescent may see that his intense preoccupation with his parents' current (and usually unconscious) hatred and lack of interest and his longing for their love and involvement are a consequence of his own regression and his deep dependency on them. This recognition and the beginning repetition of these conflicts in an individual transference may loosen the current family dependency enough for the adolescent to appreciate the conflicted nature of these issues in both his parents and himself (Shapiro, Shapiro, Zinner, and Berkowitz 1977).

Conclusions

Adolescent suicide is a multidetermined symptom. In this chapter, we have suggested that this tragic outcome may represent not only a consequence of the adolescents' ego deficits or faulty internalization but also a response to certain unconscious dynamic issues within their families. A shared family regression during the adolescence of particular children may evoke in the child unconscious connections between the early care of his or her body and current needs for parental protection. Parental regression and lack of responsiveness in interaction with the child's fantasies and ego deficits may evoke unbearable rage or feelings of abandonment that may eventuate in self-destruction.

The suicidal act, as the ultimate externalization and dramatization of the individual's internal conflicts, is a powerful metaphor—most powerful because of its presentation as a solution to a dilemma. The components of the act—the behavior itself, the conscious and unconscious fantasies involved in it, and the interpersonal responses relating to it—compose the text for a complex description of a central dynamic meaning of an individual's life.

NOTE

Presented at the World Organizing Conference of the International Society for Adolescent Psychiatry, Paris, 1985. The authors would like

to thank Drs. Michael Hollander, John Mack, and Michael Robbins for their helpful comments.

REFERENCES

Berkowitz, D. A.; Shapiro, R. L.; Zinner, J.; and Shapiro, E. R. 1974a. Family contributions to narcissistic disorders in adolescents. *International Review of Psychoanalysis* 1:353–362.

Berkowitz, D. A.; Shapiro, R. L.; Zinner, J.; and Shapiro, E. R. 1974b. Concurrent family treatment of narcissistic disorders in adolescence. *International Journal of Psychoanalytic Psychotherapy* 3:371–396.

Erlich, H. S. 1978. Adolescent suicide: maternal longing and cognitive development. *Psychoanalytic Study of the Child* 33:261–278.

Feder, L. 1980. Preconceptive ambivalence and external reality. *International Journal of Psycho-Analysis* 61:161–178.

Frankl, L. 1963. Self-preservation and the development of accident proneness in children and adolescents. *Psychoanalytic Study of the Child* 18:464–483.

Galdston, R. 1981. The domestic dimensions of violence: child abuse. *Psychoanalytic Study of the Child* 36:391–414.

Inhelder, B., and Piaget, J. 1958. *The Growth of Logical Thinking from Childhood to Adolescence*. New York: Basic.

Khantzian, E., and Mack, J. 1983. Self-preservation and the care of the self: ego instincts reconsidered. *Psychoanalytic Study of the Child* 38:209–232.

Laufer, M. E. 1981a. The adolescent's use of the transference: a comparison of borderline and narcissistic modes of functioning. *Psychoanalytic Study of the Child* 36:163–180.

Laufer, M. 1981b. The psychoanalyst and the adolescent's sexual development. *Psychoanalytic Study of the Child* 36:181–191.

Mack, J., and Hickler, H. 1981. *Vivienne*. Boston: Little, Brown.

Maltzberger, T., and Buie, D. 1980. The devices of suicide. *International Review of Psychoanalysis* 7:61–72.

Modell, A. 1975. A narcissistic defense against affects and the illusion of self-sufficiency. *International Journal of Psycho-Analysis* 56:275–282.

Robertson, J., and Robertson, J. 1967. Young children in brief separation: a fresh look. *Psychoanalytic Study of the Child* 26:264–315.

Robertson, J., and Robertson, J. 1971. Film: *Young Children in Brief Separation*. London: Tavistock.

Shapiro, E. R.; Zinner, J.; Shapiro, R. L.; and Berkowitz, D. 1975. The influence of family experience on borderline personality development. *International Review of Psycho-Analysis* 7:61–72.

Shapiro, E. R.; Shapiro, R. L.; Zinner, J.; and Berkowitz, D. 1977. The borderline ego and the working alliance: indications for family and individual treatment in adolescence. *International Journal of Psycho-Analysis* 58:77–87.

Shapiro, E. R. 1978. The psychodynamics and developmental psychology of the borderline patient: a review of the literature. *American Journal of Psychiatry* 135:1305–1315.

Shapiro, E. R. 1982a. The holding environment and family therapy with acting out adolescents. *International Journal of Psychoanalytic Psychotherapy* 9:209–226.

Shapiro, E. R. 1982b. On curiosity: intrapsychic and interpersonal boundary formation in family life. *International Journal of Family Psychiatry* 3:69–89.

Shapiro, R. L. 1963. Adolescence and the psychology of the ego. *Psychiatry* 26:77–87.

Shapiro, R. L. 1978. The adolescent, the therapist and the family: the management of external resistances to psychoanalytic therapy of adolescents. *Journal of Adolescence* 1:3–10.

Zinner, J., and Shapiro, E. R. 1975. Splitting in families of borderline adolescents. In J. Mack, ed. *Borderline States in Psychiatry*. New York: Grune & Stratton.

14 ✓ADOLESCENT DEPRESSION: A GROWTH AND DEVELOPMENT PERSPECTIVE

JAMES R. McCARTNEY

Adolescents now constitute approximately one-third of our country's population. Many of these young people are angry, despairing, cynical, and depressed. In fact, in 1968, suicide ranked fourth as a cause of death for this age group, behind accidents, neoplasm, and homicide. In the 1978 census, suicide ranked as the third leading cause of death for those fifteen to nineteen years old. The rate doubled over 1961–1975, tripled over 1956–1975 (Holinger and Offer 1982), and is still increasing. Newspaper accounts almost daily speak of this latent contagion. What is it that drives these young people to suicide or suicidal self-destructiveness and nihilism? Why is it that so many adolescents in pursuit of pleasure and happiness find instead despair and emptiness?

Universality of Adolescence

Kiell (1964) contends that adolescent turmoil and external disorder are universal and are only moderately affected by cultural determinants. He observes that, in spite of specific differences in content and degree of stress from one culture to another, "adolescent development is basically uniform in all societies." In support of this thesis, he uses over 200 autobiographies and diaries spanning the centuries. Nonetheless, while the experience is universal, there may well be harder and easier times for an adolescent to fight his way to maturity. The generation of conformity of the 1950s gave way to the generation of rebellion of the 1960s, in turn, to the indifference of the 1970s, and now to the atomic-born despair of the 1980s.

Anna Freud (1958) wrote that it is normal for the adolescent to experience turmoil and wild fluctuations in behavior. Most adolescents show fluctuations, without truly becoming pathological, as they seek to establish their own identity. This accomplishment requires successful navigation of previous crises of growth; an individual resolves the crisis of a later stage of development with the tools forged in earlier stages. In Erikson's (1959) view of growth and development, Basic Trust versus Mistrust, Autonomy versus Shame and Doubt, and Initiative versus Guilt bring the child to latency and its crisis of Industry versus Inferiority as preparation for the task of Adolescent Identity versus Identity Diffusion and Repudiation. Along with the task of identity formation goes the task of separation from parents and achievement of a secondary autonomy, aided by a firmer sense of self apart from parents and family. This struggle for secondary autonomy is a reenactment of previous struggles and requires the assistance and support of parents and cultural institutions. Unresolved residuals of previous phases of ego development are reactivated in adolescence, with its phase-specific normative tasks.

The child who was burdened by excessively demanding or rejecting, infantile parents—concerned with their own struggles and viewing the child chiefly as their entry in the sweepstakes of life—may not come to the adolescent task well prepared. If the child's society has failed to furnish a milieu that permits consistent object relations for positive identification and role modeling, that child may be similarly ill prepared. For the adolescent, establishment of an adult identity and depreciation of the parents and the relationship with them are a necessary part of distancing. To start with a negative or nonexistent relationship/identification leaves no room for distancing as a normative phase without collapse into the void of nihilism.

It is difficult enough to come to adolescence with a view of self that is clear, realistic, and positive. It is even more difficult to come to adolescence with a view of the world that is clear, realistic, and negative. Traditionally, the adolescent's self-deprecatory trends are based on his sense of betrayal by his parents, whom he once idealized. Mark Twain is alleged to have said: "When I was a boy of fourteen, my father was so ignorant I could hardly stand to have the old man around. But when I got to be twenty-one, I was astonished at how much the old man had learned in seven years." This distancing in the service of autonomy is necessary; to move from a position of dependency to autonomy, however, is a risk. The relative security of certainty in dependency must be sacrificed. This sacrifice must be supported by parents secure enough to accept the loss of confirmation by their child. While something is gained by both, something else is given up. For the child, the giving up of a dependent relationship, even a negative one, in the move to autonomy is a loss.

This accounts for many transient depressive feelings of adolescence that are part of normal adolescent crises. When one looks at normative adolescent depression as viewed by Offer and Offer (1976), one notes that only 23 percent of their sample showed smooth, continuous growth—the rest having more uneven growth or frankly turbulent development. Turmoil is not necessary to adolescent development but is certainly often present. Given a period when much was clear-cut, given relatively decent, mature parents, and given a latency period in which to rest and consolidate one's gains, one could move from something sure through loss and resultant uncertainty to something new. One could tolerate the more or less transient sense of loss. Today's children seem to grow up with too much hostility and aggression in a world filled with ambiguity and uncertainty. Many parents appear to be frightened, insecure, and immature. They seem too easily manipulated and are thus disrespected. In many broken homes, many of these children are "parentified" and pushed into pseudomaturity.

Traditional Psychoanalytic View

Schneer and Kay (1961), studying eighty-four adolescent suicides at King's County Hospital, commented on the remarkable rise in suicidal behavior in this age group. They found operative basic psychoanalytic factors such as turning of aggression against the self, killing the internalized hated object, and joining the lost object—the classical dynamics of depression described by Abraham (1911) and Freud (1917). If today's children have had difficulty making lasting object relations, even with their parents, then how can they turn hatred in on that internalized object, never adequately internalized? Fragmented object relationships are incompletely internalized and offer little support at this time of lonely struggle. As in marasmus, their detached depressed state may represent something other than hatred turned against the lost but internalized object.

JAMES R. MC CARTNEY

Changing Concept

Teicher and Jacobs (1967), studying thirty-one suicidal attempters, drew a different conclusion. They found little in these adolescents to indicate that they acted impetuously or out of aggression turned inward. Rather they acted as a consequence of a lifelong series of unwanted, sorely disruptive separations from significant people. To paraphrase Erikson, one might say they had achieved basic distrust. Teicher states: "These young people perceived as hopelessly eroded the one value which all of us hold essential; the establishment and perpetuation of meaningful social relationships. Their despair was such that they had come to believe that life was just one chronic problem and that the only relief from the pain of living was to die."

A brilliant young patient of mine, when a sixteen-year-old girl, wrote:

> One and one are two
> Two and two are four
> But shift your definitions
> And you'll find it true no more.
> Twist and bend the language
> As it suits your use—
> Consensus of opinion
> Is the only truth.
> Truths gone out of usage
> Fade and leave no mark—
> Wait, don't go away
> And leave me in the dark.

The classical universal idiom of depression of adolescence is there. She also wrote:

> Someone tell them I was a hero
>   for eleven days before I was a traitor
> Tell them I was perfectly justified
>   in my actions
> Tell them it was all predetermined
>   before I was weaned
> Tell them they wouldn't have faced
>   it either

> Folks will believe, believe, and in
> pity protect
> While in a friendly impersonal ear
> I talk away the memory of the
> face of him whom I destroyed.

Is this classical depression or is it a stance—in many ways a reaction to the perceived world?

The Effect of Our Times

Many observers have stated that today's young people are the brightest and most idealistic we have ever had. Informed, sophisticated, educated in complexities at an earlier age, it has often been indicated that they possess a certain social ease, if they are lacking in commitment. Rebellion and depression in adolescence are not new, but this is a time of doubt and social turmoil. Ours is a mobile population with some resultant uncertainties both for the young and for their parents. This uncertainty appears often to intensify family pathology. Mass communication, as much as our educational system, has made our young people better informed. No disaster, no inhumanity goes unreenacted before their very eyes in living color. They learn early that we have not lived up to our expressed values: there are not equal rights for everyone; we treat minority groups badly. Religion has lost its place as a cornerstone of family life, becoming concerned with form not substance. In education, little is clear-cut. The exceptions are taught with the rules so that children learn to think, not just to learn by rote. These ambiguities, these changes have been powerfully expressed by Schlesinger (1971). Commenting from his perspective as a historian, he states, "The dominating factor in modern life is surely the increase in the rate of change, the increase in the velocity of history."

Hendin (Epstein 1974), studying suicidal students at Columbia University and Barnard College, said:

Student suicide has traditionally been attributed to a concern with achievement and, in America, theory has been that parents pressured their children to perform. But, in the students I saw, this

212

pressure was not a crucial factor in their being suicidal. Rather, the child's relationship with his family involved developing an emotional deadness as a kind of protection against life. Their parents wanted quiescent children; they were fairly egocentric—and I think that's true of the whole culture.

Alienated, hostile, despairing, isolated, lonely—these are words that describe too many of our adolescent patients. When the world goes a way they do not wish it to, they undergo depression—not as pathology but as an inevitable response to a frustrating world.

Feeling, Life-Style, or Disease

Many are thus properly "depressed," but are they suffering from clinical depression? Depression can be a feeling, a symptom, a life-style, or a physical illness. The physical-illness depression does not seem to describe many of our patients, even those who attempt suicide. There are important differences between the physiological illness depression and the feeling depression. We all at times feel depressed. The symptom depression is at times present as part of a diagnosable neurotic or schizophrenic illness. The physiological illness depression—whether neurotic or psychotic—is characterized by definite symptoms and behavior other than the affect of depression. The symptoms of psychomotor retardation, the development of dysfunction of the autonomic nervous system, and resultant somatic symptoms are indications that the "dys-ease" has become a disease. The neurochemical state may be seen as a psychosomatic disorder finally precipitated as the result of psychodynamic factors or, in some cases, precipitated by physical factors such as exhaustion. For some, we understand there is a genetic proclivity to respond to stress with depression. While some adolescents who develop this physiological disease respond appropriately to antidepressants or electroconvulsive therapy, most do not. This can be taken as further confirmation that a correctable disease state, a neurophysiological disorder, does not exist. Pharmacotherapy or electroconvulsive therapy appears effective in restoring neurochemical balance when such an imbalance is present. Such techniques are corrective for the depressive illness but not the depressive state.

Adolescent Depressive State

Bonime (1966) describes a depressive life-style characterized by demanding, manipulative behavior, aversion to influence, unwillingness to give gratification, hostility, and anxiety. This description sounds strangely like a troubled adolescent. Neither our adult patients with a depressive life-style or personality nor our adolescent patients with depression yield to pharmacotherapy corrective for the illness "depression."

Blos (1962), in writing on what Bernfield as early as 1923 called "prolonged adolescence," describes a state where adolescent crisis is "adhered to with persistence, desperation and anxiousness," whereby the adolescent "strives to bypass the finality of choices which are exacted at the close of adolescence." While he describes their self-consciousness and ashamedness, our patients with their despair—at times culminating in suicide—are different. In Blos's words, "The difference is a remarkable resistivity against the regressive pull in conjunction with a persistent avoidance of any consolidation of the adolescent process."

Perhaps Erikson (1959) comes closest to describing our patients when he describes the borderline state and the identity diffusion that can occur at adolescence: "Symptomatically, this consists of a painfully heightened sense of isolation; a disintegration of the sense of inner continuity and sameness; a sense of overall ashamedness; an inability to derive a sense of accomplishment from any kind of activity; a feeling that life is happening to the individual rather than being lived by his initiative; a radically shortened time perspective; and finally, a basic mistrust which leaves it to the world, to society, and indeed to psychiatry to prove that the patient does exist in a psychosocial sense, i.e. can count on an invitation to become himself."

It is my thesis that this depressive state is what our adolescent patients are suffering, not the disease "Depression." There are qualitative and quantitative differences.

It appears that very few adolescents actually are suffering from clinical depression. Most of our adolescent patients are going through a type of depressive state caused by the particular tasks of the identity crisis of adolescence. There is a human proclivity to totalistic reorientation at critical stages. In Erikson's (1959) words, "The adolescent would rather be nobody, or somebody bad, or indeed dead—and this totally and by free choice—than be not quite somebody."

Kiev (Epstein 1974), while talking of suicides in general, describes adolescent suicide thus:

> The suicide rate reflects the stimulus overload in our society. We have a high degree of freedom and a multiplicity of choices to make. At the same time, traditional mechanisms like religion and custom—which serve to screen out the stimuli—have been lost and the individual has no framework within which to make choices. The stimulus overload makes it difficult for anyone to make decisions. The depressed person has great difficulties in saying no to the pressures placed upon him, in disappointing other people's expectations. When he does so, he feels guilty, worthless, confused, and even more indecisive. Suicide can seem a way of asserting control over one's life.

If the depressed state is the adolescent's psychosocial moratorium, then adolescent suicide is the ultimate closure on choice and growth.

Treatment

How do we treat this superego's triumph of depreciation, to ensure that what Erikson calls a "transitory adolescent regression to avoid a psychosocial foreclosure" remains transitory? Alexander (1956) spoke of psychotherapy as a corrective emotional experience. Life itself often supplies such opportunities. Psychotherapy is but an effort to ensure that a corrective experience takes place. If the difficulty is rooted in defective, unreliable object relationships, then a corrective object relationship is necessary.

Whether in formal family therapy or in individual therapy after family evaluation, the key to change is the relationship with the therapist. This is not a matter of mere friendship. As a patient stated after four years of treatment, "I've decided there are two things necessary for a healthy productive life; one, a sense of self, of self-respect, and where one is going, and, two, a friend with whom you can talk honestly, without any games—and you won't do." The relationship in therapy supplies a different quality on which the patient acts and to which he reacts in the process of therapy. An object relationship is established that is different. There must be no requirement of confirmation to meet the therapist's needs. More than friend and ally to the patient, the therapist is also a parent surrogate. He is tested and must not be found to be the same as those who have previously let the adolescent down. The therapist walks the line—being neither manipulated nor rejecting—as he seeks to nourish the adolescent's search for viable, reliable values and relationships. One must be honest—"tell it like it is"—yet supportive of the assets and strengths not just of the patient but also of society, against which he batters himself. The adolescent patient needs to see his parents' virtues as well as their faults. The therapist supports the adolescent's idealism and hopefulness while disagreeing with his cynicism, negativism, and effort to escape from responsibility for self. In the presence of an honest, mutually respecting relationship, disagreement without destructive conflict becomes possible. We can guide patients to a positive and responsible approach rather than join them in an orgy of narcissistic, nihilistic complaints. As Blos (1962) states in discussing treatment of prolonged adolescence, "We must not forget that the adolescent retains a readiness to identify with an adult who possesses those personality attributes in which he desires to share. The therapist's aim is to replace infantile sharing and merging by identification or, to put it differently, to replace the search for external sources of self-esteem (rescue fantasy) by the discovery of one's own resourcefulness. In fact, exploring and testing, validating and differentiating this resourcefulness in daily life constitutes a large part of the therapeutic endeavor."

As adolescents make responsible choices, they build new self- respect. Learning from their own and their parents' mistakes, they can move to something better than a mirror image of their parents' and the world's mistakes.

Conclusions

Many adolescents sail smoothly through this period of growth; many do not. Some become patients. Of these, some may have clinical depression responsive to either electroconvulsive treatment or medication, but many, if not most, are in a depressed state as a part of adolescent turmoil in a world viewed as chaotic, unreliable, and uncaring. Their therapist must offer them not simply medication but also a consistent, corrective psychotherapeutic relationship that helps them resume growth toward autonomy.

REFERENCES

Abraham, K. 1911. Notes on the psychoanalytic investigation and treatment of manic-depressive insanity and allied conditions. In *Selected Papers on Psychoanalysis*. Reprint ed., New York: Basic, 1960.

Alexander, F. 1956. Analysis of the therapeutic factors in psychoanalytic treatment. In F. Alexander and T. French, eds. *Psychoanalytic Treatment*. New York: Roland.

Blos, P. 1962. *On Adolescence*. Glencoe, Ill.: Free Press.

Bonime, W. 1966. The psychodynamics of neurotic depression. In *American Handbook of Psychiatry,* Vol. 3. New York: Basic.

Epstein, H. 1974. A sin or a right? *New York Times Magazine* (September 8), pp. 91–94.

Erikson, E. 1959. The problems of ego identity. *Psychological Issues* 1:101–164.

Freud, A. 1958. Adolescence. *Psychoanalytic Study of the Child* 13:255–278.

Freud, S. 1917. Mourning and melancholia. *Standard Edition* 14:243–258. London: Hogarth, 1961.

Holinger, P. C., and Offer, D. 1982. Prediction of adolescent suicide: a population model. *American Journal of Psychiatry* 139 (3): 302–307.

Kiell, N. 1964. *Universal Experience of Adolescence*. New York: International Universities Press.

Offer, D., and Offer, J. 1976. Three developmental routes through normal male adolescence. *Adolescent Psychiatry* 4:121–141.

Schlesinger, A. 1971. Quoted in *Off Center,* January 11.

Schneer, H. I., and Kay, P. 1961. Events and conscious ideation leading to suicidal behavior in adolescence. *Psychiatric Quarterly* 35:502–511.

Teicher, J. D., and Jacobs, J. 1967. Broken homes and social isolation in attempted suicides of adolescents. *International Journal of Social Psychiatry* 13:139–149.

PHASE-SPECIFIC SYMPTOMATIC RESPONSE
TO SIBLING LOSS IN LATE ADOLESCENCE

HELEN A. WIDEN

Recent studies on sibling loss have examined the impact of such loss
on surviving siblings and concluded that they are very much at risk
for psychosomatic and emotional disturbance (Altschul 1985; Bank and
Kahn 1982; Pollock 1985; Rosen 1985). Solnit (1985) noted the increasing incidence of violent death in adolescence and young adulthood by
murder, suicide, and automobile accidents. The victims leave behind
surviving siblings whose adolescent difficulties with mourning are exacerbated by the shocking nature of the death and often by the resulting
incapacity of their bereaved parents.

It is not surprising that phase-specific developmental tasks and normative crises of adolescence are interfered with and that preexisting
pathology is accentuated. What did surprise me was a certain specificity
in symptom response in my caseload of late adolescent males. At the
end of their review of the psychoanalytic literature on siblings, Colonna
and Newman (1983) express amazement about the noticeable lack of
writing about the specific role of the sibling relationship during adolescence. All these factors have motivated me to observe, speculate,
review the literature, and communicate with colleagues.

Case Reports

In reviewing my recent caseload for sibling loss, I found that three
cases came to mind. All three were young men of ages twenty and
twenty-one who were university students when they came to the college

mental health center for treatment. Because of the exigencies of the academic calendar and the rather transient nature of college life, their treatment inevitably bore certain characteristics and limitations of short-term dynamic psychotherapy.

To summarize the cases briefly, all three men, several years earlier in their adolescence, had lost an ambivalently admired older sibling with whom there was closeness and identification. This had happened suddenly and violently. All three had been unable to mourn and had employed varying degrees of denial, disavowal of meaning, suppression of affect, and character rigidity to defend themselves. And, in all three, there was an overdetermined and excessive preoccupation with sexuality, specifically with the issue of homosexuality. Two of the men were predominantly heterosexual, while the third, whom at this point I cite for contrast, was an active homosexual.

The first two men came for treatment at age twenty-one in an intense anxiety state that might be called homosexual panic. The idea that they might be homosexual was deeply disturbing and ego dystonic. The onset of the sexual obsession had occurred some time after the death of their brothers, when each subject was age seventeen. An exploration of their psychosexual history, their fantasies, and the dreams that occurred during treatment was soothing in that little was discovered to confirm their dread and fear. Instead, many of their dreams indicated that the death of the brother and the incapacity to mourn were the focal issues, rather than the sexual preoccupation. The twenty-eight-year-old brother of one, a physician, had been shot to death by his father as he was trying to break down a locked bedroom door to vent his rage on his mother. The twenty-year-old brother of the second patient had killed himself and a passenger in a head-on collision that his brother believed was suicidally motivated. These men had never been able to share feelings about the death with their parents.

The third man, with different sexual dynamics, was involved in his first homosexual love affair when he presented for treatment at age twenty. His homosexuality was relatively ego syntonic and, on inquiry, he revealed that he had "known" he was homosexual since age ten. This man came when a possible breakup with his lover threatened to release feelings that had been frozen since the death of an older sister in an automobile accident some years before. An important diagnostic fact is that the homosexual erotic preference in men can usually be recollected as being present from the latency years or early adolescence, that is, from ages nine to thirteen (Isay 1985). This third case, which is not discussed further, highlights the fact that the other two men were heterosexuals whose concerns about homosexuality both expressed and defended against the difficulties each was having consolidating a satisfactory heterosexual identity and moving into young adulthood. Although it is likely that both men might have had problems with this developmental task had their brothers lived, I think that the sibling loss itself was, at least, a complicating factor and, at most, a significant developmental interference.

CASE EXAMPLE 1

The first case, Kemal, was a twenty-one-year-old foreign graduate student who had arrived from abroad in September, only one month previously. He related warmly and directly, and, although English was his second language, a great deal unfolded and was expressed verbally and affectfully in the session. He had been referred by a college physician whom he had consulted about hyperventilation and chest pains. He was quick to acknowledge anxiety and psychological stress. Parenthetically, in twelve years, Kemal was the only male foreign student from a Third World country who came to see this female therapist more than two times. Because homosexual panic was inferred only after treatment ended, I shall report the first two diagnostic sessions in some detail.

Kemal began by telling me that he had married just a few weeks before leaving his homeland and that he was working through the Foreign Student's Office at the university and the American Embassy abroad to obtain a visa for his wife so she could join him. His anxiety went beyond this separation and uncertainty, however. He found himself obsessed with "paranoid" thoughts about her fidelity, both while she was alone back home and if she were to join him. He later told me he had made plans to spy on her and monitor her phone calls when she arrived. He started out by telling me about "her psychological problems"—her childishness and her distrust of men caused by "a too forceful father." However, his wife assured him she loved him and was overjoyed when he proposed marriage after they had been going together only four or five months. Kemal believed they were very well suited but was having second thoughts about their youth, impulsiveness, and timing. He then told me that sometimes, in bed with her, he became afraid that she would kill him by stabbing him with a knife.

220

At that point, I directly challenged the paranoid defense and asked whether he had been angry with her at the time. He went on to say that he had been afraid of the dark and had similar fears before he even met her. He then spontaneously introduced the subject of his brother, a medical doctor who had died "accidentally" at age twenty-eight, three years earlier. When I wondered how this death might be connected to his problems, he nodded and said, "My father killed my brother!" At that point, tears began to flow and the story unfolded with very little prompting except my readiness to listen.

Apparently, the brother had been subject to frequent attacks of rage at the mother and had at one time threatened to destroy the family. He had alternated between despair over bad relations with his parents and hopes for a happy togetherness. A week before the shooting, the brother had gotten into another rage at his mother, and his father had had him arrested. On that day, when he came home unexpectedly at midday, his mother had sent Kemal to a neighbor's house and had locked herself in her room. The brother tried to beat down the door so that she would serve a meal, and, at that point, his father shot him. Kemal heard the shots, was "in shock," and developed somatic symptoms afterward. The father had been imprisoned for two years but was now released.

There was much grief expressed over this family tragedy. Kemal then returned to the subject of his wife. Although she knew nothing about the facts of his brother's death, she and Kemal stayed with his parents for a few weeks before their marriage. When relatives came, of course, he feared a wrong word would be said. He feared her reaction. We agreed that he had problems with his marriage whether his wife stayed abroad or came to join him. He was eager to make a return appointment and indicated that he would want some advice from me in this "complicated situation" but was also "afraid to burden" me.

The next week he resumed our contact without hesitation and told me that he felt depressed at times and "optimistic" at others. He had not slept well the past few nights following a two-hour conversation with his wife. He found himself disturbed by feelings of inferiority and dependency, which he partly ascribed to her and partly accepted as his own, and, more important, he was worried and obsessed about her fidelity or betrayal of him.

The session quite naturally proceeded to discussion of his brother. They were very close and Kemal admired and missed him and still had frequent dreams of him alive. His last one had been three days earlier. He acknowledged that some of his depression was mourning for his

221

brother and also said that "it's possible" that the obsession with his wife's fidelity was connected in some way (or displaced from) this mourning process. Kemal was very close to and affectionate with his brother as a young adolescent. Later, his brother actually had instructed him about how to relate to girls. The brother had been unmarried and "somewhat cynical about women." Kemal had felt deceived about a previous lover's virginity and thought he could not trust women. In an earlier relationship with a girl his brother had rehearsed him in a breaking-up speech. Kemal wondered how honest, dependent, and vulnerable he should be with his wife and had decided to dissemble somewhat. He felt "disgust for the human being," because he himself looked at other women on the street and doubted his ability to remain faithful.

I saw Kemal six more times during autumn 1983. More facts about his history emerged in the early sessions. He had dreamed again that the four family members were together "before the event" and something happened as usual to disturb their tranquility. He found himself blaming his brother and hating him for this. He would often feel this way until the two of them were alone together, and then he would feel close to his brother and admiring of him. He recounted the family dynamics with particular emphasis on the brother-mother interaction. His brother had been diagnosed as schizophrenic. His mother often reacted to the brother's criticisms by becoming withholding and vengeful. She had recently begun to change, "but it was too late," and she suffered guilt and regrets. Kemal said that his mother always loved him more than his brother, and while he blamed her for this unfairness, he also blamed himself for not wanting to lose his mother's affection. He never mentioned his father during the sixteen sessions following the first one. Kemal had been born when his brother was ten, seemingly because his brother had wanted a sibling. Therefore, he felt he was not only his mother's favorite but also his brother's reason for being. Kemal felt himself to blame for the family problems, even though he knew he was not, and wondered why this was so.

In the process of treatment, his anxiety subsided as he brought his fears into the sessions—among them, fears about being passively victimized by some murderous intruder. He remained active during the sessions, and I found it safer to let him take the lead, because of differences in language and culture and the possible limit of time. In the first set of eight sessions, Kemal focused on issues of sexuality, guilt, anger, and "disappointment in human nature." Reactions to what he called "the event" were warded off and suppressed, but when his brother appeared in his dreams, I felt on safe enough ground to make connections. He became more easily reassured by long phone conversations with his wife and was able to begin and maintain excellent functioning in his academic work.

Kemal suddenly interrupted treatment when he brought in his young wife to meet me after her arrival. He returned in autumn 1984, three weeks after his wife had left for home. I saw him for nine sessions, which ended when he received his master's degree and returned to his homeland.

The sudden interruption was a surprise. I subsequently came to understand it as a further defense to split off "the event" and his reactions to the disturbing loss of the homosexual love object from his present sexual life in his marriage.

Kemal returned for the ninth session the following October after his wife had gone back abroad. He said he was lonely, "but I no longer have the paranoid ideas about her fidelity." Rather it was his own guilty conflict about compulsive voyeuristic sexual fantasies that disturbed him and made him feel abnormal. I believe that he still was compelled to defend by reaction formation against the homosexual issues that surrounded his brother's death. He still had not told his wife about "the event," and I tried to connect this secrecy with his expressed difficulty in integrating sexuality and tenderness in his marriage, his tormenting cycle of arousal and guilt, and the disappointment he felt in sexual relations with his loving, faithful, and responsive wife. He was still dreaming of his brother. Because I knew that we would terminate in eight weeks, I actively focused on "the event" and on what interfered with his mourning, and there was open grieving at last. When, after a few sessions, and with termination in sight, we returned to his sexual concerns, the paranoid flavor was gone. He was able to explore relationship issues, and, at my insistence, to appreciate the impact of his withholding, suppression, and secrecy on the marital relationship. In the final sessions, I departed from my usual practice and answered his personal questions, which were asked with some of the permissible curiosity of a foreigner—questions, for instance, about my marital status, age, and religion, all different from his. In retrospect, I think I was providing a model of open communication and self-disclosure. We parted warmly and with a sense that we had had a mutually satisfying relationship within the constraints of the implacable limits of time, language, and culture.

In many important respects, the case of Kemal was very similar to one that Freud (1922) cited to illustrate his paper entitled "Some Neurotic Mechanisms in Jealousy, Paranoia and Homosexuality." Freud described a young man tormented by the jealous conviction of his wife's infidelity. Although there was no sibling loss, Freud's young man also had a distant father, was his mother's favorite son, and had a homosexual attachment to an older brother. Sexual intercourse with his wife aroused both heterosexual and homosexual feelings. The latter were expressed toward her by paranoia and jealousy. Fortunately for him, Kemal's paranoid projections were still quite malleable.

CASE EXAMPLE 2

In the second case, the homosexual panic was obvious from the beginning. Therefore, the case is reported in summary form.

Ken was referred in October and was seen privately because he was assessed as needing longer and more intensive care than could be offered at the university. He requested a female therapist. Ken was then twenty-one years old and just beginning his senior year. I saw him three times weekly for the first month, then twice weekly until the end of April. At that point, termination in June because of graduation became a focal issue, and Ken failed to come for his sessions in May, although he acknowledged and paid for them and apologized for his absence. I believe that this disruption was evidence of a desperate need to defend against emotional reactions to separation and loss. Ken presented in a state of anxiety and depression so intense that it seemed likely that he would have to leave school. His parents, his therapist, and Ken himself openly wondered whether he was suicidal. He was tormented by the deeply dystonic and obsessive idea that he was homosexual. We explored his psychosexual history in detail and could find nothing to support this dreaded conviction. Neither did his interests, preferences, or dreams that developed during therapy give confirming evidence. Ken was able to feel reassured by this kind of accepting and acknowledging exploration and became dependent on the therapist. I believe that the symptom, in addition to its defensive aspects, was an expression of his sense that something was bad and/or unacceptable about himself. Within a couple of months of treatment, the anxiety subsided and Ken was able to function academically even better than before. Because of therapy, he could now understand intellectual concepts more completely at a deeper level. Throughout the year, he also gradually experimented with more emotional intimacy in friendships with both young men and young women. He became more active on the campus, proceeded actively with a job search, and graduated on time.

The symptom had begun as a part of the sequelae to the sudden, possibly suicidal, accidental death of a withdrawn, twenty-year-old brother when Ken was about seventeen. He had become emotionally frozen when this occurred. A mourning process was finally begun in the therapy, pressed in part by the therapist's reactions to his dreams of his brother. There were deep feelings of survivor guilt—anxiety about moving beyond his brother's age and achievements. These feelings were exacerbated by the inevitability of his impending graduation when he would successfully complete his senior year.

The recognition by another person of his thoughts and feelings—both disturbed and normal ones—and the experience of empathy stimulated a poignant awareness of the deficits in his entire emotional development. His devoted father had been and continued to be emotionally distant and constricted, and his depressed mother had always employed a defense of shallowness and an emphasis on appearances. We dealt with the depressive but not rageful side of these deficits during the academic year. I repeatedly chose to interpret the homosexual obsession as a defense. This initial course of therapy helped Ken to complete his college career but postponed the inevitability of a necessary and more thorough therapeutic regression.

Ken phoned me late the following autumn for a psychiatric referral, and I confirmed the name of a male psychiatrist he had received. I saw him as a guilt-ridden and depressed person, with quite a well-developed character structure but with earlier deficits in the development of a cohesive self. These were rendered more difficult by the additional emotional demands imposed by the sibling loss.

Discussion

In reviewing the literature on sibling loss, on homosexuality, and on adolescent mourning, I found no explicit mention of the connection between sibling loss and homosexual anxieties in late adolescence.

However, this connection can be inferred in the writings of a number of authors.

Ritvo (1971) discusses the developmental phase of late adolescence and emphasizes the formation and structuralization of the ego ideal during this period. He writes that one of the main genetic roots of the ego ideal is in the passive-feminine homosexual position of a negative Oedipus complex. The homosexual aspect of the ego ideal is useful in understanding the problems of homosexuality that occur in late adolescence in connection with taking steps that have a crucial impact on self-esteem. The threat of failure stems from the pressure to take steps to define identity. At such a point, the adolescent may turn to someone who represents his own ideal.

Laufer (1966) discusses object loss in adolescence and emphasizes that ambivalence toward the object is heightened in adolescence and may be kept under repression by the idealization of the lost object. Feelings that represent anger and disappointment with the object are suppressed, and this results in such "well-known pathological solutions as depression, flattening of affect, disturbances of sexuality because of guilt feelings attached to the death of the object; acting out . . ." (p. 291).

Garber (1985) discusses mourning in adolescence and adds the idea that the usual emotional responses are suppressed because the survivor is "overly concerned about being considered different or abnormal" (p. 376). The survivor reacts to a profound sense of blame and embarrassment by expending much energy to appear as normal and as appropriate as he possibly can. Garber also mentions that the intensity of sexual feelings may heighten ambivalence and intensify the need for more rigid defense.

Coen (1981) integrates the contributions of self psychology and of classical ego psychology in understanding sexualization as a predominant mode of defense. He begins his review of the literature with Kohut's view that the sexual mode is related to the need for intense feeling stimulation to reassure the self that it is alive and whole, for defense against depressive affect, and as a mode for the expression of incorporative wishes to fill in missing psychic structure. He adds Stolorow's speculation that "the degree of primitive sexualization of narcissistic reparative efforts is a measure of the degree of narcissistic vulnerability and the acuteness of the threat of narcissistic decompensation" (p. 341). Coen cites other authors who emphasize the failure of the ego's integrative and synthetic ability for neutralization of instinctual energies, especially hostile aggression, particularly during regression. He says that "defense against hostile aggression via sexualization is an explicit or implicit premise of most writing on the subject" (p. 344).

Isay (1985) speaks of the homosexual defense in heterosexual men that defends against conflicts about anger, assertiveness, and competition and expresses the unconscious wish to be a woman, that is, passive and submissive. "In such patients, homosexual fantasies are activated in late adolescence by the specific threats and dangers inherent in increasingly successful and aggressive strivings. Symptoms are largely rooted in oedipal-stage conflicts and negative-oedipal identifications as an attempted resolution of these conflicts" (p. 9). Bank and Kahn (1982), in their most complete book on the importance of sibling relations, downplay the heavy psychoanalytic emphasis on rivalry and emphasize that the "identification processes are the psychological mortar and brick of the sibling bond" (p. 85). "If one's identity is interlocked with only one sibling, it will be dislocated by the loss. With no other sibling available to continue the identity process, the survivor is truly bereft and has for a partner in the dialectical dance for self-definition only the dead sibling's ghost" (p. 272).

A reference from Freud (1922) is the most pungent and resonant statement of all. He writes that:

observation has directed my attention to several cases in which during early childhood impulses of jealousy, derived from the mother-complex and of very great intensity, arose in a boy against rivals, usually older brothers. The jealousy led to an exceedingly hostile and aggressive attitude towards these brothers which might sometimes reach the pitch of death wishes, but which could not maintain themselves. . . . These impulses yielded to repression and underwent transformation, so that the rivals of the earlier period became the first homosexual love object. . . . After a short phase of jealousy the rival became the love object.

Freud sees this as an exaggerated form of "the process which leads to the birth of the social instincts" (p. 231).

The literature indicates that one needs formulations both from self psychology and from classical drive and ego psychology in order fully to understand and integrate the clinical material. Indeed, my sessions with these men stimulated many reactions, thoughts, and questions. The following scheme presents some of the constructs and ideas that were stimulated by the cases and by the literature:

Self Psychology	*Drive (Ego) Psychology*
brother as selfobject	brother as oedipal object
structural deficit	object loss
depletion	free-floating homosexual libido
narcissistic rage	hostile aggression
shame	guilt
grandiose restitutions	regression
internalization	identification

In the sessions, I also entertained many ideas about the variety of transferences and functions of the therapeutic relationship.

When confronted with this array of complex theoretical elements, it seemed important to avoid reductionism and premature closure on the one hand and, on the other, to avoid becoming diffuse or confused. There was a need for focus, to order priorities, and to consolidate ideas in order to make balanced, appropriate, and realistic interventions. The circumstances under which treatment occurred seemed to demand the ones that were made. In part, the therapist dealt with the rigid defenses of the patients by providing a model for flexibility and awareness of complexity along with providing focus and consolidation. This occurred in each session. The therapeutic task became a paradigm of the central developmental task faced by these men in their late adolescence with their particular histories and in their particular life situations. For the patients *and* the therapist, the task was the same: that is, the formation and development of the ego ideal—composed of feelings, defenses, aspirations, ideas, and values—had to be exposed to the reality of an intimate relationship and a new integration achieved.

Conclusions

In the time-limited psychotherapy of two young men who were seen in homosexual panic at a college mental health center, the therapist chose to focus on their sibling loss. Specifically, each, at age seventeen, had suddenly lost an older brother. As was described in the case reports, the focus on sibling loss was accomplished (1) by making observations of gross defensive reactions to that event, (2) by connecting that event and its sequelae with the presenting complaints, and (3) by interpreting character resistances to mourning and to integrating that relatively recent life event into an emerging adult identity. This approach facilitated the successful completion of two college careers, but it also left more therapeutic work for the future.

It is suggestive that the recent caseload of one psychotherapist contained three cases where there was sibling loss in adolescence and where young college men were preoccupied, either overtly or by inference, with issues of homosexuality. Further case reports are needed in order to state with assurance that this connection is significant.

REFERENCES

Altschul, S. 1985. Tragedy or trauma: when does coping become pathology? Paper presented at a conference on sibling loss, Chicago, June.

Bank, S. P., and Kahn, M. D. 1982. *The Sibling Bond*. New York: Basic.

Coen, S. J. 1981. Sexualization as a predominant mode of defense. *Journal of the American Psychoanalytic Association* 29(2): 337–352.

Colonna, A. B., and Newman, L. M. 1983. The psychoanalytic literature on siblings. *Psychoanalytic Study of the Child* 38:285–309.

Freud, S. 1922. Some neurotic mechanisms in jealousy, paranoia, and homosexuality. *Standard Edition* 18:221–232. London: Hogarth, 1955.

Garber, B. 1985. Mourning in adolescence: normal and pathological. *Adolescent Psychiatry* 12:371–387.

Isay, R. A. 1985. Homosexuality in homosexual and heterosexual men: some distinctions and implications for treatment. Paper presented at a meeting of the Chicago Psychoanalytic Society, April.

Laufer, M. 1966. Object loss and mourning during adolescence. *Psychoanalytic Study of the Child* 21:269–293.

Pollock, G. 1985. Childhood sibling loss: a family tragedy. Paper presented at a conference on sibling loss, Chicago, June.

Ritvo, S. 1971. Late adolescence: developmental and clinical considerations. *Psychoanalytic Study of the Child* 26:241–263.

Rosen, H. 1985. *Unspoken Grief: Coping with Childhood Sibling Loss*. Lexington, Mass.: Lexington Books.

Solnit, A. 1985. New challenges and obstacles in adolescence. Paper presented at a meeting of the Chicago Society for Adolescent Psychiatry, February.

16   IDENTITY DIFFUSION:
A LONG-TERM FOLLOW-UP

RUTHELLEN JOSSELSON

What shall I do now? What shall I do?
I shall rush out as I am, and walk the street
With my hair down, so. What shall we do tomorrow?
What shall we ever do?

—T. S. Eliot, *The Wasteland*

Erikson was the first theoretician to attempt to understand the familiar but perplexing failure of late adolescents to resolve successfully the identity formation task, a syndrome now known as identity diffusion. The enigma of this state is perhaps reflected in the fact that Erikson has variously called the negative pole of the identity stage "role confusion," "identity diffusion," and, finally, "identity confusion." He wrestled with how best to title these phenomena and admitted to never finding a suitable term.

The state that Erikson attempted to encompass in a phrase is one in which the individual is unable to make a commitment to a chosen role or life-style. The self is poorly differentiated; identifications are total and shifting as the self cannot maintain its integrity. The capacity for work is impaired; the individual either is unable to concentrate or is immersed in task-irrelevant activity. The avoidance of choice leads to an inner vacuum, vulnerable to regressive phenomena.

Erikson (1968) discusses identity diffusion as characterized by problems in intimacy, time perspective, and industry. The young person at a loss in the process of identity formation cannot risk closeness to another, foreshortens both the future and the past, and lacks the capacity to concentrate on tasks. Erikson considers identity diffusion to be an unstable state, for where the person fails to claim an identity, society tends to provide one. Often, this failure of choice leads to the individual being labeled "deviant," and this deviance becomes his (passively) accepted negative identity. Further, Erikson (1968, p. 17) comments, "Young patients can be violent or depressed, delinquent or withdrawn, but theirs is an acute and possibly passing crisis rather than a breakdown of the kind which tends to commit a patient to all the malignant implications of fatalistic diagnosis. And as has always been the case in the history of psychoanalytic psychiatry, what was first recognized as the common dynamic pattern of a group of severe disturbances revealed itself later to be a pathological aggravation, an undue prolongation of, or a regression to, a normative crisis 'belonging' to a particular stage of individual development."

Kernberg (1976), taking issue with Erikson, believes that identity diffusion is a pathological phenomenon in adolescence. In his view, a well-integrated ego will, in adolescence, rework its relations with the psychosocial environment without undue disruption.

> Normal adolescence typically presents identity crises but not identity diffusion—two concepts which deserve to be clearly differentiated. An identity crisis involves a loss of the correspondence between the internal sense of identity at a certain stage of development and the confirmation provided by the psychosocial environment. Such a discrepancy threatens one's sense of identity as well as one's relationship to the environment and calls for their reexamination. In contrast, identity diffusion is a severe psychopathological syndrome typical of borderline personality organization. It is characterized by mutually dissociated ego states. The lack of integration extends to the superego and, even more fundamentally, the world of internalized object relations. [Kernberg 1976, p. 224]

Kernberg goes on to list three characteristics helpful in distinguishing benign emotional turmoil from the syndrome of identity diffusion: (1) the capacity for experiencing guilt and concern; (2) the capacity for establishing lasting, nonexploitative relationships where the other person is viewed realistically; and (3) a consistently expanding and deepening set of values (1976, p. 225).

While both Erikson and Kernberg regard identity diffusion as a pathological state, Erikson tends to view this as a developmental crisis while Kernberg discusses identity diffusion as an aspect of a borderline process. The DSM-III essentially follows Kernberg's model in listing "identity disorder" as an adolescent precursor to the diagnosis of "borderline personality" in adulthood. But, to date, there have been no studies that document whether those adolescents who are diffuse in identity do indeed show signs of borderline psychopathology as adults.

While Erikson elaborates the concept of identity diffusion in life histories (of Shaw and William James) and in case histories (of hospitalized young men), he at the same time stresses the need to view the processes of identity formation and identity diffusion in the life histories of "ordinary" individuals. Except for the biographical material on extraordinary individuals, there is no record in the psychological literature of what becomes of people who have manifested states of identity diffusion in adolescence. Nor is there any information on this form of failure of identity resolution as it occurs in women.[1]

Erikson's theoretical "stages of life" framework is an effort to map normal developmental crises of the human life cycle. The cases that he presents to illustrate identity diffusion are, however, all drawn from his clinical practice—that is, they were all people who were defined by themselves or others as in need of help. Kernberg's views on identity diffusion are likewise drawn from his clinical experience.

Yet identity diffusion is common on college campuses, well known even to those who are untrained in psychopathology. Among college students, the sense of identity confusion—uncertainty about goals or values—is frequently viewed as a transient state, as something that will be grown out of. Are these the same students who, viewed from a clinical perspective, are diagnosed as incipient borderlines? The present study follows longitudinally a group of eight women who were classified as "identity diffuse" in college and who were reinterviewed ten to twelve years later. The purpose is to discover the fate of their identity diffusion.

The Research Paradigm

Much research attention has been given to the identity formation problem, partly because of the availability of a powerful and conceptually valid research instrument developed by Marcia (1966) to operationalize Erikson's theory. In the past ten years, a great many studies have looked at the process of identity formation by using the Marcia interview, which divides people into four identity statuses as follows: (1) Identity Achievement: those who have made identity commitments following a period of crisis; (2) Moratorium: those in a period of crisis who are struggling to make commitments; (3) Foreclosure: those who have made identity commitments without a period of crisis, largely resting on childhood or parentally derived decisions; (4) Diffusion: those without identity commitments who are unconcerned about it and/ or not struggling to make such decisions.

These studies,[2] which mainly compare the identity statuses to each other, have found reliable and consistent covariates for each status. The authors, however, have largely been most interested in the Identity Achievements, in understanding the factors that lead to successful resolution of the identity task. The Identity Diffusion group has been treated rather perfunctorily.

The group of those who are diffuse in identity, however, has been the most predictable and, at the same time, most diverse in identity-status research. Predictability has derived from the Diffusions' consistency in being the lowest of the groups on any measure with positive valence. Therefore, they have been shown to be lowest in ego development (Hopkins 1982), intimacy (Kacerguis and Adams 1980), highest in anxiety (Schenkel and Marcia 1972), most undifferentiated in sex-role orientation (Orlofsky 1977), and most field dependent (Schenkel 1975).

The diversity of the Diffusion group, on the other hand, derives from a conceptual base. In that Diffusions are defined by the absence of characteristics—namely, crisis and commitment—they are, subsequently, a group of people who share something missing rather than something present. Since many factors can lead to the failure of the identity formation process, it is not surprising that, on closer examination, the Diffusion group would show mixed personality configurations.

Bourne's (1978a, 1978b) critical review of approximately thirty studies using the identity status paradigm concludes that the most we really know about Diffusions is that they tend to withdraw from situations. Speculating that they are "probably at the more severe end of the psychological continuum" (1978b, pp. 374–375), he urges that more research on Diffusions is necessary.

The purpose of the present study is to focus on the Identity Diffusions, to ask about what becomes of them. Is identity diffusion, as Erikson suggests, a transient state, a kind of more-severe moratorium, which people, given the right circumstances, outgrow? And if they transcend this state, what are the right circumstances? Or is it true that, as Kernberg suggests, identity diffuse individuals harbor underlying psychopathology that prevents resolution of the identity task? Do those showing signs of identity diffusion in late adolescence become adult borderlines?

Method

The present study is part of a long-term follow-up of sixty-six college-senior women who participated in an identity-status study ten to twelve years ago. Of the sixty-six, forty were located and thirty-four participated.[3] Originally, the women were students in one of four colleges or universities, three in the Northeast and one in the Midwest, two public and two private. They represented a random sample of college women and a range of social classes. Eight of the sixteen[4] women who had been classified as Identity Diffusions in the original study contributed their life stories to this study. They now live in all parts of the country and are thirty-two to thirty-five years old. All factual data have been disguised in this report, although I have made efforts to preserve the spirit of the phenomena.

The interview data from the original study consisted of a forty-five-minute identity-status interview and a two-hour recorded clinical interview (Josselson 1973) covering a wide range of topics, oriented to assessing underlying psychodynamic themes, object relationships, and significant experiences. The current data were derived from a lengthy protocol (either taped or written) that attempted to assess all aspects of their experiences in the intervening years. In-person interviews averaged three hours, and the women were permitted to stray from the structured format and to organize their accounts of their lives in the fashion that made most sense to them.

The method of data analysis was clinical and descriptive rather than hypothesis testing in order to preserve the heuristic value of phenomenologically rich data. While a between-groups study will be forthcoming, this chapter focuses on developmental aspects unique among the Diffusion group.

Identity-Diffuse Women—and What Has Become of Them

In a previous study (1973), I attempted to classify Diffusion-status women into four subgroups based on personality structure: previous developmental deficits, severe psychopathology, Moratorium Diffusions, and Foreclosed Diffusions. Several of the women in the Diffusion status appeared to be suffering from either severe psychopathology or from previous developmental deficits that prevented them from experiencing a true identity formation stage. Their preoccupation with archaic or disturbed conflicts overshadowed and obstructed work on identity issues, and, although they were functioning adequately in college, they were operating on quite a different psychological level than their peers. Several other of the Diffusion-status women were discussed as Moratorium Diffusions, women in crisis but dealing with the crisis in areas other than those of psychosocial identity issues. It was typical of these women to move in and out of active work on identity issues—to struggle for awhile, then give up only to begin anew. Finally, a number of women were thought to be Foreclosed Diffusions, women who were uncommitted and drifting with their amorphousness, but women whose parents seemed to have had equally diffuse identity resolutions. In many ways, these Foreclosed Diffusions seemed to be women who would have adopted their parents' modes of being if only their parents had given them enough structure to internalize. Lacking such clear principles to define themselves by or against, they became leaves blown about by the wind, waiting, perhaps, to be claimed by something.

Because the Diffusion group begins, then, as such a mixed group, one would expect their lives to follow very different courses after college. In one sense this is true, but what is more striking is that they continue to be predictable, to have commonality as a group.

Women who were classified as Diffusions have, without question, become the most unusual people in the sample. Their lives most frequently have the quality of gothic novels; they make more unlikely choices and try to live with them. Statistically, Diffusions, as a group, have held more jobs and moved their residences significantly more than any of the other groups. In general, they have experienced more and made more changes.

235

Five of the eight women who were in the Diffusion status at the end of college were still found to be diffuse in identity ten to twelve years later. Most of these five appear to have remained diffuse in their identity throughout that time, with brief periods of effort to define an identity for themselves. The remaining three women have made identity commitments but, as is discussed later, have done this in a way quite different from the other identity-status groups.

The Still-Diffuse Diffusions

Three women could best be classified as still-diffuse Diffusions. All had been categorized among the subtype of severe psychopathology or previous developmental deficits at the time of the analysis ten years earlier. The following case exemplifies a life history typical of this subgroup.

THE CASE OF SUSAN

COLLEGE

When first interviewed at the end of college, Susan showed the fragmented, disorganized approach to her life characteristic of the "pure" Diffusions—that is, she was diffuse in each identity category.[5] An art major, she had no plans for after graduation and felt that it was unimportant what she did as long as she did something. She did not hope to marry. "I have more fun not married," she said, "and you can spend all the money on yourself and you don't get saddled down with responsibilities."

Susan had no religious beliefs at that time. Her father had forced her to go to his church while her mother had pushed her to another. Her mother's counsel, though, was to wait until she married to choose a religion. For a while, Susan had been involved in Eastern mysticism, but "it got too weird. I kind of got into it—not that I believed in it or anything."

On politics, Susan had no ideas at all. "I don't like to vote and anyway, I don't know where to vote." Her parents never discussed political issues, and there were no issues on which she had strong opinions.

236

Susan's sexual standards were equally diffuse. Her decisions about whether to have sexual intercourse or not were related to whether she liked the man and whether he was good-looking. As she tried to define her standards, she became increasingly confused and ended up saying, "I don't know—I hide a lot—think about something else."

This identity-status interview clearly portrayed a very scattered young woman, unable to define herself on any issue and relatively untroubled about it.

Susan's parents, neither of whom were college graduates, divorced when Susan was in her late teens. She described her mother as "really nice—she'd help me out if I needed it." Although closer to her mother than to her father, Susan did not feel she could confide in her or talk to her about serious things and, as a result, saw her only rarely. The youngest of three girls, Susan saw the family dynamics as mother catering to the middle child, father to the oldest, and she being left out. She saw her mother as very conservative in her values, especially with regard to sex. "I used to believe like that. A year ago, if somebody would have told me I'd be living with a guy, I wouldn't have believed it. This last year I got messed up somewhere along the line."

With her father, Susan had had for some years "only a financial relationship." He was at work during most of the time she was growing up, and Susan had little sense of knowing her father. She was clear, however, that she wanted to be different from him in every way possible.

Susan admired her two sisters, especially their feminine qualities with regard to looks and clothes. When she was growing up, her heroes were fashion models and movie stars and Scarlett O'Hara because "she always thought about herself, always came first."

At the time of the interview, Susan's emotional energies were centered on a highly ambivalent relationship with her live-in boyfriend, whom she referred to as Dummy throughout the discussion. He mistreated her in many ways, including turning their apartment into a kind of a commune for his friends where the main activities were drugs and sex. She was fitfully trying to summon the resources to leave him.

Susan's previous experiences with men had been largely fantasy dominated, with many crushes on unavailable men. Her few previous real involvements ended abruptly when the man "split."

In general, Susan presented a portrait of great emotional impoverishment. Her earliest memory was, "Probably singing to the cows.

That must have been age six or seven. I always showed the cows everything I got new, plus I'd sing to them." In this memory is expressed both the difficulties in object relationships as well as the narcissism revealed more directly in her movie-star fantasies. The other issues Susan showed in the projective material were centered on themes of abandonment, loss, and destruction. Her defenses were mainly magical thinking and denial, all interwoven with romantic fantasies of happy endings.

Although, clinically, Susan appeared to be suffering from borderline psychopathology, she was nevertheless functioning. Her impulsive, self-indulgent, and self-protective approach to life was under enough ego control to make it possible for her to continue to college without psychotherapeutic intervention. The clinician, however, would, at the time, have questioned her ability to organize herself and would have wondered about the fate of her underlying anger and self-destructive relationships with men.

ADULTHOOD—TWELVE YEARS LATER

Upon her graduation from college, Susan's aunt found her her first job—teaching art in an alternative school for which an education degree was not necessary. Susan very much enjoyed this job, but it was short-lived because the school closed for lack of funds. She then moved to Arizona, where she had a friend, and unsuccessfully looked for another teaching job. Since then, she has knocked about, trying a variety of relatively unskilled jobs and, for the past five years, has been working as a cashier back in her hometown.

Susan continued her pattern of unpredictable relationships with men who mistreated her in one way or another until two years ago when she found a special man whom she felt would change her life and whom she wanted to marry. She began converting to Catholicism in preparation for their marriage when he abruptly left her after she announced to him that she was pregnant. Susan had decided to have the baby even though she was in no financial position to care for it. Tragically, however, the baby was born with severe congenital defects and lived only three months. This very difficult time of stress led to a religious mystical experience, including visions, and Susan became a devout Catholic.

The church has become, at least for now, the center of Susan's life. She answered many of the current questions in terms of her religious

238

beliefs, as though she had truly experienced her conversion as a rebirth. Christ, she says, and her priest are the most important people in her life.

At present, Susan is living with her mother because the unsteadiness of her work does not allow her enough money to live on her own. Her mother is also helping her to manage money, something Susan has never done very well. Susan still wishes for a career, instead of these "measly jobs," but seems to have no idea how to go about this. Despite this rather depressing picture, Susan does not seem depressed (at least superficially). She has a number of friends with whom she enjoys good times, and the major good experiences in her life have centered on pleasurable interactions with friends. Of her life goals now, Susan summarizes, reflectively, "Here I am—I'm still thinking—I'll get a job, then I'll get married. That's terrible . . . I'm still thinking . . . that really is."

Susan's romantic fantasies have not come true. The overall feeling about her is of a very childlike person, wandering among the fragments of her life.

Like the other two still-diffuse Diffusions, Susan has difficulty being reflective or adding up her life. Meaning exists at the moment. One of the other still-diffuse women is currently engaged in an effort to research careers and figure out what she wants to do. This sounded very promising, largely because of her enthusiasm, but further probing unearthed that she has embarked on such projects before, only to have them end in failure. The style of these women is impulsive. Great energy may be invested in an undertaking, but the plan always sours. This is in part because they do not look too closely at things and greet each opportunity as salvation. Despite disappointments, they remain hopeful that the next thing that comes along will fulfill their dreams.

What the three still-diffuse Diffusions share is a lack of personality structure, making them dependent on external egos. All of them have found friends or family members to organize around internally and who also help to organize them externally. The deficits that underlay their identity diffusion in college have not mended themselves. It is, in fact, hard to perceive growth or development in these women. Their external circumstances change; they are buffeted or supported by the Fates, but they, internally, remain essentially unchanged.

It is striking that these women all welcomed the interview—as an external structuring agent to think about issues they do not usually think about. Interestingly, two of them (including Susan) had brief (two to three months) passes at psychotherapy, which they found "helpful." To them, therapy was one more process that was "tried."

What is hardest to find in these women is the source of ego strength that keeps them going. Overall, they seem not to take life too seriously and to be able to lose themselves in a "good time." As one of the other women put it, "I'm doing the things I want to do"—mainly sports, recreation, being with friends; she is not troubled about working in a job far below her potential.

All of these three women have had unusual experiences which they elevate to the status of personal myth (such as Susan's very elaborate telling of the loss of her child). They are colorful, if tragically so, and would, no doubt, be viewed by others as likable eccentrics. While they take risks, they are the risks of impulse rather than growth, and life becomes a process of living with the consequences of hastily formed decisions. But, whatever the degree of underlying psychopathology, depression does not overwhelm them. They have their ups and downs but bounce back.

The three still-diffuse Diffusions share a history of difficulties in relationships with men. With what appears to be deeply rooted fears of men, they all choose unusual partners and have a checkered and disappointing series of experiences. One of the women has found consistency and stability in a long-distance relationship, one way of dealing with her fears of intimacy. Failure of the intimacy task seems to coexist with the failure of the identity-formation process. Unable to define a sense of self, these women remain unable to commit themselves to another, unless there are certain safeguards of distance or difficulty that would prevent the much-feared closeness and commitment. None of them wishes to marry or have children, but they do not rule out its "happening."

In their views of their lives, only what is present is real for these women. Unlike women in the other identity statuses, the still-diffuse Diffusions could give only hazy outlines of what occurred in their lives up until the present issues and struggles. The future is unimaginable, and the past is largely lost. They are not self-analytic women, and the questions they ask of life are basically concrete: How can I get a higher-paying or more secure job? Shall I live alone or share an apartment?

These women stand in contrast to another form of continuing identity diffuseness, which is much more probing, philosophical, and aware. In the earlier study, these women were subclassified as Moratorium Diffusions, and their form of identity diffusion is quite different from that already described.

Still Diffuse; Trying to Settle Down

THE CASE OF DEBBIE

COLLEGE

Of all the women in the college sample, Debbie was the most articulate. On occupation: "I don't know what I want to do—join the circus, a gypsy camp, I don't know. Yesterday I was thinking of starting a day care center in Vermont. I guess I'm about 50 percent serious about it. I'm terrible at planning. I can't do long-range things very well. When the time comes, I'll do something." On religion: "I've always believed in God, but God has changed." On politics: "I got involved like everyone else in petitions and marches, then I thought it was all absurd and I don't bother with it anymore." On sexual standards: "The first time I see a person, if I want to sleep with him, something clicks—the vibrations he gives off . . . I just trust my instincts."

Throughout her college interview, Debbie focused on her fascination with possibility, her experimentation with altering her consciousness and perceiving reality through varied lenses. She was drawn to cosmic experiences, feelings of unification with the universe that allowed her to feel that she could be whatever she wanted to be. At the same time, however, Debbie maintained a cynical view of her mystical heights and felt unable to commit herself fully to "being in the clouds."

Debbie was struggling painfully with the contrast between her earlier self and her current one. She saw herself as having been a good girl who believed all that her parents taught her and thought the crossroads of the world were on the local corner.

"Then I came to college and there were all these people who came from all different places and there were really rich people and smart people and freaky people and people who didn't believe in God and there were so many things—drugs, sex, hippies. It was all very confusing.

"I have no idea about the future. There are possibilities open to me and what it has done has totally confused me. In the old days, it was so easy. Either you were going to get married or you weren't going to

241

get married. You were going to be a teacher or a nurse. But now you can go anywhere and do anything and there are so many possibilities that—I don't know. I could be doing something I couldn't name because I don't know it exists yet."

Debbie described her parents as having been opposite in character. Her mother was warm, soft, and quiet while her father was loud, aggressive, and demanding. She felt she had elements of both in her nature. Although she described her family as having been close, she seemed to have little emotional investment in them. She recalled, at age thirteen, telling her parents that she did not need parents anymore except for food and shelter. Debbie had always been very involved in peer culture, and when her parents tried to impose restrictions about hours or friends, she fought them until they relented.

From an early time, Debbie had the sense of being very special. She and her sisters were the smartest pupils in their school, and her father had great pride in and expectations of his daughters. While Debbie always admired her mother, she always felt different from her. She saw her mother as gentle, sure of herself, peaceful, and calm. In contrast, Debbie felt in herself an aggressiveness and adventurousness that never left her satisfied with herself, her friends, or her world.

For Debbie, as for the other two women in this subgroup of the college Diffusions, struggle with important questions was central to her life. Although conflict did not focus specifically on psychosocial identity issues—at least, not the ones used to define the statuses—these women were not passively resigning themselves to amorphousness. Their lives tended to be marked by movement between moratorium and diffusion states as they tried new modes of being, searched for answers, quested for meaning, and then gave up for awhile only to begin again.

These women seemed not, however, to be involved in the separation-autonomy struggle that has been found to be central to Moratorium women (Josselson 1973). On the contrary, they had rejected their parents and their life-styles and were conscious of no conflict about this. They had disowned their pasts and had decided what they were not going to be. Conflict was handled largely by repression or denial. They behaved as though the superego, internalized long ago, could simply be turned off. Their impulsivity was in the service of keeping the superego out of service, and it is no wonder that none of the avenues they chose felt right to them. Choices tended to be the choices of parts of themselves while the remaining parts were left to object. In this vein, Debbie spoke of feeling "incomplete." What they had of their ego-ideal was its tone, to be something very special, but the goals they aspired to were unrealistic and did not take account of the people they had already been.

The parents of these women all seemed to have had high expectations of their daughters (particularly the fathers). Yet these expectations of greatness and specialness tended to have an amorphous tone, such that these women never seemed to have a concrete sense of what they were supposed to have been. This ego-ideal, given its vagueness, also appeared to have been immune to the experiences in reality that tend to force revisions. As Debbie expressed it, they could have their own reality—at least for a time. These women had lived a kind of double life, existing and coping in reality while maintaining a strong investment in a private world. Like Debbie, they tended to search for totalistic experiences where they could exist at a pinnacle, at one with the romanticized ego-ideal. These experiences took them outside the social mainstream, which required too much compromise and delivered too little emotional pitch.

There was a striking developmental theme among these women in regard to their mothers. After having idealized their mothers, they discovered in latency that they were completely unlike them. They spoke of having always wished to be like their mothers, who were warm, loving, giving, and extremely talented domestically or artistically. And they felt great disappointment when they found that they did not have their mothers' gifts. Again reality did not provide what had been wished for.

Toward their fathers, these women felt intense ambivalence, and some of their inner difficulties were traceable to conflicts in this relationship. Unable to be like their mothers and wishing to be less like their fathers, these women seemed to have no other recourse besides casting around among the multitude of possibilities in the larger society for a totally new mode of being. Lacking solid and trusted introjects against which to test "what they really are," they found their quest a difficult one.

TWELVE YEARS LATER

In the twelve years since her graduation from college, Debbie very much followed her fantasy of going anywhere and doing anything. At present, as she looks back at herself in college, she judges herself to

243

have been "naive." On leaving college, she felt less interested in pursuing an occupation and more bent on "living my life" or, in one of her preferred phrases, "unfolding as a person." She took several jobs where she could pursue her interest in "helping people," but these jobs did not fulfill her hopes of what it would be like. "I filled out form after form [as a case worker]. Indeed, it was a job of form with no content. After three months, I quit, giving my reason for leaving—that the job was uninteresting and irrelevant."

Shortly thereafter, a year after college, she met and married an artist and they began traveling the world together. It was a relationship built on intensity, often drug-induced:

> We met while doing LSD. That's the kind of relationship he and I had. Everything was very magical and energized and high—very all possibilities—and everything was very adventurous and open and everything was like sparks flying and nerve-ends opening and life happening [deep sigh] and then what happened, I think, is that we both began to grow. I became tired or something and I began to want to build my ego up again. I didn't want to be smashed into a million fragments. . . . In those days, anything intense was very real and meaningful to me. It didn't seem to matter whether the intensity was in the direction of pain or joy.

For six years, this increasingly ambivalent relationship absorbed her. She found it difficult to break her vows in the marriage and felt that her husband, Brett, had become her family. Interestingly, they had had a very traditional church wedding with a large reception.

Debbie's marriage to Brett seems to have continued two patterns apparent at the end of college. First of all, it may have been an effort to unite the two sides of herself—the traditional, family-rooted Debbie of domesticity and the mystical adventurer—the traditional in the act of getting married and meaning it, taking it seriously, and the sensation-seeking in her choice of husband.

The second resonating pattern was her disillusionment with ego-shattering experiences. In her college interview, Debbie spoke poignantly of her bruising returns to reality after flights in the clouds. At this time, it seemed as though she had learned something she could integrate. Yet her marriage seemed to be one more effort to reach for this peak of experience, and again her reaction was similar—to tire of it, to wish to be back on the ground.

244

The separation and divorce from Brett marked a very painful period for Debbie. Living, at the time, far from her family and former friends, Debbie resisted her parents' urging to return home and set out to "make myself anew." She deliberately took part-time jobs with little responsibility, the better to focus on an inner search for her "true self." As in college, she turned to Eastern mysticism and spent much time meditating and keeping a journal. "I was emptying myself so I could get to the core of me and my life and then re-create myself."

During this time she became closer to one of Brett's friends, also an artist, but more settled, less scattered. (It seems likely, from Debbie's description, that Brett was schizophrenic.)

After a somewhat longer period of being together, Debbie married this new man, Bob, with whom she still feels she has excellent communication. "Although both of us are older and some of our views have tempered, we both feel it's important to remain open and questioning, and we are both trying to look at ourselves and see who we are and grow into all that we might be—perhaps." What they share, as Debbie puts it, is "being into exploring with life."

One outcome of Debbie's almost monastic inner searching was a decision to enter teaching in a radical education school, one focused on "guiding children to their true selves." She had, at the time of the interview, been teaching for a year and found it satisfying, challenging, and creative—the first such work experience she has had.

Overall, at present, Debbie gives the impression of trying to settle into her occupational and marriage commitments. She and Bob are trying to conceive, in order to "experience family anew." But at the same time that she sounds more reality-bound, she remains determined to cling to her sense of possibility. To most questions related to the future, Debbie says, "I don't know how with what life offers me, I will react." Asked what she would like to do in the future, she replied, "I might write someday—or become a counselor—or something else I haven't even thought of yet." The same words she had used in college.

This summary does not adequately capture the raggedness of Debbie's life before her marriage to Bob. She had had, for example, four abortions, many unusual relationships with unusual people, brushes with death of those close to her. Throughout this time, she again became close to her mother and two sisters, although her relationship with her father has continued to be ambivalent and difficult.

There is a vagueness and fluidity about Debbie, saved by the almost poetic expression of her acute perceptions. Her commitments are to

experience itself. Everything, however, is elevated to a higher plane—
she takes nothing for granted. She is still fascinated with merger, with
the wish to lose herself in another, which she did for a time with Brett
and is probably also doing with Bob, but less so. But, having merged,
she then needs to withdraw and regroup, redraw her ego boundaries.
The paradox of Debbie is that, with all the ego indefiniteness, with the
search for other states of consciousness, the energy of playing with
her own mind—all this exists in a context of some fundamental strength
that keeps her together at the same time that she is going over the
edge.

While Debbie defines herself by her internal focus, she is most related
to reality by her connectedness to others. It is as though, lacking inner
structure, she reaches out to others for the pieces she is missing.

It is impossible to predict the success of Debbie's current commitments—they are too new and she is too impulsive and volatile. What
one sees is her struggle—a continuation of the college struggle—to find
firm ground on which to stake herself without betraying other aspects
of her self, without foreclosing possibility, change, and growth. Unlike
the other still-diffuse Diffusions discussed earlier, Debbie has an internal focus. It is not an insightful one, but she does experiment with
her own malleability. In contrast to Susan, for example, who picks
herself up after getting knocked down by life, Debbie tries to understand her life, to find its meaning, and to look inward for answers.

Settled and Committed

Three of the Diffusion women have made life commitments and are,
at present, leading lives with clearly defined goals. They have, however,
embraced their choices totalistically—without ambivalence or struggle—and all of these choices rest on an external agent. Of the three
who are discussed here, two were judged to be Foreclosed Diffusions
at the end of college. One was a Moratorium Diffusion (as was Debbie)
but followed a very different course.

THE CASE OF EVELYN

In her college interview, Evelyn was viewed by the clinical interviewer as being covered with open wounds, living perilously close to
raw and painful feelings. She was emerging from a serious depression,

for which she was in psychotherapy, and in retreat from her involvement in the drug culture. Desperately low in self-esteem, Evelyn had tried fruitlessly to win the love and approval of her distant, critical father whom she adored. She had grown up in the shadow of a gifted older sister whom she idealized. Her mother had been largely emotionally unavailable when she needed her. Evelyn was so deeply in the throes of working through old family conflicts and disappointments that she was not much able to participate in the expansive aspects of college. Rebellious and angry, she was involved in pointless sexual experiences, drug-induced emotional states, mysticism, and philosophical questions. She had no idea what she wanted to do with her life or what she believed in but seemed, at the time of the interview, to be trying to get herself organized.

> I dropped out of school after sophomore year. I was sick of studying and went to work and that was so awful I went back to school. And then I got into drugs until one day when I had a really bad trip and my whole self-image shattered, I realized I wasn't what I thought I was. I realized I was really alone and had never really let anyone know me. I had had an image of myself as a strong-willed individual who did everything correctly. And there I was— a terrified little girl. So I stopped drugs and started therapy. I was brought up to think you don't have problems and I'm just starting now to confront some of them.

It was quite a different person who came to be interviewed twelve years later. This Evelyn, though she vaguely remembered the interviewer, was guarded and distant; she took a long time to relax and talk freely. Her wounds had healed and her feelings had submerged. In contrast to her college experience, she was leading a constricted and narrowed life and doing it with apparent contentment.

After graduation from college, Evelyn decided to take whatever job was highest paying, which turned out to be a responsible clerical job in the corporation where her mother had a secretarial job. She has been with the company ever since, moving up through the ranks of jobs with increasing administrative responsibility. This job hierarchy has provided a structure to organize herself, as she plots each new promotion, studies the politics, and increases her skills. "Upward mobility," as she puts it, is what is central in her life. Her political views have grown more conservative, but she has involved herself in local issues and has strong opinions about national and world events. She reads a great deal and generally feels connected to society.

Evelyn had had a very disappointing love affair with a man she met shortly before graduating from college. They were involved for five years, but he abruptly broke off the relationship when they were unable to reconcile their differing views of marriage. She came away feeling deeply and personally rejected. Since then, Evelyn has not found anyone to care about as seriously. She is philosophical about the possibility of marriage. "If it happens, it happens," but she seems not to fret about it and is not actively looking for someone.

Her father died four years ago, and Evelyn's mother has come to live with her. Her mother has become her best friend and they share a mutual and close relationship. The rest of Evelyn's time is focused on caring for her house (which she owns and has learned to repair herself), on activities with companions (who are clearly more companions than friends), and on a number of—mainly solitary—hobbies and interests.

In response to a question about the main good experiences of the past ten years, Evelyn focused on things she owns and is proud of owning. Bad experiences involve her losses in relationships—her boyfriend and her father. Her hopes for the future center on more things she would like to have.

Evelyn appears to have closed off much that had been in turmoil during college, as though it had threatened to overwhelm her and she decided it was better buried. She dismisses these experiences as having been a bad time and, in retrospect, did not feel her therapy was helpful (she remained in therapy only a few months). "I had to do it on my own," she says.

At present, Evelyn does not appear to be depressed. Looking over the past twelve years, Evelyn is proud of "getting to be the person that I am—getting as far as I have in my job. It wasn't easy and I did that on my own. I don't think I'm doing that badly."

This last statement seems to be the best summary of her psychological state. It is as though the shadow of her crisis experience remains with her. She had touched bottom and has now reorganized in quite a different direction. Remembering her turmoil, she can be pleased with the tranquility she has achieved and does not ask more of life than that.

Evelyn had been in a Moratorium Diffusion state during college and has developed into a Foreclosure pattern of identity. Although her path is an unusual one, she has much in common with the now-committed women who were Foreclosed Diffusions during college.

THE CASE OF DARLENE

Darlene was raised on the West Coast, and her parents were both highly educated. They were both intellectually committed, but people who discussed everything and believed in nothing. Since her parents were involved in a variety of social and professional activities, she thought she might like to go back there and see what there was for her to do.

Religiously, Darlene's parents were "very open" and never raised her any particular way. She believed in "some kind of Being which could fit any religion" but felt that she, like her father, had more questions than answers. Her political convictions were similar.

With respect to sex, Darlene denied that it could in any way be a moral issue, feeling that what was important was a person's emotions. As a result, she had no set standards and did what "feels right." Her parents had discussed this with her quite a bit; their views were that one should have a "relationship" prior to sexual involvement. To Darlene, this implied a certain cautiousness, which she could not manage in her own behavior, but she admitted to not being sure what was meant by a "relationship." For example, Darlene had described that the previous week she had had intercourse with a casual friend, "because I had kissed him, and if I went that far. . . ." When she thought about this later, she had some initial doubts about her action, then decided that since she had done it, it must have been right at the time, and if it was right at the time, then it must still be right. Her father had warned her that people can get "screwed up" by sex. Darlene felt that it was important not to be screwed up by sex, so she never allowed herself to feel any conflict about these matters.

Darlene was very much rooted in the present, wishing to forget the past and unable to envision a future. Always very active in causes, groups, and friends, she seemed to have gained momentary pleasure from these activities, but none had a lasting effect.

Darlene was quite vague about her history. The interviewer felt that she truly could not remember very much rather than that she was being evasive. She had few friends when young, preferring the company of her family and their friends. Much of this period of her life focused on social appearances, and she was, like her family, most concerned with being at the "right" places with the "right" people. These social pleasantries had a faddishness about them, such that something new was always "in."

There was an emotional emptiness in both Darlene and her recounting of her life. Her relationships seemed stereotyped and distant. One of her dreams suggested her sense of being an observer in life as well as her deep unconscious fear of being abandoned:

It was a huge Coliseum, filled up with all the people I've known in my life. And there was a big dinner. My boyfriend was with me and my parents were there. There was a wedding ceremony going on. It was very proper, waltz-type dancing. There were trapezes all over the place, but everyone was waltzing. My boyfriend was dancing, and I was sitting on the sidelines and I felt he was leaving me completely alone.

At the end of college, Darlene, and others who were Foreclosed Diffusions, seemed to experience themselves as leaves waiting for a gust of wind. They suffered from atrophy of the will, acting for the moment but unable to define a consistent direction.

These were women whose parents always left decisions up to them, never pushed them into or out of anything. Yet these daughters seemed to have sensed that their parents, rather than encouraging them to be independent, were merely expressing their own lack of convictions and inability to make decisions. Such vacillation seems to have induced their daughters to cling even tighter to them for some small measure of security. These women shared a kind of fatalistic passivity, feeling that they had so little control over their own lives that there was no point in trying to plan.

THE PRESENT: TWELVE YEARS LATER

As she had mentioned in her college interview, Darlene did return home to see what there was for her to do. Her mother found her a job in a related agency where she began to do social service work. She enrolled for further training in social work, though she never completed a degree, and began specializing in group work. Because of many moves around the country, Darlene has held a variety of jobs. She says, "My strength is in enabling others to become more whole and I, too, benefit from such facilitating relationships."

Darlene spent the first five postcollege years involved with a man with whom she ultimately broke off. A month after this, she met the husband she married two months later. She describes her husband as being very much like her father; they are both in the same profession. And Darlene is in an occupation very much like her mother's. She now has two young children who are her first priority. Although she has temporarily suspended her career, doing only very occasional volunteer projects, she maintains her interest and enthusiasm for working and intends to return to more active involvement as soon as the children need her less.

Despite the fact that Darlene has been creative and effective in her work—she has written one book and is in the planning stages with a second one—she has organized her life around her husband's career path. A number of times, she has made geographic moves because of his advancement, but she expressed no resentment about this. She does, however, feel burdened by the constant demands of her children and longs for time to herself. It is not clear why she has forgone her career so much for her family, except a feeling that this is what she is expected to do.

The center of Darlene's life is her relationships with others—especially her husband and children. Her work is also people oriented, and what she enjoys about it is the opportunity to discuss personally relevant issues.

Darlene expresses great joy and pride at how well she and her husband have managed their lives. They have made some difficult transitions but have moved smoothly. One of the most effusively happy women in the whole sample, Darlene seems delighted with all aspects of her life, except the complaints about feeling too tied down to the children. But even her complaints have a good-natured quality. Of both her children and her parents, she says, "I think we have quite an extraordinary family." She admires and respects her parents and still feels very close to them. She continues to have an intensely loving relationship with her husband. She has many friends.

On one level, Darlene seems quite healthy—focused and settled but still alive and growing. She is attempting to find creative solutions to

251

the career/family conflict while deliberately choosing to give priority to her family. On the other hand, Darlene's picture of her life has something of the quality of protesting too much—everything is *very* rosy.

Darlene is clearly more integrated than she was in college; the fortuitous first job gave her a feeling of success and helped her build a career commitment. The romanticized, idealized relationship to her husband gave structure to the rest of her life. It is evident, from a distance, however, that Darlene has recreated in her own life the life of her parents. She and her husband are doing the same things that her mother and father did. In terms of values and ideals, they are identical. She is not consciously aware of this, of course, but she says that she sees herself as "very much the product of my family."

In this sense, Darlene, like Evelyn, has "gone home again." College, for them, was a period of experimentation, but their lives have followed the threads of their precollege selves.

Before I summarize the themes common to the life trajectories of the Diffusions, brief mention should be made of the last now-committed Diffusion. This woman, Gretchen, was much like Darlene in her college interview. She also had been grouped as a Foreclosed Diffusion, embedded in her family network, uncertain of her own goals or beliefs but organizing herself via a relationship with her boyfriend. Gretchen took her first job based on where her boyfriend was located and soon discovered in herself a talent for photography. Her boyfriend became her husband, but she continued to pursue and succeed at her photographic work. Giving priority to her career, she was working in a different city from her husband, although they maintained a commuter relationship. During this time, however, both became involved in extramarital sexual relationships and considerable drug experimentation. At the point when they came close to divorce, they together became "reborn" through involvement in an Eastern religious sect. Gretchen, on advice from her spiritual leader, took up residence with her husband and together they began to live out a life of spirituality and meditation. They now have three children, but Gretchen is pursuing her photography part of the time. Most of the decisions in Gretchen's life are now made by her spiritual leader who is the most important person in her life. She feels now that she has found the "true path" and has organized her life around it.

In Gretchen, we see another form of foreclosure, this time not on aspects of her family of origin, but in a totalistic system which answers all of her questions and to which she can adjust in toto. In spite of her fortunate discovery of a talent, which led to a successful career, Gretchen had been unable to organize the rest of her life. Her lack of inner structure was exacting its price. It seems that Gretchen was in need of external discipline and, once it was provided, has been able to settle into a goal-oriented, if constricted, way of life.

The final Diffuse woman on whom I have data is one who was overwhelmed by the lack of external structure following college. Six years after graduation, she committed suicide. This was a woman whose identity diffusion in college has been seen to result from previous developmental deficits—deficits which were held in check by the relatively safe, structured world of college. One of the brightest and most thoughtful women in the sample, this young woman, as best as can be reconstructed from an interview with a family member, was unable to take hold of any life plan. And nothing appeared to claim her or to rescue her. She lapsed into a deepening depression that, by the time psychotherapists intervened, had gone beyond help.

Discussion

As in the previous study (Josselson 1973), Diffusions remain a diverse group. Yet there are themes that unite them. My major conclusion at that time was this: "What seems to be most salient is the failure of internalization of objects." This conclusion appears to be borne out by the follow-up investigation.

Of course, it is not correct to say that the Diffusions had failed totally at internalizing objects. They are not, after all, schizophrenic. The problem with the particular form of internalization evident in this group is that it does not lead to personality structuralization. Inner experiences do not fit together with other inner experiences, and self-representations can fluctuate widely. It is the synthetic function of the ego that is impaired. As a result, the self has little autonomy and the individual remains at the mercy of impulses and environmental forces. The process of identity formation, in its essence, is to forge the synthesis that eludes the Diffusions (Josselson 1980).

What is common to the still-diffuse and the now-committed Diffusions is the underlying personality fragmentation. Those who have made commitments are ones who allowed themselves to be "claimed." Evelyn, Darlene, and Gretchen, each in somewhat different ways, are using external egos to organize themselves. They each accept narrowing and limits as a way of controlling the impulsivity and confusion that is beneath the surface. They are women who have learned the dangers of trusting oneself or following an inner direction and have found themselves benign jailors.

Although the committed Diffusions profess to be satisfied with their lives and are, indeed, a great deal more optimistic and emotionally balanced than at the end of college, one wonders if they have paid too high a price. Evelyn and Gretchen are achieving in the work world and we can expect Darlene to achieve again. Both Gretchen and Darlene are experiencing their generativity, having settled—for better in Darlene's case, for worse in Gretchen's—the intimacy tasks. Yet one senses that there is more in these women that is being kept suppressed. One wonders how their children will experience them as mothers.

Several of this group of women have spoken of their interest in helping others to be whole. This is, perhaps, an externalized effort to repair their own sense of fragmentation. Except for Debbie, none of these women can think very clearly about how they wish to grow as a person, although many have plans for what they wish to do. Debbie thinks about who she is as a person, but not clearly. The solution to the Diffusion dilemma, then, seems to be not to solve it. Get something (a job or a religion) or someone (a husband) to tell you how to live your life and accept that authority. This settles things but does not seem to lead to ego development.

Erikson discusses the propensity for "totalistic" solutions to be found, especially among identity diffuse adolescents. He traces this to super-ego pathology—specifically, a superego that remains infantile and primitive in its "categoric" attitude. One aspect common to these women as they appeared in college was their general effort to disavow the superego, which reflected their incapacity to modify or integrate its functions. The committed Diffusions are women who have made peace with the superego by accepting its demands for total "goodness." As a result, they suffer neither ambivalence nor guilt. And it is perhaps the lack of moral ambiguity, of superego tension, that makes them seem so static.

The still-diffuse Diffusions are, in a sense, in search of the organizing principles that the others have found. They are people in search of an authority. Susan is trying to do what Gretchen has done (i.e., embrace religion). Debbie is trying to make experience itself an organizing principle. Why the still-diffuse Diffusions have not been able to find such authority thus far remains a puzzle. They are perhaps somewhat more fragmented than the others, have fewer foreclosing possibilities open to them. But this cannot be predicted from the earlier data.

It is tempting to suggest that the general upheaval in the roles of women contributed to the difficulty of these women in smoothly identifying with clear modes of being. Erikson views the lack of well-defined rituals and passages as a strain on a weak ego attempting to formulate an identity. These women grew into womanhood at the height of the turmoil in the Women's Movement, having graduated from college in 1972 and 1973. But, if they were affected by it, it was not consciously. Sex-role conflicts seem to be an individual rather than a socially determined area of concern for these women.

The social forces that most strongly color their lives are the ones that make anything possible. The lack of social taboos, the sense of "anything goes" are social phenomena that did seem to have increased the pressure, by expanding the choices, on the ego capacities of these women. Having largely escaped parental influence by the conclusion of college, they were not bound by pleasing parents or conforming to standards by which they were raised. Moves far from home are commonplace among this group, thereby making it possible for someone like Debbie to "recreate" herself far from a self that was known and recognized as a self with a history. Gretchen was able to experiment with a commuter marriage, with social approbation, but was unable to control herself in the absence of spousal restraint. Susan found social support for having a baby without a husband or income while Evelyn lives a highly independent, nonintimate life without criticism from others.

The social freedom of the past ten years has required inner structuralization from these women. A decrease in restriction and an increase in freedom are factors that necessitate the work of the ego's synthetic function. The "successful" Diffusions seem to be the ones who have found the social anchors to, in Erich Fromm's phrase, escape from these freedoms.

When I reported on the Diffusions as college seniors, I commented on their romanticized ego-ideal. Unable to temper their idealizations with reality, they seemed then to be in search of whatever salvation happened to appear. When this failed for them at the time, they simply sought salvation in something else. The follow-up data confirm the predilection to idealization and the quest for existence in an idealized state. It is striking, for example, that four of the seven had periods of involvement in Eastern mysticism, an embodiment of oceanic, ideal unity. Gretchen, in her religious commitment, and Darlene, in her family life, both present their lives as idealized, as having found the true, perfect path, as though they experience themselves as living out their ego-ideals. Debbie elevates all of her experience to a higher plane. Existential limitations are experienced by the Diffusions as unacceptable boundaries. They remain, as in college, mesmerized by possibility.

It is, of course, reckless to generalize from such a small sample, and more extensive research is clearly mandated. Some confirmatory evidence is available from a related longitudinal study of identity formation. Marcia (1976), in a six-year follow-up of men, found that six out of seven Identity Diffuse men in his sample remained diffuse in identity or were Foreclosed Diffusions six years later.

What is clear from these data is that identity diffusion in college is not a transitory state and should be taken seriously as a signal of an ego in distress. Several women in this group (Evelyn in college, Susan after the death of her child, Debbie when her marriage was breaking up, and another still-diffuse woman) have had brief brushes with psychotherapy. It appears that each time, the therapy was directed to the presenting symptom or crisis and did not attempt to address the underlying ego structure.

From my own clinical experience with women who would be rated as Identity Diffusions were they to be in such a study, the effort to address aspects of personality structure, especially failures of internalization, is a lengthy and difficult one. However, it appears, based on these long-term findings, that it is an effort that must be made where identity diffusion is present. Diffusions are people who will quickly and easily accept external ego support in a crisis, declare themselves cured, and move on, leaving everyone with the impression that the "therapy" was helpful. From this vantage point, however, such "help" only perpetuates the Diffusion yearning for external structure. It does not address the difficulties in internally structuring, which is the core of the Diffusion dilemma.

It is of interest that the majority of these women, when reflecting on their college experience, express the regret that they were not more focused on things or that they did not take their studies or occupational planning more seriously. All except Evelyn found the college years to be stimulating and expanding and stress the new possibilities that were opened to them. As we have seen, however, these Diffusion women, because of their personality structure, were not much able to make use of these possibilities or of the opportunity for psychosocial growth. Either they became overwhelmed by the options, lost in the sea of choice after having severed their moorings, or else they swam to a safe shore to avoid drowning.

We have no good theoretical yardsticks by which to measure these lives. All of these Diffusion women have found ways of functioning that reflect reasonable if not optimal mental health. Yet one wonders if, with good psychotherapeutic intervention, they could not have formed more flexible and more freely chosen identities.

For half of these women who were Diffusions in college, identity is no longer a central concern. Their lives are oriented to implementing the choices they have made. For the other half, ten to twelve years later, identity formation remains an as yet unsolved life task and they appear to be as far from settling these issues as they were in college.

Conclusions

To return to the questions raised at the beginning of this chapter, it appears that identity diffusion in college is neither a unitary syndrome nor predictive of early adult functioning in any linear way. Of the eight women in the study, two could be classified as borderline (Susan and the deceased woman), but they would have been classified as borderline even in college. The remaining six would not meet the criteria for the DSM-III borderline diagnosis, nor would they meet Kernberg's criteria. One who would have been diagnosed as borderline in her late adolescence (Evelyn) would not be diagnosed as such today.

Identity diffusion, then, cannot be considered a preborderline syndrome, although such people are at some risk. Fortunate life circumstances, external events that offer identity-forming possibilities have a significant ameliorative effect on identity diffusion. At this point, not enough is known about the internal factors that predispose some identity diffuse individuals to outcomes of reasonable mental health and further research is strongly warranted.

NOTES

1. There is very little longitudinal information of any sort on women who have been followed in depth.

2. See Bourne (1978a, 1978b) and Marcia (1980) for complete reviews of this literature.

3. Changes in surnames and frequent changes in address made it very difficult to locate subjects after such a long time.

4. Two are deceased, and they are the only ones of the original sample known to be deceased.

5. Identity categories are Occupation, Religion, Politics, and Sexual Standards/Values. See Marcia (1966) and Schenkel and Marcia (1972).

REFERENCES

Bourne, E. 1978a. The state of research on ego identity: a review and appraisal. Part I. *Journal of Youth and Adolescence* 7:223–252.

Bourne, E. 1978b. The state of research on ego identity: review and appraisal. Part II. *Journal of Youth and Adolescence* 7:371–392.

Erikson, E. H. 1968. *Identity: Youth and Crisis.* New York: Norton.

Hopkins, L. 1982. Assessment of identity status in college women using outer space and inner space interviews. *Sex Roles* 8:557–565.

Josselson, R. L. 1973. Psychodynamic aspects of identity formation in college women. *Journal of Youth and Adolescence* 2:3–52.

Josselson, R. 1980. Ego development in adolescence. In J. Adelson, ed. *Handbook of Adolescent Psychology.* New York: Wiley.

Kacerguis, M. A., and Adams, G. R. 1980. Erikson stage resolution: the relationship between identity and intimacy. *Journal of Youth and Adolescence* 9:117–126.

Kernberg, O. 1976. *Object-Relations Theory and Clinical Psychoanalysis.* New York: Jason Aronson.

Marcia, J. E. 1966. Development and validation of ego identity status. *Journal of Personality and Social Psychology* 3:551–558.

Marcia, J. E. 1976. Identity six years after: follow-up study. *Journal of Youth and Adolescence* 5:145–160.

Marcia, J. E. 1980. Identity in adolescence. In J. Adelson, ed. *Handbook of Adolescent Psychology.* New York: Wiley.

Orlofsky, J. L. 1977. Sex-role orientation, identity formation, and self-esteem in college men and women. *Sex Roles* 6:561–575.

Schenkel, S. 1975. Relationship among ego identity status, field-independence, and traditional femininity. *Journal of Youth and Adolescence* 4:73–82.

Schenkel, S., and Marcia, J. E. 1972. Attitudes toward premarital intercourse in determining ego identity status in college women. *Journal of Personality* 3:472–482.

17   THE ADOLESCENT IN THE
REMARRIAGE FAMILY

ALLAN Z. SCHWARTZBERG

The rate of divorce in the United States continues to increase. A record of 1.2 million divorces was set in 1981. According to Visher and Visher (1982), the annual divorce rate has increased every year during the past two decades for a total increase of approximately 300 percent. Four-fifths of all divorced couples will remarry within five years. Sixty percent of these couples have children. It is estimated that at present approximately one out of six children is a member of a stepfamily.

In view of the large numbers of children, stepmothers, and stepfathers involved, it is surprising that relatively little attention has been paid to the problems of stepfamilies by either mental health or public health professionals or the public. The most common pattern in stepfamilies is for the new stepfather to join a unit in which the children have been living with their natural mother.

Review of Literature

Research on stepfamily relationships is limited. Several prominent works in the field include Visher and Visher (1980), Messinger, Walker, and Freeman (1978), and Sager, Brown, Crohn, Engel, Rodstein, and Walker (1983). Walker, Rogers, and Messinger (1977), in a critique of the research literature, commented that very few of the many research studies are based on procedures that permit a clear assessment of their validity, reliability, and generalization. They concluded that the greatest need is for longitudinal studies that permit analysis of the remarriage family system over time.

It is the purpose of this chapter to review the adolescent developmental tasks in the remarriage family, to summarize clinical observations of adolescents in remarried families, and finally to address issues in the treatment of these adolescents and their families.

The Process of Transition: Separation, Divorce, Remarriage

It is useful to conceptualize the divorce process as a transitional phase during the cycle of first marriage formation, eventual breakdown and disorganization, the single-parent family, dating, and often remarriage. Individuals, couples, and families intersect at different developmental stages and different phases of the life cycle.

There are significant differences between the nuclear biological family and the reconstituted family. In the nuclear family, there is a gradual development of roles, shared histories, and developed family boundaries. The reconstituted family, by contrast, has no shared family histories, traditions, or models. As Visher and Visher (1980) have noted, "All individuals have experienced significant losses not only of parents, but frequently of grandparents, friends, community supports, and the loss of the dream of an ideal family." Stepchildren also have biological parents elsewhere and are members of two households. The legal relationship between stepparents and stepchildren is often ambiguous or nonexistent. While the breakdown of the first marriage involved a process of loosening the existing boundaries and roles, the building of a new household involves a gradual process of redefining and clarifying roles and boundaries. A major task of adolescents and stepfamilies is to learn to negotiate, to accept differences of styles, values, and preferences. This quality is crucial in achieving both the consolidation of the couple's relationship as well as a cohesive sense of family.

Adolescent Developmental Tasks and the Remarriage Family

Adolescent developmental tasks in the remarriage family involve (1) working through grief and loss; (2) progressive separation-individuation leading to the development of healthy identity formation; (3) the ability to develop self-control and integration of feelings and impulses including sexual and aggressive drives; (4) the development of peer and heterosexual relationships; and (5) integration into the remarriage family. In contrast to the adolescent in the biological family faced with a single termination process, the adolescent in the reconstituted family faces a double termination process—loss of the role and status as a child combined with the loss of the nuclear family while a new adolescent role in the family has begun as well as entry into the new remarriage family system. Additionally, the adolescent in the remarriage family experiences greater difficulty with separation, since the reconstituted family attempts to move toward consolidation and family cohesiveness at the very time that the adolescent is seeking to move away, a major challenge for the remarriage family. Sager et al. (1983) have noted that "The challenge for the remarriage family is to integrate the adolescent as an adolescent and not as a child or adult."

Barriers to the achievement of adolescent developmental tasks in remarriage families include (1) incomplete mourning and (2) persistence of defense mechanisms of denial, repression, projection, introjection, and acting out. Depression and acting-out behavior are commonly encountered. When conflict has been severe and persistent without resolution, the adolescent is often extruded. The extruded adolescent syndrome has been described by Sager et al. (1983).

Marital and Stepfamily Developmental Tasks

In remarriage, Sager et al. (1983) have commented that while the couple is evolving through their marital life-cycle, the family subsystem is evolving through its life cycle and individuals are progressing through their personal life cycles. Conceptually, members of the remarriage couple who were previously married have a new marital life-cycle track, while the original life cycle with the former spouse or spouses continues, especially around parenting tasks.

The most important task of the reconstituted family is to achieve integration, consolidation, and cohesiveness. Visher and Visher (1980), Lewis, Beavers, Gossett, and Phillips (1976), and Messinger et al. (1978) are all in agreement that a key to the achievement of family cohesiveness is the development of strong couple bonding. Developmental tasks include (1) working through of loss of nuclear families for remarried spouses as well as development of realistic expectations for the first-time spouse; (2) the development of new family traditions; (3) the cultivation of new stepparent-stepchild relationships while maintaining established parent-child relationships in both custodial and noncustodial situations. These tasks are very much aided by individual working through of the inevitable losses associated with separation, divorce, and remarriage.

Adolescent Reactions to Remarriage

Adolescent reactions to remarriage vary depending on the age, stage of emotional development, ego strength, sex, amount of stress previously experienced, relationship with biological parents, relationship with stepparents, and the current relationship between parent and stepparent. Additional variables are present depending on the loss of the biological parent by death or divorce, previous marriage of stepparent, presence and number of stepsiblings, and so forth. Major problems that children and adolescents need to deal with involve (1) working through of loss; (2) jealousy and competition; (3) loyalty conflicts; (4) guilt and anger; (5) discipline conflicts; and (6) conflicts surrounding household boundaries, roles, and expectations. These problems can be illustrated by a review of some of the effects of the remarriage process on adolescents seen in psychiatric practice.

Methodology

Twenty-six adolescents who were members of reconstituted families were seen in private psychiatric practice. For the purpose of discussion, the terms "reconstituted," "blended," and "remarried" are all used synonymously. All adolescents were living in suburban middle-class homes. Information was obtained from one or more consultation interviews or through ongoing psychotherapy. In all instances, at least one biological parent was seen either in consultation or in ongoing individual or couple therapy. Psychological test data were also available in a number of cases. Eight girls and eighteen boys were seen. The average age was 15 at the time of consultation, 7.2 at separation, and 11 at remarriage. Thus, while psychiatric consultation occurred in early adolescence, the loss was typically sustained during latency.

Results

Twenty of the adolescents (80 percent) were brought to consultation because of academic underachievement, which was most distressing

262

to the custodial parent. Nearly two-thirds exhibited moderate to severe depressive symptoms, characterized by sadness, mood swings, impaired concentration, isolation, withdrawal, and often insomnia. Depression frequently alternated with acting-out behavior. Prominent defenses included repression, denial, acting out, and projection. Passive-aggressive personality features were commonly reflected in lack of interest in and attention to homework assignments, frequent episodes of truancy and tardiness, indifference, emotional withdrawal, and oppositional behavior at home, exemplified by an "I don't care attitude." Eight adolescents had individual therapy prior to consultation. Nearly all had been poorly prepared for the remarriage. Alcoholism in either a biological parent or a stepparent was involved in six of the families. Four adolescents suffered loss of a parent by death. All children, without exception, experienced loyalty conflicts, anger, and grief. The best adaptations were made by six adolescents presenting basically with adjustment reactions; these teenagers had access to both biological parents on a regular basis, with reasonably good communication present between parents. In these adolescents, ego strength was good, with no major preexisting conflict.

In general, three groups of adolescents emerged from the study: (1) those with adjustment reactions with transient dysfunction; (2) those with moderate impairment; and (3) those with severe impairment. The latter group was primarily associated with hospitalization, borderline personality disorders, and conduct disorders. Primary diagnoses included Adjustment Reaction (6), Borderline Personality Disorders (5), Conduct Disorders (5), Dysthymic Disorders (10). Ten adolescents were hospitalized, seven for suicide attempts. Many adolescents presented with dual diagnoses.

Major themes in working with these adolescents involved working through of loss and dealing with conflicts involving jealousy, loyalty, guilt, anger, and discipline.

Loss

As has previously been recorded with initial reactions to separation (Schwartzberg 1980), the initial reactions to plans for remarriage were frequently disappointment, anger, and a high degree of stress. This was especially difficult in those single-parent families that had become closed systems with longstanding mother-child bonds developing prior to the advent of the prospective spouse. The greatest degree of problems were experienced by adolescent boys who had experienced loss of a parent prior to age six with no contact with the biological father. These adolescents maintained fantasies at the time of the father's remarriage.

Jealousy and Competition

Competition for affection and attention was present in all of the adolescents. Most commonly, there was competition between stepfather and stepson for the mother's attention. Numerous triangles were observed, such as between biological parent, natural child, and stepchild; triangles between custodial parent, noncustodial parent, and child; and often rivalry between biological child, stepchild, and children born into the reconstituted family. These triangles triggered much jealousy, competition, resentment, and repeated tests of loyalty and love. A key dynamic was the existence of an alliance between biological parent and child against the stepparent. This relationship, predating the remarriage, often served as a persistent stumbling block to the development of a strong couple relationship. The examination of these alliances was a repeated focus of therapy.

Loyalty Conflicts

All adolescents experienced significant loyalty conflicts. If they were on good terms with the noncustodial parent, they often felt very conflicted about establishing a positive relationship with the stepparent—viewing this as an act of disloyalty. Many conflicts surfaced, especially during holidays, involving the amount of time spent with the stepfamily versus the noncustodial parent. Working through of loyalty conflict was a major task of therapy.

Anger and Guilt

Anger was evidenced by defiance, oppositional behavior, and acting out. The latter behavior was exemplified by vandalism, shoplifting, drug abuse, and hostile behavior with peers, parents, and siblings. Guilt feelings were especially noteworthy in those adolescents who sustained loss of the biological parent before the age of six. Guilt was also a prominent motivating factor not only for many stepfathers who had left their families but also for the one-third of the mothers who had left their marriages. Guilt feelings often triggered overly generous settlements with former spouses and became the cause of resentment for some married couples. Guilt feelings were often severe in some stepfathers, making them reluctant to invest emotionally in the relationship with stepchildren because of guilt about depriving their biological children. Many adolescents were aware of their anger and manipulative behavior and felt guilty about it, but they also felt a sense of entitlement exemplified by one teenager who cried, "You owe me for all you've put me through."

Discipline

Many adolescents reported little discipline during the single-parent stage. Therefore, they were shocked and resentful when the stepparent and/or the biological parent attempted to impose discipline and structure. Resentful of the remarriage, these adolescents often displaced their anger from biological parents onto stepparents. Many adolescents expected that a peerlike relationship would continue with the biological parent. When these expectations did not develop, the adolescents were often furious and felt betrayed. There was constant testing by the adolescent to reestablish the relationship prior to the remarriage.

Treatment Issues

Treatment of the adolescent in the remarried family utilized a family-systems perspective combined with insights on adolescent development, life cycle development, and psychodynamics. The treatment approach chosen depended on the nature and severity of the conflict, the developmental stage of the adolescent, the motivation for treatment, the ego strength of individual family members, and the commitment of the family to the therapeutic process. A systems orientation allowed the therapist deeper understanding of the differing needs of family members at different stages of the life cycle. It is important for the therapist to feel comfortable relating both with different members of the family system and subsystem and with the use of different therapeutic modalities.

Therapeutic Modalities

Therapeutic modalities included individual, group, couples, family, and multifamily therapy. Each approach presented its own indications. Often several modalities were used in combination. Many questions arose concerning what therapeutic modalities to use, when, whom to include, and the duration of treatment and goals. Flexibility, sensitivity, and an ability to shift therapeutic activity level were essential.

Individual therapy aided in the development of a good working alliance and allowed the teenager to work further through the mourning process, to ventilate, and to gain ego support. Couples therapy was useful when the relationship was strained by adolescent acting-out behavior, and when couple communication was distorted. Couples therapy helped facilitate clear communication and assisted with mourning for the lost spouses, while educating the couple about realistic expectations for the remarriage family. Couples groups were especially useful in providing support, appropriate role modeling, and corrective emotional experiences. Close collaboration between therapists working with different family members was often helpful. When the same therapist was employed for both individual therapy of the adolescent and family therapy, special attention was paid to issues of confidentiality.

The timing and readiness for family therapy were gauged by the nature and circumstances of the presenting problem, the presence of beginning alliances with the adolescent and family members, and a willingness of the family to meet to explore the current dynamics and communication patterns. Involvement of both sets of parents, though stressful, was especially useful in helping to lessen loyalty conflicts and splitting. Multiple-family therapy groups with a cotherapist were very useful with heightened resistance, severe conflict, and for hospitalized adolescents. These groups provided a good deal of support and helped clarify and confront family dynamics and interactional patterns. They also facilitated awareness and practice of alternative ways of interacting and resolving conflicts. Utilization and awareness of crossed transferences were important here. The adolescent and stepparents were noted to be more willing to listen to different parents and teenagers than members of their own families. In addition to mutual support, these groups often provided clarification, ventilation, role modeling, and corrective emotional experiences.

Case Example: Moderate Impairment

Jane, a sixteen-year-old girl, lived with her mother for two years following separation and subsequently for two years with her father. The father, forty-four, a chronically depressed, obsessional man, indulged her, and there was often role reversal with inconsistent discipline. Jane assumed the role as temporary head of the household when father was hospitalized with a severe depression. When he subsequently responded dramatically to antidepressants, his fiancée of six months moved into the family home. Within one week of hospital discharge, the father opted suddenly for marriage but did not tell the daughter until after the ceremony. Jane reacted to this sudden decision with intense anger, defiance, and feelings of betrayal. She refused to talk with her father other than to request money and withdrew from family meals. Her grades significantly declined, and she withdrew from peers. Reluctantly, she agreed to see a therapist and subsequently to be involved in family therapy sessions. Individual therapy allowed her to ventilate her tremendous anger and disappointment as well as to begin to gain an ally. The father was angered by the daughter's behavior and began to relate to her in a sarcastic and hostile fashion, which dismayed his new wife, who, paradoxically, began to relate better to the daughter. The new marriage relationship was threatened.

Couple therapy was accepted with a collaborative therapist concurrently with family therapy. During family therapy sessions, Jane indicated repeatedly that she did not want to live at home and have to relate to her father. She resented the fact that before the marriage, "we were friends, now you're the boss." Couple therapy stressed the need to consolidate the relationship and to present a united front to Jane and her brother, twenty, a manipulative, willful young man. During the family therapy sessions, Jane continued to be angry and provocative. As the father reclaimed his role as head of the household, he allowed Jane a choice either to live by household rules or to live elsewhere by a set date. A dramatic change in behavior was noted in her twenty-year-old brother, who interrupted his defiant behavior when given an ultimatum. Father persuaded his new wife about the need to present a united front. At a family meeting, he reactivated long-dormant authority and stated that Jane was welcome to live in the house provided she adhered to house "ground rules." When she continued to balk, an agreement ensued for Jane to live in an apartment for her senior year of high school. Father, stepmother, and both therapists agreed that Jane appeared to be mature enough to cope with this new arrangement. With continuing therapy and tension abatement, Jane was secretly relieved that the couple's communication and relationship improved. Jane could realize that she was not being extruded but had chosen to leave and would accept responsibility for her choice. Thus, a planned extrusion with ongoing therapy was instrumental in reduction of family tension.

Discussion

Three clusters of adolescents emerged from this study: adolescents with (1) adjustment disorders, (2) moderate impairment, and (3) severe impairment. The best coping responses in this group of adolescents were from those who demonstrated prior good ego strength, had good relationships with the custodial parent and stepparent, and had regular access to the biological, noncustodial parent. These adolescents were diagnosed as having adjustment disorders with transient dysfunction. This finding is reminiscent of similar research by Wallerstein and Kelly (1980) and Schwartzberg (1980), who observed that adolescents who did best had regular access to both parents and maintained a strategic distance from both parents to lessen loyalty conflicts.

The large number (46 percent) of hospitalized adolescents may represent a skewed sample, since, for an eight-month period, I was an attending psychiatrist on an adolescent inpatient service. Approximately two-thirds of these adolescents came from separated, divorced, or remarried families. Many of these hospitalized adolescents presented with borderline personality disorders, conduct disorders, and severe depression.

Conclusions

The incidence and prevalence of adolescents in the reconstituted family have been reviewed as well as some of the highlights of the research literature. Development tasks of both adolescents and stepfamilies were reviewed. Role expectations among stepfamilies were highlighted along with some of the differences between nuclear and stepfamilies.

ALLAN Z. SCHWARTZBERG

A clinical series of twenty-six adolescents in reconstituted families was reviewed. Eighty percent presented with significant academic underachievement. Three groups emerged from the research: (1) adolescents with adjustment disorders; (2) moderately impaired adolescents; and (3) severely impaired adolescents. The latter group was associated primarily with conduct disorders and borderline personality organization. The three most common symptoms were depression, academic underachievement, and varying degrees of belligerent behavior. Passive-aggressive personality features were very common. Ten of the adolescents (46 percent) were hospitalized. Two-thirds of the adolescents exhibited moderate to severe depression. Basic therapeutic issues related to loss, jealousy, competition, loyalty conflicts, guilt, anger, and discipline. The best coping responses in this group were shown by adolescents who demonstrated prior good ego strength, had good relationships with the custodial parent and stepparent, and had regular access to the biological, noncustodial parent. This group presented with adjustment reactions. Therapeutic strategies for dealing with these adolescents were discussed, with special emphasis on flexibility and a multifamily-systems approach. A variety of therapeutic modalities were utilized including individual, group, family, couple, and multifamily therapy.

Research on stepchildren in reconstituted families is still in its infancy. Well-controlled, longitudinal studies of stepchildren in the reconstituted families are needed if mental health professionals are to be of maximum assistance not only in the prevention of emotional disorders but also in their effective treatment.

REFERENCES

Lewis, J. M.; Beavers, W. R.; Gossett, J. T.; and Phillips, V. A. 1976. *No Single Thread: Psychological Health and Family Systems.* New York: Brunner/Mazel.
Messinger, L.; Walker, K. N.; and Freeman, S. J. 1978. Preparation for remarriage following divorce: the use of group techniques. *American Journal of Ortho-Psychiatry* 48(2): 263–272.
Sager, C. J.; Brown, H. S.; Crohn, J.; Engel, T.; Rodstein, E.; and Walker, L. 1983. *Treating the Remarried Family.* New York: Brunner/Mazel.

Schwartzberg, A. Z. 1980. Adolescent reactions to divorce. *Adolescent Psychiatry* 8:379–392.

Visher, E. B., and Visher, J. S. 1980. *Step Families*. Secaucus, N.J.: Citadel Press.

Visher, E. B., and Visher, J. S. 1982. Conference on Family Systems Theory and Therapy. The Psychiatric Institute of Washington, D.C., June 4.

Walker, K. N.; Rogers, J.; and Messinger, L. 1977. Remarriage after divorce: a review. *Social Case Work* 58:276–285.

Wallerstein, J., and Kelly, J. 1980. *Surviving the Breakup: How Children and Parents Cope with Divorce*. New York: Basic.

18 JOHN WESLEY HARDIN, ADOLESCENT KILLER: THE EMERGENCE OF A NARCISSISTIC BEHAVIOR DISORDER

RICHARD C. MAROHN

The myth of the Western hero and villain—the cowboy, rancher, miner, prospector, gunfighter, outlaw, lawman, and vigilante—has permeated twentieth-century American culture. He (usually he) appears in our folklore, literature, radio, movies, and television. More than any other aspect of United States history, this epoch has captured the imagination of America, youths and adults as well. The paradigm of this now-classic struggle between the Western hero and outlaw, between oversimplified good and bad, is the pursuit of Billy the Kid by Garrett (1882). At one time Billy and the author were buddies, but as the Kid involved himself in the contagion of a feud and could not contain himself, he was pursued and eventually shot by Garrett, the man who brought law and order to New Mexico Territory. Strangely, the Kid became in many ways a greater folk hero than Garrett. Part of his appeal is the adolescent quality of his devotion to one of the principals in the feud, his boyish appearance, and the fact that he, like a "true" adolescent, refused to bend to the constraints of authority. The story of the Kid and Garrett is a favorite theme of Western history, fiction, and movies (Adams 1960).

The symbolism is of one man, good or bad, making a difference. Rarely is his activity sexual but more often self-assertive in nature. He is appealing because in him is reflected our own disowned or consciously-held grandiosity for omnipotent control, symbolized in his use of the Colt or Winchester. He often typifies high ideals and values of loyalty, integrity, honesty, commitment, and self-sufficiency, which are portrayed in sharp definition in the simple Western movies of the 1930s, 1940s, and 1950s. More recently, movies have begun to appreciate both the Western hero and villain as more complex and human.

The details of the life of Billy the Kid have been fairly well reconstructed (Cline 1984), but what we know of his adolescence and his personality is derived from others' descriptions and reactions. He wrote nothing and said nothing that remains with us; we know nothing of his ideas and feelings, perhaps because he died around the age of twenty-one and really never reflected on his life and experiences. Consequently, the early life of the classic adolescent Western gunfighter and killer eludes us.

However, largely because he survived into adulthood, John Wesley Hardin's life and personality can be studied in detail. His violence first shows in adolescence, and he left us with a legacy of his written ideas, beliefs, explanations, and feelings. He was notorious, having killed forty-two people in eight years. He appears in American folklore, the subject of many Texas tales and myths—such as "John Wesley Hardin Shot a Man, Just for Snorin' " (Trachtman 1974) and an album and song *John Wesley Harding* by Bob Dylan (Columbia Records, 1968) in which he erroneously portrays Hardin as a kind of Robin Hood. He appears frequently in print in virtually every history of the West, in some Western novels, and in his own autobiography (Hardin 1896). He appears in a Hollywood production, *The Shootist* (Sonnichsen 1979). Often, however, he is presented as a stereotype, for example, "despite his efforts to reform, gambling, drink, and women got the best of him."

Wasn't he, after all, fairly complex? Perhaps, we can discover the answer in Hardin's written legacy—notes and verses in his photo album, about 120 letters from prison, letters to newspapers, and his autobiography. Because he spent sixteen adult years in the penitentiary, he lived long enough to reflect and write about himself.

I recognize the limitations of psychobiography. We cannot interview Hardin nor can we analyze together his transference reactions in a controlled treatment situation. Nonetheless, we can infer from his writings parallels to what we already know about other people, their adolescent development, propensities for violence, transformations of narcissism, and the emergence of the adult personality structure.

272

Sketch of Hardin's Life

John Wesley Hardin[1] was born May 26, 1853 in Bonham, Texas, the son of a Methodist circuit preacher who became a lawyer when Hardin was eight. His parents hoped that he would become a preacher and teacher like his father. He showed early promise, being a good student, but he also displayed a flair for adventure—and violence. At age eleven, he wounded another boy in the chest and back during a knife fight. At fifteen, he shot and killed a former slave and then ambushed and killed three soldiers who were trying to arrest him. At eighteen, in Abilene, Kansas, while on a cattle drive, he had an armed standoff with the legendary Wild Bill Hickok, whom he idolized. Later, he allegedly shot and killed a man for snoring and disturbing his sleep. More than likely, Hardin's explanation for the episode is more accurate—he was awakened from sleep in a rooming house by a man who was going through his pants' pockets and shot him. Obviously, legends were already beginning to develop about Wes Hardin. For example, in September 1874, a Texas Ranger (Parsons 1985) sent to track Hardin wrote: ". . . I had heard of him before I ever came to Texas. He kills men just to see them kick . . . he can take two six-shooters and turn them like wheels in his hands and fire a shot from each at every revolution . . . he is said to have killed thirty men and is a dead shot. . . ."

Hardin married Jane Bowen in 1872, when he was eighteen and she sixteen. They had three children, Mollie (born in 1873), John Wesley, Jr. (born in 1875), and Jane or Jennie (born in 1877). He liked to gamble, drink, and race horses. He continued his violent ways, such that he is said to have killed about forty-two men. In 1874, he killed a deputy sheriff, probably in self-defense, was indicted for murder, and fled to Florida but was captured by the Texas Rangers in 1877. He was returned to Texas, tried and convicted of second-degree murder, sentenced to twenty-five years imprisonment, and began serving his sentence on October 5, 1878.

Almost immediately, Hardin plotted to escape and made one or two attempts, which were foiled. During his imprisonment, Hardin wrote many letters to his wife, Jane, and other relatives and friends, which provide a fascinating look into his personality. His wife died on November 6, 1892, before he was released on February 7, 1894, after serving almost sixteen years. While in the penitentiary, he studied literature, religion, and the law, and, later, because of his own efforts to have his civil rights restored, he was pardoned and passed the Texas State Bar on July 21, 1894.

He resumed gambling, tried his hand at politics, and attempted to establish a law practice. On January 8, 1895, he married fourteen-year-old Callie Lewis. One story is that Hardin had won her from her father in a poker game; however, she left Hardin after a week or two of marriage.

Lawyer Hardin then traveled to El Paso to assist his cousin in the prosecution of a case. On April 7, 1895, the *El Paso Times* reported an item, which had probably been paid for and inserted by Hardin himself:

Among the many leading citizens of Pecos City who are now in El Paso, is John Wesley Harden, Esq., a leading member of the Pecos City bar. In his younger days Mr. Harden was as wild as the broad western plains upon which he was raised. But he was a generous, brave-hearted youth and got into no small amount of trouble for the sake of his friends, and soon gained a reputation for being tempered and a dead shot. In those days when one man insulted another, one of the two died then and there. Young Harden, having a reputation for being a man who never took water, was picked out by every bad man who wanted to make a reputation, and there is where the "bad men" made a mistake, for the young westerner still survives many warm and tragic encounters. Forty-one years has steadied the impetuous cowboy down to a quiet, dignified, reasonable man of business. Mr. Harden is a modest gentleman of pleasant address. But underneath the modest dignity is a firmness that never yields except to reason and the law. He is a man who makes friends of all who come in close contact with him. He is here as associate attorney for the prosecution in the case of the state vs. Bud Frazier, charged with assault with intent to kill. Mr. Harden is known all over Texas. He was born and raised in this state.

Hardin's El Paso law practice did not thrive. He resumed drinking and gambling and reacted violently when he felt cheated in a crap game at the Gem Saloon on May 1, 1895. After being called a "jail rat" by the dealer, Hardin drew his Colt revolver "from under his vest" and "presented it in my face. He kept his pistol pointed at me until he walked around the table and I had counted out $95, which he took and put up his pistol and walked out" (Marohn 1979).

At first, after the robbery, the newspapers were afraid to mention Hardin by name, calling him "a visitor to the city" and "the stranger" for fear that he was on the verge of a rampage. Then, the papers criticized city officials for not arresting Hardin: El Paso "has lost her nerve." On May 4, 1895, Hardin wrote to the *El Paso Times* and the *El Paso Tribune* and described his holdup of the Gem:

To the people of El Paso and to everyone to whom it may concern: I have noticed several articles in the *Times* and *Tribune* reflecting on my character as a man. I wish to announce right now that in the past my own ambition has been to be a man and you bet I draw my own idea, and while I have not always come up to my standard, yet I have no kick to make against myself for default. My present and my future ambition is no higher than it has been in the past, and I wish to say right now that whether in a gambling house or a saloon, and El Paso seems to be crowded with these places, my only aim is to acquit myself manly and bravely. . . . As to the Gem holdup on craps, after I had lost a considerable sum, I was grossly insulted by the dealer in a hurrah manner, hence, I told him he could not win my money and hurrah me too, and that as he had undertook to hurrah me he could deliver me the money I had played, and you bet he did it. And when he had counted out the $95 I said that is all I want, just my money and no more. He said all right Mr. Hardin, and when I left the room and had gotten half way down the stairs, I returned, hearing words of condemnation to my play. I said to everyone in the house and connected with the play, I understand from the reflective remarks that some of you disapprove my play. Now if this be so, be men and get in line and show your manhood, to which no one made any reply, but others nodded that I was right and that they approved my play. Now someone has asked for my pedigree. Well, he is too gross to notice, but I wish to say right here once and for all, that I admire pluck, push and virtue wherever found. Yet I contempt and despise a coward and assassin of character, whether he be a reporter, a journalist or a gambler. And while I came to El Paso to prosecute Bud Frazier and did do it on as high a plane as

275

possible, I am here now to stay. I have bought an interest in the Wigwam Saloon, and you, who, whether in El Paso or elsewhere, that admire pluck, that desire fair play, are cordially invited to call at the Wigwam where you will have everything done to make it pleasant for you. All are especially invited to our blowout on the evening of the 4th. Now I have no apology to make to any one for my acts over a jackpot or a crap game, but solicit everybody's custom and guarantee fair play.

Hardin was finally arrested for carrying a pistol and for gambling. He was fined, relieved of his revolver, and his legal appeals failed. During this period, Hardin did not neglect gunplay. He shot holes through playing cards to amuse others and to show his skill with a six-shooter. In an interview published in the *El Paso Herald* on August 23, 1895, Hardin's landlady said:

Yes, Mr. Hardin was certainly a quick man with his guns. I have seen him unload his guns, put them in his pockets, walk across the room and then suddenly spring to one side facing around and quick as a flash he would have a gun in each hand clicking so fast the clicks sounded like a rattle machine. He would place his guns inside his breeches in front with the muzzles out. Then he would jerk them out by the muzzle and with a toss as quick as lightning grasp them by the handle and have them clicking in unison. He showed me how he once killed two men in that way. They demanded his guns and he extended them, one in each hand, he holding the muzzle as if to surrender, and when the men reached for the guns he tossed the pistols over, catching the handles, and killed both men while their hands were yet extended for the weapons. Oh, he was a wonderful man. He practiced with his guns daily, and I liked to see him handle them when they were empty.

One of the people Hardin encountered during his practice was Martin Mrose, a cattle rustler from Texas and New Mexico, who was hiding in Juarez, Mexico, to escape prosecution. When his wife, Beulah, a onetime prostitute, approached Hardin in El Paso for his legal services to defend her husband, they became lovers and participated with three El Paso lawmen in the ambush of her husband. Hardin and Beulah had a stormy relationship. On one occasion, she had him arrested for assaulting her while he had been drinking. They then lived separately but continued to be intimate. Once, when Hardin was out of town, Beulah was arrested for being drunk and disorderly. When Hardin returned, he threatened the arresting officer, whose father, also an El Paso law-man, shot Hardin in the back of the head on August 19, 1895, while he was throwing dice at the bar of the Acme Saloon.

Hardin's funeral was a festive occasion as crowds tried to get a look at him. The *El Paso Herald* of August 21, 1895, reported: "The body was photographed . . . in the morning, and in the afternoon photos found a big sale on the street. . . . The saloon where the killing occurred was an object of curiosity all day, as hundreds of people wanted to see where Hardin was shot, and look at the bullet marks on the floor. . . ." Hardin's death was noted by newspapers throughout the United States.

About 2,500 copies of *The Life of John Wesley Hardin: From the Original Manuscript, As Written by Himself* were published by Smith and Moore, in 1896. The book was later republished in 1926 and then in 1961 by the University of Oklahoma Press. Adams (1969), a noted authority on western history and literature, describes the book as "carefully written," and Nordyke (1957), a later biographer of Hardin, says that all the facts Hardin states can be verified. Hardin probably began writing the book late in 1894, during his stay in prison. He had written to Jane that he would some day write such a book and asked her to save his letters, which she did, and Hardin had these with him in El Paso when he was killed. In 1877, Hardin's mother, Elizabeth, wrote to him on two occasions about the "true" story of the Webb killing that his father had planned to write; but the Reverend Hardin had died a few months before his son's arrest in Florida, apparently grieved by his son's fugitive status and the hanging of another son, Joe, in retaliation for Wes's violence:

> . . . I have a true statement of the killing of Webb written by your
> Pa. How we all were treated and how your poor Pa was destroyed.
> He intended to have it published but died before he accomplished
> it. He said if he did not live to carry it out he hoped his friend
> would consult your lawyers and if they think it would do you any
> good will sent it to you or them. . . .

Hardin's plan to write his autobiography may represent an identifi-cation with his dead father as well as an effort to vindicate his actions.

Early in 1895 and before his marriage to Callie Lewis, Hardin contacted a publisher about the costs of publishing a book. Later, Hardin borrowed $1,575 from Beulah Mrose, using the manuscript as collateral. She had helped Hardin write some of the book, and they apparently planned to leave El Paso and move to Austin, where he was making arrangements for its publication when he was killed. On August 26, 1895, the *El Paso Daily Herald* reported: ". . . she had all the data with her with which to complete the unwritten parts. . . . She says she was very much attached to Hardin, and did not fear him except when he was drinking and jealous, and that when he was sober he treated her better than she was ever treated before in her life. . . ." She said that Hardin had requested not to be buried in the ground but "in the ocean and she would have taken his body and deposited it there, if she had been here." From the day of Hardin's burial on August 21, 1895, until September 29, 1965, Hardin's grave was left unmarked (Sonnichsen 1979) because cemetery officials feared it would attract tourists, vandals, and sensation-seekers.

Narcissism and Narcissistic Behavior Disorders

John Wesley Hardin exhibited significant problems in the narcissistic realm of his personality and typifies a narcissistic behavior disorder.[2] Significant transformations of primitive narcissistic structures took place during his imprisonment, and after release he experienced a significant regression to the point that, in part, he provoked his own killing. On a few occasions during his life he seems to have fragmented, and one can trace the emergence of the narcissistic personality structure during his adolescence.

The person experiencing a narcissistic personality disorder is beset with problems in self-esteem regulation. He has not been able developmentally to attenuate primitive narcissistic structures, grandiosity, and the need to idealize in the direction of ambitions and respect/admiration for others and ideals/values. He has difficulties with empathy, creativity, accepting his transience, and has no humor about himself or his limitations. He readily rages about his or others' mistakes and failures. His feelings are easily hurt; he needs to be perfect but usually feels imperfect and damaged. He desperately needs the involvement of another (a selfobject) to complete himself or to soothe, comfort, and regulate himself. He may feel listless, unmotivated, bored, unenthusiastic, tired, and with little energy for work or relationships. He has never reached his potential. Nonetheless, he seems to function well, has friends, works hard, and appears happy. At times, he may become overstimulated and energized by a success or a personal encounter, feeling elated and euphoric. He may welcome challenges because to master them revitalizes and excites him.

The narcissistic personality disorder seeks to maintain equilibrium by attachment to other people, selfobjects, who provide certain psychological functions that he cannot provide for himself. Every successful adolescent and adult selfobject experience resonates with the most primitive selfobject/parenting experiences of childhood, adequate or inadequate, and thus by transference we relive our earlier lives. While the narcissistic personality disorder requires, from time to time, contact with a selfobject, when self-cohesion or self-esteem is threatened, the narcissistic behavior disorder substitutes some kind of behavior for contact with a selfobject. One boy, when insulted by his girlfriend, may seek the solace and comfort of a friend, or talk to Mom or Dad, or find another girl. He may have a narcissistic personality disorder, if this is a recurrent and disabling pattern, or he may be "normal." Another boy may go out and steal a car to restore his self-esteem, get drunk to regulate his feelings, or get into a fight to prove his prowess, because he cannot readily call on other selfobject representations to restore himself.

The "psychopath" or "sociopath," of earlier diagnostic manuals and psychiatric lore, is insensitive to the needs of others and seems to be without a conscience. Others, like Cleckley (1964), have shown that this person may be very disturbed, even psychotic, in the face of limits, failure, and confrontation. These labels do not describe adequately the real nature of psychic life. For example, the psychopath does have contact with other people and may even in a very astute way be aware of what another person needs or wants; in fact, it is often on that basis that he manipulates the other person. The psychopath usually gives evidence of a primitive narcissistic fixation at a developmental level where the other person exists simply to serve his own needs; the other is like a piece of furniture or a toy, to be moved about and used as he sees fit. This is not an issue of morality or conscience but of meeting this patient at the level at which he is functioning. In order to treat him, we must meet him—or her—at that primitive level, create a controlling structured environment where the usual character or personality defenses are not allowed to operate smoothly, and try to provide a human environment that will serve as selfobjects to give the psychopath the psychological functions he lacks and cannot provide for himself. This is not done easily, or cheaply, or in a short time. We have known since the days of Aichhorn (1925) and Friedlander (1960) that we need to provide limits; and now we know (Marohn, Dalle-Molle, McCarter, and Linn 1980) how important it is for residential or hospital milieu staff to provide important psychological functions, especially tension regulation, help with identifying affect, channeling and controlling affect and behavior, organizing and planning, verbalizing, and the like.

The borderline personality tries to use other people to complete the self and provide the psychological functions he lacks. Because he is fragmented and lacks a cohesive self, he cannot in a stable and consistent manner make use of another to secure his own stability. The schizoid and paranoid personalities are really variations of the borderline. The schizoid fears the inevitable pain and fragmentation of involvement with another and stays away, while the paranoid sees involvement as dangerous and damaging and projects onto the outside world his own inner fears of disintegration and destruction.

In the course of growing up, the child turns to the parents, the original and primary selfobjects, for a variety of narcissistic affirmations. In the face of inevitable parental failure—part of normal, expectable development—the child develops compensatory or defensive structures to deal with narcissistic injuries. Defensive structures are psychological operations designed to keep from one's awareness and experience the painful narcissistic injuries. Compensatory structures are psychological operations designed to heal the narcissistic wounds. For example, a mother who becomes severely depressed after a miscarriage may also become emotionally unavailable to respond to her eight-year-old daughter. The daughter might defend herself against the pain of rejection by a retreat into fantasy where she is a princess, or she might compensate for the pain by focusing on her father's work as a teacher and pursue her studies vigorously.

The personality and the character structure are heirs to the closure of adolescence (Marohn 1981). The adolescent has been beset by increased tensions and has responded to these pressures by experimenting with and developing various and new ways of coping. The adolescent attempts to integrate genitality into the personality and to achieve psychological separation from the parents of childhood. He

RICHARD C. MAROHN

shifts to peer relationships to replace the selfobject functions of parents, and various narcissistic and libidinal claims and wishes are frustrated. If these frustrations are tolerable and can be mastered, they are reintegrated into the personality as functions that the adolescent now performs for himself. Those functions that peers—same sex and opposite sex—provide for the adolescent are eventually replaced by small accretions of psychic structure. Hopefully, the adolescent now learns how to modulate and channel urges, to calm and soothe the self, to regulate self-esteem, to judge performance realistically, to plan ways of fulfilling ambitions, and to revere and respect important people without being swept away by crushes. The multiple infatuations of the fickle adolescent eventually give way to a capacity for intimacy. This can derive only from a relatively intact and cohesive personality that has suffered the threats of adolescent fragmentation, integrated genital urges as parts of the self rather than as foreign temptations, begun to be regulated by his own ideals and values rather than those of parents or society, and experienced himself as someone with a continuous past and prospective future. The interpersonal experiences of adolescence provide rich opportunities for the maturation and growth of psychological skills, but the kinds of experiences that many adolescents have reflect, rather than cause, the internal shifts and growths that are occurring. For example, it is not bad kids that cause Johnny to become a delinquent (unless Johnny is a borderline who clings to whomever he can attach himself), but Johnny's attraction for delinquent kids reflects something about his own inner psychological world and he is displaying it, actualizing it, and practicing it by his involvement in a gang.

It is in the course of adolescence that the earlier preoedipal, oedipal, and latency solutions to inner psychic conflict and narcissistic injury are reworked, and by the close of adolescence we begin to see the character, the personality, the way the person will more or less look for the rest of life.

It is from this matrix that personality disorders emerge. Because the personality is not completely established until the close of adolescence, it is contradictory to speak of adolescent personality disorders. The very presence of a personality disorder in an adolescent suggests a premature closure of adolescence or a failure to experience adolescent experimentation and maturation. Yet we can speak of some fairly well established behavioral patterns among adolescents that could be called personality disorders. Delinquent adolescents typically show such pat-

281

terning. Offer, Marohn, and Ostrov (1979) found four parameters of nonpsychotic adolescent delinquent behavior—impulsive, narcissistic, depressed borderline, and empty borderline—demonstrating the possibility of understanding rather than simply describing deviant adolescent behavior and showing that pervasive behavior patterns and psychodynamic formulations can be inferred, from which generalizations about assessment and treatment can be made.

Hardin's Psychology and Psychopathology

John Wesley Hardin gives evidence of significant narcissistic problems, a narcissistic behavior disorder, but, at least in terms of his self-cohesion, no evidence of borderline, paranoid, schizoid, or psychotic psychopathology. He had some difficulty regulating self-esteem, attenuating primitive grandiosity to more reality-based ambition, and modifying primitive idealizations to a set of personal values and ideals. There are many instances of Hardin struggling to accomplish these transformations. At times it was difficult for him to empathize with others, such as when he wondered why some citizens might fear him and, as a result, want him out of the way. Another example was his defensive anger and inability to understand his wife's accusation that he had deserted her and the children when he had not written for several years. He reconciled with her out of his desperate need for her comforting rather than concern for her feelings. He showed a fearless bravado in his exploits, as if he anticipated immortality, but later shifted, in part, to leaving his legacy through telling his story. He gives little evidence of a sense of humor, except at the expense of others. His efforts at creativity—in writing verse or his autobiography—came later. Occasionally, he seemed to experience out-of-control narcissistic rages, but more often than not his rage was controlled and resulted in deliberate action and long-standing grudges. For example, his feelings might be hurt if he were losing at craps and the dealer "hurrahed" him by calling him a "jail rat" or someone questioned his "manhood," but he also bore a persistent determination to avenge his brother's hanging and to vindicate his own acts.

He needs to be perfect and, in his letters, preaches to his wife about child rearing and to his children about virtue, school studies, and their writing skills. Often he would feel damaged and imperfect. For example, on January 22, 1888, Hardin wrote to his wife:

Teach them [the children] to be temperate in their habits and to control their passion, their desires and their appetites, the last is necessary and essential to a happy prosperous life. I know their tempers are high but teach them that their happiness in this life will greatly depend upon how they control their passions, drives and etc. George Washington has a high temper but his strength, his excellence was the more conspicuous because he controlled it. . . . Now Sweet Jane it becomes at last my duty to speak plainly to you. My knowledge of wayward, forward men and women is that they lead wicked miserable lives and die wretched deaths. The gambler . . . the prostitute . . . the thief . . . the robber . . . the murderer . . . yes each of his or her kind beget children who make men and women of corresponding habits of vice and crime . . . by your love, your courage, patience and by your perservering industry and your wisdom you may and can reverse this general rule and snatch our loved ones from those who have broken many mothers hearts by leading their daughters and sons astray and who gladly look forward to the day when they can lead your children into the paths of [oblivion]. . . .

Hardin is clearly asking Jane to protect their children from his example and his personality.

He showed a persistent and imperative need for selfobjects—for their mirroring functions, especially the women in his life, his mother, Jane, Callie Lewis, and Beulah Mrose; for functioning as twinships and idealized others, such as his father, Wild Bill Hickok, and his cousin, Mannen Clements; and for the mirroring and feeding of his own grandiosity and exhibitionism provided by his "fans" and by his family and friends who wrote him and wished him well or who asked for his picture. In 1877, his mother wrote him: ". . . my darling sweet boy . . . John I am proud to tell strangers that I am the Mother of John Wesley Hardin though you are published as the notorious J. W. Hardin, a thief and a murderer and all this yet I know that you are an honest man and those that know you best say that you are honest, honorable and high minded. . . ."

He was a charismatic character whose skill, "pluck," and daring attracted many and still do. His difficulties in soothing himself and regulating strong affect caused him to turn to others for help, as one would expect of a narcissistic personality disorder. His affective needs, on other occasions, would often be managed by his behavior. He would drink to comfort himself or gamble in an effort to try to master either the external world his grandiosity demanded he control or his inner world of unexpected overstimulation. Gambling was an effort to try repeatedly to master the unpredictable.

He may have had several fragmentation experiences. In fall 1869, at age sixteen, Hardin shot and killed Jim Bradly, who allegedly fired at him first. After Hardin had hit him from a distance of five or six feet in the heart and head, "I could not stop. I was shooting because I did not want to take chances on a reaction." Although Hardin justifies his repeated firing, there is a suggestion here that he had lost control; yet he successfully eluded a mob and then escaped from a posse that had captured him. He seems to have reintegrated quickly. Excitement and activity, especially frantic activity, often help the narcissistic behaviorally disordered person reintegrate or prevent fragmentation.

In 1877, in the Austin jail, when his mother and his wife had a falling out, he writes desperate, disorganized, frantic, and frequent letters to them both to try to effect a reconciliation:

> Answer at once. I think it is a dam shame on all excuse, I am mad for the first time in one year. . . . Jane Dear, have you got me foul . . . never was I troubled before. I am bound to distraction at your hands. . . . Dear Ma, you and Jane's troubles are foolishness. . . . Consider my interest, looks like someone allways unintentionally is doing me harm.

Later, in the Huntsville Penitentiary, when his efforts to escape fail, a movement toward fragmentation may have been heralded by many and persistent somatic complaints, although these may have been the result of prison beatings. On August 26, 1885, he wrote to Superintendent McCulloch that he might have "cancer of the stomache Brights Desease Heart Desease or what else but whatever it is it give me much pain both mentaly and physicaly beyond Description at this present time . . . that my heart longuis liver and kidneys are affected I have little doubt." He lost over twenty pounds during this period. He appears also to have experienced recurrent depressions, which suggests enough internal structure to forestall a severely fragmented regression. In 1881, he again wrote to Jane, after a gap of about two years, giving credit to Superintendent McCulloch for his renewed correspondence. He says that he wanted her to be free to seek her happiness with someone else, that he would never be ". . . allowed my liberty . . . for at that time my heart was filled with such desperate ideas that I knew not what moment my end would be in this world by some rash act of mine and how it ever turned out as it has I cannot account only by God's mercies for only death I did not bear it nor did I have any dread for the grave . . . despaired, I . . . refused to write to anyone for a long time . . . I failed to write you in my degraded state."

His personality seems to have been organized (1) around the pole of the grandiose self—with his exhibitionism, bravado, "pluck," daring, propensity to get revenge, motivation to remove all obstacles in his path, and impulse to destroy (not in uncontrolled, psychoticlike rage but with deliberate and purposeful narcissistic rage) using his talents and skills, his intellect, his ability to express himself in writing, his cunning and cleverness, his dexterity with a revolver, and his good looks; and (2) around the pole of idealized figures and values—with his reverence for his father as preacher, teacher, and lawyer, for Hickok as gunfighter, and for certain religious and moral values including a strong allegiance to family and friends that he frequently espoused. The need for selfobject contact persisted throughout his life, as his writings attest. He always needed to be reassured that others were on his side. His wife Jane was paramount, and their correspondence may have sustained him during prison, along with the selfobject/ representation of his God. Later, after Jane's death, he tried unsuccessfully to connect with other women—Callie Lewis, in an impulsive effort to recapture his adolescence, and Beulah Mrose, whose attention may have sustained him to some extent in the writing of his autobiography but whose own behavioral difficulties complicated Hardin's life in El Paso. In his later years, there was a transformation from idealized men to an emphasis on values, but the need for female contact persists. Nonetheless, these efforts at selfobject contact continued to fail him, and his behavior demonstrates efforts at reestablishing psychological equilibrium by drinking, gambling, and gunplay.

Significant Transformations in Prison

In the office or hospital treatment of narcissistically disordered patients, the treatment involves the creation of an empathic selfobject milieu, wherein missing psychological functions are provided by the other (or others), and with the emergence of mirroring, twinship, or idealizing transferences, dosed and tolerable frustrations are mastered by the patient and replaced by the accretion of internal psychological structures, whereby the patient now performs these heretofore missing functions for himself. In psychotherapy and psychoanalysis, the appropriate frustration is usually accomplished by interpreting rather than gratifying the transference wishes. In the hospital, ward staff provide important selfobject functions and, in so doing, provide enough psychological structure to facilitate the experiencing of transferences in the psychotherapy relationship. Of course, such "transmuting internalizations" could perhaps also be accomplished in a setting other than the treatment milieu; often, healthy relationships may provide such psychological growth, as does proper parenting. Despite its often dehumanizing conditions, the prison can, and for many frequently does, provide important psychological functions and meaningful relationships (Marohn 1967); change during imprisonment results from such dynamics, not from simple fear of punishment or fleeting identifications with the aggressor-jailer.

For Hardin, the prison may have provided important regulating and controlling functions, which he alludes to when he preaches to his wife about helping their children with their own passions and drives and when he begins describing in his letters changes in his attitudes toward his jailers. We know, for example, that he probably had intense personal relationships with the penitentiary staff; for example, early on, one prison guard helped Hardin out with contraband money and letters; and later, Hardin's relationship with the Huntsville Superintendent, Captain B. E. McCulloch, had its therapeutic aspects. Hardin writes to Jane in 1881 about resuming letter writing:

> . . . it was only by the persuasion of my respective and worthy superintendent that I again begin to write. . . . I have long ago gave up any disposition on my part to get out of this by any other means than by legal process of law as I believe I would be better off to say nothing of those I love . . . would rather spend the balance of my life in a dungeon than be the outlaw I might be ever I to gain my liberty by any other means than by law. . . . Dear I am getting along splendid and of late have no trouble and believe that the keepers of this place are above treating a man confined to their care with anything else than with humanity and kindness.

As to my treatment when (I tried to escape) I alone was to blame, but when I have conducted myself in a conscientious way, they have ever been ready to assist me, and even when I did not, I can look upon these officers as being my friends and who would refrain from doing anyone intrusted to their care an injustice. My work is the shoe, and am admired by all acquainted with the shoe and boot business as being a splendid filler, that is doing all the stitching on boots, shoes, gators and fixing them ready for the last. Jane I really admire the work I am following. . . .

This was written some two-and-one-half years after Hardin had received the maximum thirty-nine lashes for his escape plot. McCulloch's daughter later wrote (Hicks no date) that ". . . when his term had expired Hardin came to us, thanked us for all we did, asked forgiveness for all past faults and told Father this: 'Capt. McCulloch, you will never hear of me being in the pen again. I will try not to kill another man.' "

There is evidence that Hardin's self-esteem regulation shifts from various expressions of grandiose ambition and control to emphasis on work, in making boots and shoes and sending them to his children; to the development and promulgation of ideas, as he reacts to ideas, practices with them, and then tries to teach them in the penitentiary Sunday School and to his children by letter; and to increasingly obvious efforts at being creative and developing as an attorney, in writing letters, pursuing legal remedies, and writing his autobiography.

Hardin's Postimprisonment Regression

After his wife Jane's death, Hardin seems to have experienced grief, but newly developed structural transformations continued to function and to grow. He continued his legal appeals, studying the law, and writing to and admonishing his children. All of this persists within the probably supportive prison milieu, as well as through the many meaningful relationships with relatives and friends. Superintendent McCulloch's efforts may have been important in this regard.

After his release from prison, this equilibrium was initially maintained and supported by the greeting and adulation he received from children, family, and friends, by the temporary persistence of newly developed psychological functions, and by encountering no obstacles in the beginning. He tried to use his newly found identification as an attorney and did legal work to try to master the external and internal environments and used his newly developed expertise as a writer to complete the challenge first laid down by his parents: to write the true story of the killing, as his father had begun to do. He got a few law cases and was paid in kind; he tried to enter politics but failed; he wrote his life story but was not yet ready to publish it. He left his children and found a new woman—a child herself—to marry, who is so embarrassed by her infatuation with a man almost thirty years her senior that she flees. Temporarily, Hardin is supported by contact with another relative who calls on him for legal help, but the case falters and Hardin does not thrive as a lawyer in El Paso. He can attract women, however, and he does, this time separating Beulah Mrose from her husband and taking his money in the process. Beulah helps him with the book, but her own propensity for impulsivity and drink only supports his further regression. He gambles, drinks, responds in rage to insult, loss, or defeat, steals, and threatens violence; he does so in his behavior and presence, which the citizens and newspapers of El Paso recognized and felt, despite Hardin's professions to the opposite.

His explanation of the Gem Saloon holdup clearly depicts Hardin as someone whose pride is readily injured, who will attack when it is injured, who is protective of his "manhood" and "pedigree," who admires "pluck, push and virtue," and who assaults a problem head on, attempting to master whatever the difficulty—a crap-game loss, an insult, or doubts about his character. At the same time, he practiced his skill as a gunfighter, as described by his landlady. Thus it was that Hardin continued to confront some inner sense of danger—possibly his "passions" getting the best of him—by trying to control the outer world and the threats of others, by trying to calm himself with drink, and by trying to prepare for the unexpected.

He insults two former El Paso lawmen, probably while drunk, but has the good sense to back down when confronted by each of them and apologizes publicly. It may be that their firmness, like Father's and McCulloch's, helped him reestablish controls. Apparently he could not do the same with John Selman and his son. Why, we cannot say, but it may have had to do with the son threatening Hardin's crucial relationship with Beulah and, on the day of Hardin's death, Beulah's absence from El Paso. She had that day wired him about her fear that he was in danger. Indeed he was, as he could no longer control himself without her presence despite his efforts at self-healing by drinking and gambling. It seems that Hardin (and Beulah) planned to leave El Paso, to publish his book, and to find happiness elsewhere. Perhaps Hardin recognized that El Paso did not provide a supportive and therapeutic milieu, as Jane and even prison had, but rather proved to be a stimulating, provocative, and therefore dangerous atmosphere. For example, people tested and insulted him. Others were themselves out of control, and there were complex contradictions and delinquent, even criminal, undercurrents in El Paso. The rules about not carrying and using firearms were being violated routinely and enforced selectively; the newly imposed prohibition of gambling was controversial, and Hardin participated in challenging it on May 1, its first day of application. Lawmen, or former lawmen, participated in criminal ventures. Selman's acquittal after killing Hardin demonstrates the disorganization of the criminal justice system. As Hardin lost control, he threatened violence, telling Selman that he would shoot him up and make him run scared.

Hardin's autobiography might have become his way out, as well as representing an identification with his father, perhaps a return to a more successful, though personal, regulating system. Shooting holes in playing cards and passing them out showed his willingness to capitalize on his fame and notoriety—a public relations venture, possibly connected with his saloon business and his persistent identification as a gunfighter and killer. The book too would have been a successful public relations venture and a vindication of Hardin and his life.

Selman killed Hardin out of his own fear and rage, and El Paso citizens experienced relief, for they feared him, they idealized him. No one protested the killing, yet they viewed Hardin's body with awe. The reactions of the citizenry reflected the paradoxes of Hardin's narcissistic problems, his instability, and his charisma.

Hardin's Adolescence and the Emergence of Adult Pathology

John Wesley Hardin's childhood development resulted in certain well-internalized narcissistic structures. His grandiose self asserted itself readily in various academic and behavioral activities, tolerating no affront and fearing little. He idealized certain virtues, as exemplified in his father and his assertive friends, to whom he was fiercely loyal.

He would even challenge authority when he thought it wrong and showed no automatic respect for or compliance to authority. He began showing a willingness to be violent to defend his pride, and his gun becomes a tool and means thereto. Thus, he maintains his self-esteem by fighting, he helps his friends, and he challenges authorities—the teacher and the "bully."

In his autobiography, Hardin (1896) emphasizes:

> The way you bend a twig, that is the way it will grow, is an old saying, and a true one. . . . Our parents had taught us from our infancy to be honest, truthful, and brave, and we were taught that no brave boy would let another call him a liar with impunity, consequently we had lots of battles with other boys at school. I was naturally active and strong and always came out best, though sometimes with a bleeding nose, scratched face, or a black eye; but true to my early training, I would try, try, try again. . . . I always tried to excel in my studies, and generally stood at the head. Being playful by nature, I was generally first on the playground at recess and noon. Marbles, rolly hole, cat, bull pen, and town ball were our principal games, and I was considered by my schoolmates an expert. I knew how to knock the middle man, throw a hot ball, and ply the bat.

In 1931, Attorney W. B. Teagarden, a childhood friend and schoolmate of Hardin, wrote to Mollie after her brother and sister had died (Hardin et al. 1870–95). He described their lifelong friendship, her father's commitment to a friend, and how Hardin often protected him from older bullies and:

> on one occasion he stepped out into the aisle of the large school room, with open knife in his hand, and met the irate teacher coming with hickory in hand to whip me unjustly, and told him that he would kill him if he struck me with that stick. The teacher retreated and that was the end of it; he knew, and everybody in the school room knew, that John meant what he said. . . . Any decent man could always get along with him without any trouble, and so could any man who treated him fairly. He was always frank and honorable in all things, but he would not brook any kind of an insult from anybody. His sensitive, resentful disposition would not stand for it.

Hardin describes the knife fight he had at fourteen as justified and a matter of pride: as the other boy "wanted to be the boss among the boys, of course I stood in his way." The other boy accused Wes of writing on the school wall some obscene rhyme about a girl classmate, when in fact the other boy had done it: "I at once denied it and proved it up on him. He came over to my seat in the school room, struck me and drew his knife. I stabbed him twice almost fatally in the breast and back." Hardin was exonerated.

Of his adventurous childhood, Hardin writes: "Here I wish to tell my readers that if there is any power to save a man, woman, or child from harm, outside the power of the Living God, it is this thing called pluck. I never was afraid of anything except ghosts, and I have lived that down now and they have no terrors for me . . . if you wish to be successful in life, be temperate and control your passions; if you don't, ruin and death is the inevitable result."

Obviously, he was concerned about regulating and controlling the intensity of the strong affects he would experience, and his writings from prison showed evidence of a beginning ability to tame his rages and to embrace both religion and law.

In November 1868, at fifteen, he went to visit an uncle near Moscow, "carrying my pistol of course." A cousin of his matched the two of them in a wrestling match against a "large, powerful" former slave named Mage, "and we were but two boys." Nonetheless, they threw him twice, and Mage became enraged, threatened to beat Hardin, and went for his gun. Hardin went to get his own Colt revolver, but his uncle intervened and ordered Wes to stay in the house and the black man off the plantation. The next day, on the way home, he encountered Mage, who threatened to kill Hardin and attacked him with a big stick, even though Hardin told him that he was only "playing with him . . . and did not intend to hurt him." When Mage struck, Hardin shot him several times, wounding him fatally. "If it had not been for my uncle, I would have shot him again. . . . This was the first man I ever killed, and it nearly distracted my father and mother when I told them."

He then used his Colt to kill one black and two white soldiers who were after him because "I had no mercy on men whom I knew only wanted to get my body to torture and kill. It was war to the knife with me, and I brought it on by opening the fight with a double-barreled shotgun and ending it was a cap-and-ball six-shooter."

Shortly thereafter, in January 1869, while still fifteen, Hardin helped his father teach school for about three months but did not accept the

291

offer to continue because he wanted to become a cowboy. He was becoming addicted to gambling, perhaps expressing externally some sort of inner struggle that he was trying to master. Clearly, Hardin was trying to gain some sense of mastery over his impulses; the gambling suggests an intense need to control and master, and the target seems to be impudence and bullying, perhaps grandiosity and power urges.

Mage, Hardin's first victim, may himself have been enraged and out of control. Hardin's killing Mage may have truly been in self-defense—to defend himself against an out-of-control rage with which he himself was burdened, an external representation of Hardin's internal struggle; otherwise, he might have fled the encounter with Mage. He then tried to stay close to Father, who told him to hide, and Father's regulation seems to work temporarily while Hardin helps Father teach school. Then, the typical adolescent separation/individuation and displacement from the infantile objects to older heroes and then peers takes effect; "Wes" invests in cousin Mannen Clements and his cattle drives and begins to display in his "action language"—the internal issues of trying to master strong affect and impulses. He races horses, gambles, drinks, and cavorts with his adolescent buddies and engages in gun play. Often he is trying to punish "bullies"—again perhaps the grandiose bully inside.

His first killing, that of a freed slave, is an extension of his challenge of authority, as is, more obviously, its aftermath—the killing of three soldiers hunting him. Simultaneously he experiences considerable difficulty with self-regulation and is readily stimulated to act and to rage and readily overstimulated, sometimes to the point of near fragmentation. These problems become more evident as Hardin concludes his adolescence. For awhile, his self-esteem and idealizations are fulfilled by intellectual pursuits like his father's teaching, but the needs to discharge strong affects and to master strong affects through action, like his cousins and his cowboy friends, come to the foreground. He gambles and engages in gunplay and displaces his attachments to peer relationships and other idealizations, such as Wild Bill Hickok.

There is a shift of attachment from Mother to Jane Bowen, and this works off and on. The history of their marriage is of frequent separations, as Hardin goes off to play with the boys, returning every now and then for narcissistic refueling with Jane. His mother no longer serves as a soothing selfobject, though he seeks such regulation in his wife and later in other women. His father no longer serves as an idealized selfobject, but peer and other displacements do, until later in prison he returns to the pursuits of his father—studying, teaching, and writing. These later adult transformations occur in prison but are maintained only for awhile after his release. Substitute maternal selfobjects fail him, gambling and drink fail him, and he dies before his written autobiography can help him with one final attempt to organize his crumbling self.

Of course, one could say that Hardin never ceased being a troubled adolescent and that, except for a quiscent period in prison, he continued the same delinquent career, tenuous relationships with selfobjects, the threatened fragmentations, and the propensity for narcissistic rage that he showed prior to his flight to Florida. On the contrary, there is evidence in his letters from prison that significant transformations developed—he began to write, to express himself, to experiment with ideas, to try to teach others, to think about his impact on his children, to use legal recourse instead of violence, and to tell the world about his life. This adjustment was tenuous, however, and stable selfobjects and a supportive milieu were needed to assure his survival. He did not survive but died a violent death, just as do a high percentage of juvenile delinquents (Marohn 1982; Marohn, Locke, Rosenthal, and Curtiss 1982).

Conclusions

John Wesley Hardin's capacity to regulate internal tensions and strong affects were not securely established when he emerged from adolescence, and he frequently sought solace from maternal selfobjects and their substitutes. The idealization of his father and his virtues were more stable factors around which to organize his self, and as he emerged from his teenage years, he displaced such attachments to male peers and older male heroes. He would attempt to master internal chaos by behaving violently, but when he was overstimulated, he would just as likely become violent. The adult Hardin manifested a narcissistic behavior disorder, as he behaved in order to regulate himself, restore his self-esteem, and maintain his self-cohesion. Often he needed contact with selfobjects, such as his wife or his heroes, or with selfobject substitutes, such as drink and gambling, to restore himself. In prison he gained new internal regulating systems, other than behavior and action, and these could be maintained for awhile after his release. Then, as his self-regulation fails, and as his selfobjects fail him, he displays and provokes violence and falls victim.

Hardin's (1896) own evaluation of his violent career, written shortly before he was killed in 1895, tells us again of his propensity for narcissistic rage:

> While I write this, I say from the deepest depths of my heart that my desire for revenge is not satisfied, and if I live another year, I promise my friends and my God to make another of my brother's murderers bite the dust. Just as long as I can find one of them and know for certain that he participated in the murder of my brother, just that and nothing more, right there, be the consequences what they may, I propose to take life. . . . True, it is almost as bad to kill as to be killed. It drove my father to an early grave; it almost distracted my mother; . . . I do say, however, that the man who does not exercise the first law of nature—that of self preservation— is not worthy of living and breathing the breath of life.

NOTES

1. This history of Hardin's life is based on Hardin (1896), Hardin et al. (1870–95), Metz (1966), Nordyke (1957), and Parsons (1978).

2. For a discussion of these issues, see Kohut (1971, 1977, 1984) and Ornstein (1978).

REFERENCES

Adams, R. F. 1960. *A Fitting Death for Billy the Kid*. Norman: University of Oklahoma Press.

Adams, R. F. 1969. *Six-Guns and Saddle Leather*. Norman: University of Oklahoma Press.

Aichhorn, A. 1925. *Wayward Youth*. New York: Viking Press, 1935.

Cleckley, H. 1964. *The Mask of Sanity*. St. Louis: C. V. Mosby.

Cline, D. 1984. Secret life of Billy the Kid. *True West*, April, pp. 12–17, 62.

Friedlander, K. 1960. *The Psycho-Analytical Approach to Juvenile Delinquency: Theory, Case Studies, Treatment*. New York: International Universities Press.

Garrett, P. F. 1882. *Life of Billy the Kid*. Norman: University of Oklahoma Press, 1974.

Hardin, J. W. 1896. *The Life of John Wesley Hardin: As Written by Himself*. Norman: University of Oklahoma Press, 1961.

Hardin, J. W., et al. 1870–95. Hardin Papers. Southwest Texas State University, San Marcos, Texas.

Hicks, A. M. No date. Letter to the Editor. *Collier's*.

Kohut, H. 1971. *The Analysis of the Self*. New York: International Universities Press.

Kohut, H. 1977. *The Restoration of the Self*. New York: International Universities Press.

Kohut, H. 1984. *How Does Analysis Cure?* Chicago: University of Chicago Press.

Marohn, R. C. 1967. The unit meeting: its implications for a therapeutic correctional community. *International Journal of Group Psychotherapy* 17:159–167.

Marohn, R. C. 1979. El Paso has lost her nerve. *Westerners Brand Book* 35:49–51, 56.

Marohn, R. C. 1981. Personality disorders and adolescence. In J. R. Lion, ed. *Personality Disorders*. Baltimore: Williams & Wilkins.

Marohn, R. C. 1982. Adolescent violence: causes and treatment. *Journal of the American Academy of Child Psychiatry* 21:354–360.

Marohn, R. C.; Dalle-Molle, D.; McCarter, E.; and Linn, D. 1980. *Juvenile Delinquents: Psychodynamic Assessment and Hospital Treatment*. New York: Brunner/Mazel.

Marohn, R. C.; Locke, E.; Rosenthal, R.; and Curtiss, G. 1982. Juvenile delinquents and violent death. *Adolescent Psychiatry* 10:147–170.

Metz, L. C. 1966. *John Selman, Texas Gunfighter*. New York: Hastings House.

Nordyke, L. 1957. *John Wesley Hardin, Texas Gunman*. New York: William Morrow.

Offer, D.; Marohn, R. C.; and Ostrov, E. 1979. *The Psychological World of the Juvenile Delinquent*. New York: Basic.

Ornstein, P., ed. 1978. *The Search for the Self, the Collected Papers of Heinz Kohut*, 2 vols. New York: International Universities Press.

Parsons, C. 1978. *The Capture of John Wesley Hardin*. College Station, Tex.: Creative.

295

Parsons, C. 1985. *"Pidge," A Texas Ranger from Virginia*. Wolfe City, Tex.: Henington.

Sonnichsen, C. L. 1979. *The Grave of John Wesley Hardin; Three Essays on Grassroots History*. College Station: Texas A&M University Press.

Trachtman, P. 1974. *The Old West, The Gunfighters*. New York: Time-Life Books.

PART IV

PSYCHOTHERAPEUTIC ISSUES IN ADOLESCENT PSYCHIATRY

EDITORS' INTRODUCTION

The dynamic psychiatric treatment of the adolescent—particularly of the severely disturbed adolescent—is a complex, difficult, and often frustrating process. The adolescent's action orientation, his intense self-preoccupation, and his propensity to recapitulate aspects of his troubled family relationships in the therapeutic context all conspire to impose special demands on those who seek to help young people and on the techniques they seek to employ in doing so. Psychotherapy may be rendered in a variety of settings. While the majority of psychiatrists see patients in an office setting, increasingly adolescent psychiatrists find themselves treating adolescents in specialized hospital facilities necessitating not only an appreciation of the specific psychotherapeutic issues involved but also the importance of working with the family and developing effective alliances that can be utilized for aftercare. Innovative use of treatment parameters may also be judiciously used when circumstances do not permit ongoing therapy. The following chapters describe interesting aspects of the vicissitudes of the therapeutic alliance, including the candid consideration of therapeutic failure.

François Ladame describes a number of therapeutic failures among adolescents owing to pathological narcissism. These illustrate what he considers a structural defect—a malignant divorce between narcissism and object cathexis—and he questions its reversibility since these patients manifest a negative therapeutic reaction. Ladame comments that, with these adolescents, a "missing piece" is absent from the psychic functional organization that normally would be internalized. He concludes that the question of the efficiency of the analytic method in this type of disorder remains open.

Linda Greenberg, Susan Haiman, and Aaron Esman view the acute psychiatric hospitalization of an adolescent as a crisis point during which unresolved developmental, intrapsychic, intrafamilial, and social conflicts arc in evidence. They believe that the treating interdisciplinary staff needs to develop an awareness of countertransference issues as well as a method with which to monitor these phenomena. They found the division of evaluation from treatment as arbitrary and see the first stages of an acute hospitalization as an important step toward the establishment of a therapeutic alliance and the later stages as vulnerable to withdrawal by staff as sadness over separation increases. The authors conclude that an integrating theory that addresses both intrapsychic factors and their behavioral manifestations can be utilized to address milieu problems from the patient's perspective as well as to provide for staff an environment conducive to resolving countertransference issues.

Joan Tolchin reviews the use of the telephone as a therapeutic parameter in mental health care, with special attention to adolescents. She describes its use in clinical situations where face-to-face availability is impaired and discusses some of the technical difficulties to be handled. The author concludes that it may be useful to let adolescent patients know that the therapist is available by phone if any significant problem arises out of session or during a brief separation or interruption. Even a brief telephone contact can be reassuring and decrease anxiety as part of a supportive, therapeutic alliance.

Glen T. Pearson discusses his experiences with long-term treatment and follow-up of severely disturbed adolescents. He focuses on aspects of the physician-patient relationship as they bear on specific needs during the course of treatment. The author believes that the key to the physician's ability to meet these needs is the provision of a stable, long-term object relationship and traces the development of the relationship through the various phases of treatment including aftercare and final termination.

300

19 DEPRESSIVE ADOLESCENTS, PATHOLOGICAL NARCISSISM, AND THERAPEUTIC FAILURES

FRANÇOIS LADAME

Rather than discuss the general problem of normal or pathological depression and the narcissistic tribulations of adolescents, I shall limit myself to the study of a group of depressive adolescents who have experienced a breakdown in their development according to the definition of Laufer and Laufer (1984). These adolescents may undertake treatment, but the treatment frequently fails. I have become increasingly aware of the predominant role of the activation of archaic and pathological narcissistic mechanisms in some of these difficult cases.[1]

Being a therapist, I know it is not easy to speak of therapeutic failures, but this eventuality is part of our daily work and deserves more attention than we usually give it. Of course, this problem includes the role that the therapist may play in the failure through conscious and unconscious reactions activated by the patient's transference.

No doubt, the negative therapeutic reaction that Riviere (1936), half a century ago, considered a defense against an unconscious depressive reaction is relevant to the problem of interruption of treatment and failure. But most authors who describe the negative therapeutic reaction characterize it only by transitory periods of negativism and a risk of therapeutic deadlock (Bégoin and Bégoin 1981; Grunert 1981). For Schwaber (1979), the negative therapeutic reaction expresses fear of feeling annihilated—a state of nothingness.

In many cases of therapeutic failure with adolescents who are severely disturbed, narcissistic stances are in the foreground (Novick

301

1980) and acting in direct opposition to the prospect of treatment. For the depressive patients I have in mind, the need to keep absolute control and maintain the idealized image of an omnipotent loving object fused with a partial self-image should not be challenged. The fear of rejection and the dependency needs are hidden thanks to the illusion of self-sufficiency (Modell 1975). When these needs emerge, the illusion can be preserved by turning the passive into active, rejecting the other, and making the object (part-object) fail.

I shall illustrate my theme by clinical examples, although this will undoubtedly raise more questions than offer solutions.

Case Example 1

Ingrid entered my consultation room after having run away for three days. This young patient is seventeen years old. She wants to be helped, but she is afraid that I will not be able to reach her. Until now, the only person she has been able to relate to is her girlfriend, S, a perfect duplicate of herself (or, more exactly, complementary half) with whom she functions mainly through heavy projective identifications.

Usually, Ingrid is aware of what is going on in her mind. Suddenly, though, the "*krach*" occurred—something unexplainable, thoughts and affects that she could neither "think" nor "feel." She had to act out to be able to think and to feel again. She explains her running away as a challenge to herself, but she recognizes that she had no choice. Anything could have happened to her and she would not have been afraid; it would have only confirmed how "horrible" she is.

Ingrid is overwhelmed by feelings of badness; she thinks she may be a witch or have one inside her. Yet she denies any conscious suicidal thoughts because she values herself too much. Now, however, sado-masochistic tendencies quickly appear—a kind of delight in the idea of being hurt. But the question is how to hurt herself; she could not allow anyone to do it (a sign of her omnipotent narcissism).

The "shrinks" are all stupid, she says. They read all the books and only repeat what they have learned, without understanding anything. So, after the second session of assessment, she is faced with the dilemma of either seeing me as a devalued, typical bookworm from whom she has nothing to expect or as someone who understands, who is able to make sense and help to clarify—thus challenging her fantasies of omnipotency and self-sufficiency.

Ingrid probably broke down early in her adolescence, but she has found some compromises that have allowed her to keep contact with the outside reality through splitting and denial. If she gives her body to her boyfriend, letting him use it as he wants, she refuses to give him her "mind," saving it for her only friend, S. Symptoms, however, have developed, and she has had depression for several months, truancy, and anorexia. Now, sexuality is abandoned and refused. But Ingrid is upset because her absolute need for control of herself and others is challenged. She feels more and more passive toward what is happening to her.

After recognizing that I understand her and that she can show me a part of her feelings, a more negative reaction appears with an emotional withdrawal. She feels an anxiety and an unexplainable fear concerning me, but the fears are "unthinkable." Ingrid is very reluctant to go on with the interviews. She talks about a schoolmate's suicidal attempt, showing herself emotionally incongruous. The only difference, she says, between this friend who attempted suicide—the madness—and herself is that she is still "in control."

Soon afterward, when I had arrived at the end of my assessment, I told her my concern about her future and about the rigidity of her defense mechanisms that leave her without a choice. Her humiliation and shame to have to accept help were recognized, as well as her conviction that all persecution comes from men. The demands of the treatment were specified with Ingrid and with her parents. Eventually, the patient was relieved by my taking sides clearly.

Ingrid interrupted treatment after less than ten sessions. The denial of her dependency quickly activated a defensive self-sufficiency. If her therapist is not available, "she has herself" and that is enough. In fact, a part of her refuses all help. She can only be reached at the level of a false self, a level characterized by superficiality and banality. Giving me access to her internal life makes her fear that I could depossess her of something more "authentic" or use it to attack her. Two missed sessions are linked with dreams and daydreams where the splitting and denial were fading away, provoking narcissistic mortification. But this breach, thus half-opened, is unbearable. The therapist knows too much about her. She has shown him too much, that is, how important he is to her.

The session right before the breaking off is characterized by a strange atmosphere where I feel "engulfed." The patient confirms that she has taken the "environment" inside herself. She is rather silent—to speak would confirm that we are two separated and differentiated beings. The conflict between the wish and fear of fusion and feelings of persecution, on the one side, and the fear of narcissistic breakdown and loss of the feeling of continuity of the self, on the other side, is at a peak.

Eventually, Ingrid incorporated me as a selfobject (or narcissistic object). Working through and clarification put her in front of the reality of separateness and differentiation between her and me and created terrifying anxieties that could not be contained within the therapeutic setting. Since I have had many experiences with patients showing similar problems—paniclike fears coming from a deficient cohesiveness of the self-representation—I do think that the solution to the problem of continuing the treatment or abandoning it depends mainly on the strength of the defensive claim to maintain the illusion of a grandiose self-sufficiency. To demask affects means to need objects. It is that precise need that has to be denied. Ingrid told me, "During separations, I have myself." Her answer can be understood as her need to be, for herself, a better mothering object than her therapist could be (repeating, of course, her past history)—a manifestation of her identification to a preoedipal, omnipotent, and unfailing mother (Modell 1975). To hold on to that primary identification is the only way to ward off the fear of a catastrophic disintegration of the self.

At this point it may seem important to state precisely that the modalities of psychic functioning that have been described have nothing in common with those observable in normal adolescents or in adolescents showing a transient crisis without any lasting sequels for future development. The heightening of narcissistic defenses is usual during adolescence and may be accompanied by denial, but these mechanisms manifest themselves in a benign and transitory way. (The same is probably true during specific phases of psychoanalytical treatment of neurotic adults.) In these cases, there is not that malignant divorce between narcissism and object cathexis—libidinal and aggressive. To put it in a different way, self-representations and object representations are sufficiently separated and stabilized so that object closeness and awareness of instinctual needs for the object world do not release unbearable annihilation, intrusion, or engulfment anxieties.

With depressive and narcissistic adolescents, we are faced with a structural defect. A kind of interpolated piece is missing whose function is to regulate inward and outward movements; originally concrete movements eventually become psychic introjective/projective rhythms. When the ego is functional, there is no more fear of total draining out or of intrusion-persecution. From a structural point of view, that harmonious dynamic can work only if the self-representations and the object representations are clearly separated and if there are identificatory possibilities, other than archaic primary identifications, where self and object are more or less fused.

I do not discuss the question of the origin of that structural defect because it appears to me to be a false problem. What we observe during adolescence is the existence of that structural defect, and the only relevant question is about its reversibility. Are we able or not to undo the pathology and reestablish the process of growing up? The frame of reference is not the same as the one we are working with when there are internal conflicts between structuralized internal agencies.

Case Example 2

The topic of the "missing piece" or the "hole" to be filled in the organization of the ego is illustrated with the case of David. The dramatic issue also raises the question of the limits of therapy.

I met David for the first time when he was seventeen and had just graduated from high school. He wanted to go abroad to college. A few weeks before, the young man had been hospitalized briefly in a psychiatric clinic after his parents had discovered that he had taken heroin for several months. At that time, David complained about anxiety and psychasthenia, which he attempted more or less successfully to relieve with alcohol. The phobic mechanisms and behaviors were important, the narcissistic, omnipotent defenses quite obvious. A few spaced interviews convinced me that treatment was necessary but motivation was still uncertain, especially considering the narcissistic defenses. I encouraged David to go into treatment in the foreign country where he was studying.

Two years later, I found the patient back in my consultation room. David asked me to start the treatment I had once suggested. Now, the complaints are about deep depressive states, alternating with periods of elation. When he is depressed, he is overwhelmed by a feeling of nonvalue, of absolute failure. Then the manic defenses allow him to deny, very briefly, his preceding state of mind. He was afraid to become mad or to be a schizophrenic. He doubted the integrity of his body, and he had recurring suicidal thoughts. Without treatment, he said, "something" catastrophic would happen to him. During the two years of college (with scholastic success) he drank excessively.

A new assessment brought to light not only the breakdown of the defenses and compromises used to fight the developmental breakdown at puberty but also the permanence of narcissistic, archaic features—all-powerful control, refusal to be a "beginner," refusal of dependency (I am invested in my functions but not as a whole subject), shame to admit the need for a therapist, and an inability to trust others. Differing from the first patient, David seemed to function partially owing to a peculiar way of splitting and projection. In submission to a gratifying environment, he could avoid painful feelings of persecution. The alcoholism had two opposite aims: it allowed him to establish relations but to avoid the far too dangerous dual relationship. As usual, heroin offered the advantage of subduing all the affects of rage, violence, hostility, and helplessness.

Rapidly, even before any final decision about treatment, there was an occurrence of transference elements of a clinging or sticking type, with an attitude of compliance whose aim was to blur differences between the patient and me. Simultaneously, David was very persistent in his efforts to be in control of the situation, trying among other things to set a time limit for the therapy.

Acting out followed, with the patient again using heroin during separations, which released painful and unbearable feelings of abandonment and loss of self. The subject does not "lose the object," but the subject is "lost physically and mentally by the object" (Bégoin and Bégoin 1981). David was escaping more and more from the relationship with his therapist, provoking massively, and showing himself unable to take over responsibility for his actions.

At that time, David was hospitalized. The hospital stay allowed us to go on with the work of clarification and interpretation, allowing the abandonment depression, against which he was defending himself, to come out into the open. The patient felt totally miserable, and he revolted against this state, of which he accused me of responsibility. Obviously, I was included in the heroin "shoots" but in a split way: the union/fusion fantasy with me was kept more or less conscious, and the hostile aspect of the "poison-providing object" was denied. Through projective identification and turning passive into active, David made efforts to make me as helpless and impotent as he felt himself to be.

He had to attack me and triumph over me, making me feel my defeat. My capacity of synthesis and integration, my "equidistant" attitude to all his dissociated parts made him feel envious, furious, and humiliated. At this stage, I was wondering if the secondary benefits of the archaic mechanisms and of splitting would make it possible to renounce them. Nevertheless, the moments of fusion were still felt ambivalently and provoked more a panic of undifferentiation than clear, psychotic, egosyntonic behavior.

After the hospitalization, David was able to recognize that his depression had been there for years. But, in therapy, he constantly needed to see me act in one way or another to confirm his omnipotency. It was an alternating, double-sided "master to slave" dialectic: he-patient, "inferior," and I-doctor, "superior."

Later, there was a period when the daily relationship of David with his father became more conflictual. The only real sign of father's love would be if he let David use his fortune as he wanted—that he be allowed to model himself after this rich and generous parental imago who withholds all sources of gratification and treasures. David accused his father of letting him "starve." To become a suicide would signify, on the conscious level, a reproach to his father—a punishment to a frustrating father who was completely confused with the primitive parental imago.

All those who took care of him only brought him derisory help. To be taking heroin again had the meaning of punishing everyone who was around him. It expressed also his denial that I helped him, his refusal to be a patient and be treated, and his triumph over me. At the same time, David began to realize clearly that his treatment (the time limit of which he wanted initially to set) would be a very long one. Christmas was not far off. David had the aim to be magically "clean," free from any drug, and to participate in the holidays with his family as the immaculate child. It was at this time that David committed suicide.

A suicidal attempt, fatal or not, follows a complex and multifactorial dynamic and presupposes this "coalition" of the inside and the outside (Ladame 1981). To separate the narcissistic mechanisms from other factors can look like a reductive process. Nevertheless it is true that archaic narcissistic constellations are always at work and that they sometimes play a primary role. David believed that I possessed a magical solution but refused to communicate it to him. This same image had been projected onto many significant others—and they were nu-

307

merous—in his daily environment. Surely this was one of the important suicide-promoting factors.

His action was probably the only means he had to free himself not only from the analyst-mother but from the whole world of objects (objects who had all become identical with a hostile split imago). At the moment of the suicide, David was fully aware that the duration of his treatment would be out of his control. At this or another moment in therapy, other patients of this type have to be able to "abandon" themselves with trust and to try the symbiosis with the analyst as a selfobject (Grunert 1981). Only from this moment onward is there a possibility of growth and correction of structural defect. At his stage, such a perspective would mean, for David, total surrender. The catastrophic reversal of passive into active had been precipitated, so I think, by the revival of old painful feelings of frustration in the bodily relationship with his mother (handling and holding were impaired during six weeks in an incubator after birth, followed by an evident lack of gratification of the mother in giving care to her child). At the same time, the movement of triumphant self-sufficiency was also the expression of the effort to preserve the split part of the archaic loving/giving/gratifying imago to which the psychic self is totally identified. Whatever it takes to make the object-analyst fail is probably linked with the need to keep intact the idealized image of a loving, all-powerful mother and the fantasy of a narcissistic union with this totally gratifying mother.

Case Example 3

Suzan was referred for treatment by her social worker, who, over the years, had become a "friend" to her. The patient is nineteen. She does not feel well; she is tired and she complains of pains in the back and legs (so-called *rheumatismus,* which was thoroughly investigated but nothing pathological could be found). She has lost weight and can hardly fall asleep. Above all, she is unable to graduate from high school. She passes her time, locked up at home, with books and records. She has contact only with her girlfriend, Z, who regulates all contacts with her peers. Suzan holds all her affects back, while the therapist quickly feels burdened by depressive feelings.[2]

Suzan was in foster homes until the age of four. She remembers bad bodily treatment and claims to have been burnt on her chest. She did not do very well at school. There were a succession of failures, second chances, and school removals until she decided to prepare for a high school diploma by correspondence (an effort she abandoned after three months). The patient has obtained many rejections and mobilized her teachers frequently. She was brilliant in matters where she felt superior to others, but she could not bear being in the situation of someone who did not know everything and had to learn. The intensity of her contempt is fascinating. She feels contempt for everyone—parents, schoolmates, doctors, and teachers. Sexuality does not exist for her, but she does not consider it a problem.

The following assessment interviews confirm the weight of the narcissistic disorder. Early frustrations partly explain the enormous rage linked with omnipotency and self-sufficiency. Her personality was organized around the goal to be for herself a better mothering agency than her own mother was able to be. Suzan cannot rely on anyone and primary identifications were not remodeled. Z, her girlfriend, is the only survivor of the universal contempt; she is the ideal duplicate of herself, a princess of blue blood, a monument of strength, who nevertheless hides a fragility to which only Suzan has access. Together, the two girls are able to bear isolation and suffering while they go on admiring and idealizing each other. Z and Suzan attended the funeral of an old schoolmate's father. Both "impeccable," they did not show the least emotion, although the young orphan fell crying into Suzan's arms.

In spite of the obvious risk of premature negative reactions and breaking off, I encouraged my colleague to start treatment because the patient was clearly in a deadlock. Moreover, Suzan asked for treatment, even though she was aware that some hidden pain might come to surface.

The therapist, invested in the function of listening but not as an individual, is soon seen as the holder of some dangerous and destructive powers. She cannot but destroy Suzan, "taking a robot apart and putting it together wrongly," and attack the system Suzan has patiently built up. A teacher once understood perfectly Suzan's way of functioning: he never asked questions and stopped walking two meters from her. "People who approach go right through, because I am not there anymore." Suzan compares herself to an isolated castle surrounded by swamp: the others stay on the shore; she would have to throw a rope to her therapist, but she doesn't have one; even if she had one, she could not do it. The therapist has no rope either; the swamp will never be explored.

Interpretations were mostly aimed at the underlying anxiety and the link between despair, helplessness, and omnipotency. Sessions are like a tennis match where it is most pressing to send back the ball as quickly as possible; if the ball "enters," it arouses rage, hate, and impotency. The therapist is devaluated; anything she says is turned into ridicule; her interpretations are "plainly naive."

Suzan broke off after three months of treatment at the culminating point of her negativism. Before that, she had made a few new arrangements in her external reality. She insisted the therapist should have known that it would end that way (with failure), even before she came and saw her for the first time. The therapist was a stage in her life—controlled by her and used as she wanted. Anything else is much too frightening.

THE NEGATIVE THERAPEUTIC REACTION

Negative therapeutic motivation (Novick 1980) or the motivation to make the treatment fail is especially obvious here. That motivation for failure is clearly linked to a double aim: to keep control of the situation and to maintain unchanged an idealized image of an omnipotent loving mother, which is an integral part of the self-image. At the last session, Suzan stated precisely for her therapist, "You will be *the* psychologist of my life." Like Ingrid, the first patient, Suzan has probably incorporated a part of her short therapeutic experience into the narcissistic archaic constellation, which is defensive, and she has fled before it could be challenged ("Any other thing is too frightening").

Riviere's (1936) thoughts about the negative therapeutic reaction seem especially relevant here. For Riviere, the motive of the negative therapeutic reaction was the need to maintain a status quo—a state of things that were bearable until now—and avoid the panic created by any prospect of change. The defense is aimed primarily against an unconscious depressive situation where all those who are loved inside are either dead or destroyed. The resistance represses again the awareness of what lies in the depth of the psyche; the worst disasters have already happened and still that obvious situation is unthinkable. How near we are to Winnicott (1974) and his "fear of breakdown."

Suzan states clearly, "The swamp will never be explored." It is out of the question to venture into the internal world where the ghosts of the first objects are lying—beloved and hated, attacked and attacking. Ghosts that are always able to rise again as persecutors spouting out of the abyss where the patient's own drives have sent them to sleep forever—sealing at the same time an everlasting pact of allegiance.

Most authors who have used the concept of negative therapeutic reaction describe clinical situations characterized by transitory periods of negativism and risk of therapeutic deadlock. In the cases presented here, however, it was always a failure, up to the more dramatic one— suicide—with no possibility of going beyond the negative reaction and ahead with the treatment. Nevertheless, the failures depicted show many similar features to the negative therapeutic reaction. And, like Novick, I do think that the phenomenon is more visible in certain types of severely disturbed adult patients or at certain ages in adolescents.

It is also true that these situations raise many unsolved questions for our daily work and our theoretical understanding. How far is it possible, from the point of view of technique, to interrupt a movement toward breaking off? What are the ingredients at work in these situations that could be influenced by a savoir faire instead of knowledge (once we are sure, of course, that unsolved countertransferential issues are not dominant)? Is it primarily a problem of assessment and indication? The three adolescent patients that I have presented were surely in a developmental deadlock and at risk of chronic pathology as adults. But we know too that ill patients are not all treatable, and we have to face this fact. What should be our therapeutic aims and how are we able to fill developmental or structural gaps and reestablish an interrupted development?

Should we simply accept the fact that the patient has the freedom to go into treatment and to interrupt it? This conclusion is not satisfactory to me, because it presumes that these patients actually had an alternative, which generally is not the case with the very ill adolescent. The narcissistic constellations I have described are at work in many treatments but do not always lead to a failure or an interruption. The question is then about the real chances of curing. But what do we mean by "curing"? What are our criteria? My impression is that we are always torn between a clinical realism—taking into account individual pathology—and an ideal view of mental health.

Case Example 4

At this point I shall discuss a brief clinical vignette, perhaps to prevent the discouragement that might arise from a study centered only on failures.

Michel went into analysis many years ago, when he was eighteen. He had just graduated from high school and was in a developmental deadlock. The first phase of treatment here too was characterized by the appearance of narcissistic, archaic, and omnipotent mechanisms: fear of mortification, paniclike anxieties of falling forever, liquefaction, nothingness, and annihilation.

My first comment to Michel was very unskillful and surely motivated by my own painful feeling of having no reality for him as a subject. The patient talked and talked interminably, not to present himself to me but to prevent me from saying anything and from seeing the cloudiness and confusion behind his speech. I interrupted him without sensitivity, and my comments baffled and abraded him. Seemingly all cards were dealt for a negative therapeutic reaction and a possible premature breaking off. Yet Michel was able, afterward, to live moments of quiet fusion when "the one is the other and the other is the one." This treatment was characterized by an alternation of symbiosis and persecution with phases of negativism.

With the years, Michel drew great benefit from his treatment. Nevertheless, the archaic narcissistic constellations are still mostly unchanged. "The reality that my mother did not belong to me was not true," Michel told me once, which highlights the strength of denial and how far adolescents can distort reality. The beloved "possession" is his "treasure." "She is my flesh and I am her flesh." The idea of losing this treasure creates paniclike anxieties, as in any case of sticky identifications where the self-image is fused with the image of the idealized, all-loving, and omnipotent parent. Nevertheless, the conflict in Michel is still alive. His mother belongs so much to him that it becomes frightening. Fusion is not a peaceful fulfillment; it creates a panic of engulfment and dedifferentiation, and survival of the self is threatened.

That Michel has not broken off his treatment prematurely, like Ingrid and Suzan, is probably due to the fact that he could quickly project into me the idealized, omnipotent, and gratifying narcissistic constellation. At that stage, the risk was no longer of interruption but of interminable analysis (the risk of termination without working through the central core).

Schwaber (1979) sees the negative therapeutic reaction as a manifestation of the fear of nothingness, of a state of annihilation. For the patient, the threat to the feeling of continuity of the self arises from the failure to receive empathy from the therapist or the failure of the object-analyst to offer himself as a self-object or narcissistic object.

312

From the point of view of the patient, negativism through a *nego ergo sum* is far better than dreadful nothingness.

A narcissistic transference experienced on its positive side (idealization, grandiosity) is absolutely necessary at one time or another during treatment. Nevertheless, the dilemma is caused by the fact that failures of empathy are no less necessary if a really therapeutic process is to be promoted (like the defects in any "good enough" mothering). We must also remember that the persecutory feelings may serve as a defense against a real positive transference (on a genetically different level) and protect against a narcissistic mortification. As long as narcissism and object libido are divorced, acknowledgment of the need of objects and dependency on them exposes oneself to the risk of disintegration of the self-sufficiency illusion.

It is much easier to recognize what we should not do in therapy than to indicate what should be done. Among other things, I think that the therapist should avoid idealization and the promotion of a kind of pleasure-dyad where one feels at ease and nothing really progresses. With an adolescent who has broken down in his development, we have no right not to make particular demands. I consider it a mistake to show ourselves "available" and let him, for instance, come when he wishes. I agree totally with the Laufers (1984) that such an attitude would ignore his pathology and his capability to overcome it. The hazard of an interruption of treatment, even if premature, seems to me less risky. Indeed, we may hope that the patient has heard what we have communicated to him and that he is not prisoner for life of an inexorable destiny.

As far as the group of adolescents I have presented here is concerned, I think it advisable to point out directly their suspicion and mistrust and to emphasize quickly the humiliation of needing treatment and the anxiety aroused by closeness, attachment, and dependency. We have to accept the idea that there is no reason to trust a priori. In these cases, trust must be considered an outcome of treatment and not as a prerequisite. (After many years of treatment, Michel was able to tell me, "Trust, I *learned* it here.")

Conclusions

I have developed a specific aspect of the difficulties we have to face when treating ill adolescents. It is, of course, a fragmentary point of view that has to be put in the more general context of psychoanalytical

313

treatment at adolescence. My center of interest was the activation of pathological, archaic, narcissistic mechanisms among depressive adolescents and their role in therapeutic failures. I have described some specific defensive constellations and their protective function against deep annihilation or agonic anxieties, but I have not discussed an important aspect of the problem—what relates to the near indefeasible link to the bad internal split objects. These bad objects lie dormant in the depth of the psyche and seem, so paradoxically, to warrant the lastingness of being.

Adopting another point of view, we might consider that these defensive structures act against envy and the awareness of the outcome of envy, depressive marasmus, and internal desert where every loved one has been annihilated. In any case, it seems important to me to be aware that with these adolescents we are confronted with a structural defect, a "missing piece" in the psychic functional organization that should have been internalized during development. The question of the efficiency of the analytic method to help in this kind of disorder remains open for discussion. Obviously, we meet with archaic narcissistic defense mechanisms in many other patients who do not break off treatment. The questions raised in this chapter need more discussion and research.

NOTES

1. A version of the paper was read at a Conference on Psychoanalytical Treatment in Adolescence at the University of Paris VII, Paris, October 22, 1982.

2. I wish to thank my colleague M.-J. Haenni for her authorization to use this case, which I supervised.

REFERENCES

Bégoin, J., and Bégoin, F. 1981. Réaction thérapeutique négative, envie et angoisse catastrophique. *Bulletin de la Fédération Européenne de Psychanalyse* 16:4–16.

Grunert, U. 1981. La réaction thérapeutique négative pour redonner vie à un processus de détachement dans le transfert. *Bulletin de la Fédération Européenne de Psychanalyse* 16:17–32.

Ladame, F. 1981. *Les tentatives de suicide des adolescents*. Paris: Masson.

Laufer, M., and Laufer, E. 1984. *Adolescence and Developmental Breakdown*. New Haven, Conn.: Yale University Press.

Modell, A. H. 1975. A narcissistic defence against affects and the illusion of self-sufficiency. *International Journal of Psycho-Analysis* 56:275–282.

Novick, J. 1980. Negative therapeutic motivation and negative therapeutic alliance. *Psychoanalytic Study of the Child* 35:299–320.

Riviere, J. 1936. A contribution to the analysis of the negative therapeutic reaction. *International Journal of Psycho-Analysis* 17:304–320.

Schwaber, E. 1979. On the "self" within the matrix of analytic theory: some clinical reflexions and reconsiderations. *International Journal of Psycho-Analysis* 60:467–479.

Winnicott, D. W. 1974. Fear of breakdown. *International Review of Psycho-Analysis* 1:103–107.

20 COUNTERTRANSFERENCE DURING THE
ACUTE PSYCHIATRIC HOSPITALIZATION
OF THE ADOLESCENT

LINDA GREENBERG, SUSAN HAIMAN, AND AARON H. ESMAN

The acute psychiatric hospitalization of an adolescent can be viewed as a crisis point during which unresolved developmental, intrapsychic, intrafamilial, and social conflicts all are in evidence. In order for these conflicts to be addressed speedily and therapeutically within an acute hospitalization, we believe that the treating interdisciplinary staff needs to develop an awareness of countertransference issues as well as a method to monitor these phenomena.

This chapter presents a review of the literature on countertransference with the hospitalized adolescent and delineates particular aspects of this phenomenon among interdisciplinary staff. Theory is clarified with a clinical vignette in which the outcome can be seen to be, at least in part, the result of the staff's lack of awareness of and, therefore, inability to monitor countertransference. In conclusion, we offer guidelines to acute inpatient settings to facilitate the recognition and modification of countertransference so that brief hospitalization may become a more therapeutic intervention.

Gartner (1985) has noted a dearth of literature on countertransference reactions to adolescents as opposed to adults. Halperin, Lauro, Muscone, Rebhan, Schnabolk, and Schachter (1981) have indicated that discussions of countertransference regarding children and adolescents are rare for residential treatment programs and "almost nonexistent" for transitional treatment centers. To the best of our knowledge, there have been no reports in the literature about staff countertransference during the acute psychiatric hospitalization of the adolescent. Halperin et al. (1981) view brief stays as protective against the emergence of countertransference, assuming that the short-term nature of an acute stay does not allow staff to develop relationships that lead to unconscious reactions or intense affect. They argue that staff objectivity is more easily maintained in a short-term setting. On the contrary, we have found that equally intense countertransference evolves within staff who work with adolescents during an acute hospitalization. Furthermore, we believe that the unique constraints and demands of a brief hospitalization may actually heighten the intensity of countertransference reactions.

Adolescents who are initially separated from their families during the beginning of a brief hospital stay tend to experience a two-week "honeymoon" period, which is characterized by a diminution of acting-out behavior and symptomatology. This "calm before the storm" is a phase of hospitalization in which the staff's loving feelings predominate, marking the positive countertransference phase. The adolescent's poor impulse control, low frustration tolerance, and rapidly fluctuating behavior and symptomatology gradually evolve after the calm, which can trigger the emergence of staff negative countertransference or what Maltzberger and Buie (1974) have described as "countertransference hate." The adolescent's acting-out behavior (the precipitant to the family seeking his or her admission to a psychiatric hospital) may create a replication of the pathological familial equilibrium. As Hinsie and Campbell (1970) have indicated, "although behavior patterns originate in family situations, the patient preserves that pattern throughout life." If staff members lack awareness of their unconscious positive and negative reactions to such adolescents' vulnerability and acting out, they are more likely to become engaged with the adolescent as proxy parents in a repetition of the pathogenic behavior that contributed to the patient's difficulties prior to hospitalization.

We believe it is crucial that countertransference reactions be addressed in a brief setting, since a psychiatric hospitalization can be seen as a crisis point in which specific but brief help given at a "strategic time is sometimes more effective than more extensive help given at a time of less emotional accessibility" (Rapoport 1962, p. 49). We view the division of evaluation and treatment as arbitrary and see the first stages of an acute hospitalization as an important step toward the establishment of a therapeutic alliance. It is during this phase that a and thoughts expressed about the self and the others were coherent and structured. It was rated as disturbed if thoughts and feelings of the self and others appeared somewhat incoherent. Too much internal structure was inferred if the subject presented as excessively defended and rigid, while too little structure was inferred if the subject presented with an "as if" quality and with unstable, empty, or amorphous features.

2. MAINTENANCE OF IDENTITY

Maintenance of identity was assessed as competent if the subject demonstrated an ability to maintain an organized independent inner world that allowed for the retention of an accurate perception of self and others in varied relationships and in varied circumstances. Disturbed maintenance of identity implied excessive fluctuation in mental representations of self and others in varied relationships and in varied circumstances.

3. RELATEDNESS

Relatedness was judged to be competent if the subject demonstrated some satisfying emotional involvement with others. In addition, some capacity for empathy and some ability to be sensitive to small and subtle cues in others while retaining self-differentiation was required. Relatedness was considered to be disturbed if the subject demonstrated an inability to establish or maintain satisfying emotional involvement with others. An impaired capacity for empathy with some inability to be sensitive to small and subtle cues in others also was required. Subjects with disturbed relatedness usually presented as either withdrawn from emotional relationships or as chameleonlike, with a tendency to merge with the needs or demands of others.

4. SELF-ESTEEM

Self-esteem was rated as competent if the subject demonstrated feelings of adequacy, worthfulness, self-acceptance, and self-confidence. It was rated as disturbed if the adolescent presented with feelings of inadequacy, self-doubt, self-depreciation, and worthlessness in the context of most relationships. For some adolescents, disturbance in self-esteem presented paradoxically with overestimation of the self.

369

5. VERBAL COMMUNICATION

Communication was rated as competent if the subject usually was able to communicate about the self and others with some coherence, precision, and discrimination. It was rated as disturbed if the subject demonstrated significant difficulty with communication about self and others. Disturbed communication appeared as sparse, inefficient, confused, garbled, illogical or, alternatively, as pedantic, overly precise, or repetitive.

6. REALITY TESTING REGARDING SELF AND OTHERS

Reality testing was rated as competent if the subject demonstrated a moderately developed awareness of the feelings and thoughts of self and others. The subject was expected to show an ability to differentiate his or her own thoughts and feelings from those of important others. Reality testing was rated as disturbed if the subject demonstrated moderate to marked distortion regarding the thoughts and feelings of others and/or moderate to marked difficulty with the accurate awareness of a personal, internal world of feelings, impulses, and fantasies.

7. ROLE ASSUMPTION

Competence in role assumption reflected an average degree of flexibility in assuming a variety of roles (student, child, employee, friend, etc.). The subject was expected to show a usual degree of willingness to assume age-appropriate roles. Developed role aspirations were required to be moderately realistic for age, capabilities, and social context. Role assumption was rated as disturbed if the subject demonstrated moderate to marked difficulty with role flexibility, an unwillingness to assume age-appropriate roles, and inappropriate role aspirations. Subjects with disturbed role assumption appeared either as ineffectual, that is, somewhat lacking in the ability to function, or as stereotypical, that is, "playing" a role or expecting others to "play" expected roles.

Reliability

The interrater reliability of ratings on these items was derived using the statistic Kappa (Cohen 1960). All items yielded a Kappa indicating that agreements were significantly greater than chance, with an average Kappa of 0.63. Since all children were rated by both psychiatrists, the ultimate rating used was their average score.

Data Analysis

Differences between the three groups of adolescents and changes over time were examined with multivariate analyses of variance with repeated measures (group × sex × year). Significant multivariate differences were followed using univariate analyses of variance with repeated measures (group × sex × year). Consistency over time on specific scales was assessed using Pearson product-moment correlations between scores obtained at age thirteen and at age sixteen. Association between the group status of the adolescents at age thirteen and age sixteen was determined using a chi-square test.

Results

The present report examines personality functioning in a nonclinical sample of teenagers during middle adolescence (age sixteen). Ratings of these functions enabled personality classification into the following three categories: clear of disturbance, some disturbance, or marked disturbance. The results of this classification are reported for middle adolescence. In addition, consistencies and changes from early adolescence to middle adolesence are highlighted.

CLASSIFICATION INTO PERSONALITY FUNCTIONING GROUPS

The presence of disturbance in personality functioning was determined on the basis of ratings on the seven items in the Personality Functions Rating Scale. These seven items were found to constitute an internally consistent scale (Cronbach's alpha = 0.92). For each child, the number of functions rated as disturbed was determined. Subsequently, the distribution of scores on these seven functions was examined (0 indicating no disturbance in personality functions and 7 indicating disturbance in all areas). Children obtaining scores of 1 or 0 were classified as clear of personality function disturbance. Those with scores between 2 and 5 were classified as showing some disturbance, while those with scores of 6 or 7 were classified as showing marked personality function disturbance.

PREVALENCE OF PERSONALITY DISTURBANCE AT AGE SIXTEEN

The distribution of scores of the middle adolescents on the seven items described above is presented in figure 1. The prevalence of personality functions disturbance in the sample and the estimates for the sampling population are presented in table 2.

These results indicate that during middle adolescence, the majority—about two-thirds of the sample—were found to be clear of personality function disturbance. The remaining one-third were divided almost evenly between a group that manifested some disturbance and a group displaying marked disturbance.

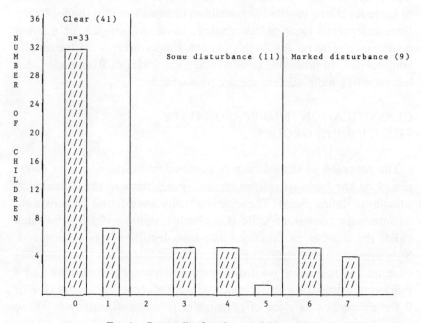

FIG. 1.—Personality functions variable scores

TABLE 2
PREVALENCE OF PERSONALITY FUNCTIONING DISTURBANCE
IN MIDDLE ADOLESCENCE

| | PERSONALITY CLASSIFICATION | | |
	Clear (%)	Some Disturbance (%)	Marked Disturbance (%)
Sample proportion (N = 61)	67.2	18.0	14.8
Population estimate (N = 540)	68.6	15.8	15.6

CONSISTENCY OR CHANGE IN PERSONALITY FUNCTIONING STATUS BETWEEN AGES THIRTEEN AND SIXTEEN

The overall level of competence in personality functioning was compared between early and middle adolescence. The group as a whole demonstrated significantly greater competence during middle adolescence than in early adolescence, as measured by the total personality functions scale scores ($F[1,59] = 9.32, p > .003$). The average total scores on the personality functions scale assessed at the two ages are presented in table 3.

It is noteworthy that the increase in competence indicated by the change in total scores is also reflected by the number of subjects assessed to be clear of personality disturbance during middle adolescence. At age sixteen, 67 percent of the sample were clear of disturbance, compared to only 54 percent that were so assessed at age thirteen.

Comparisons were also made of specific personality functions assessed at both ages thirteen and sixteen; these results are presented in table 4.

TABLE 3
TOTAL SCORES ON THE PERSONALITY
FUNCTION SCALE

| | 1979 | | 1982 | |
	Mean	SD	Mean	SD
Whole sample	26.8	5.4	28.7	4.7
Male	26.0	5.5	27.6	4.9
Female	27.8	5.1	29.7	4.2

NOTE.—Scores range from 0 to 35, with a high score indicating competence in personality functioning.

TABLE 4

COMPARISONS OF PERSONALITY FUNCTIONS IN 1979 AND 1982

	1979		1982		
VARIABLE	Mean	SD	Mean	SD	SIGNIFICANCE
Maintenance of identity	3.9	1.0	4.2	.9	.046
Reality testing	3.9	1.0	4.3	.9	.011
Relatedness	3.9	.9	4.2	.7	.037
Verbal communication	3.9	.8	4.2	.7	.002
Self-esteem	3.8	.8	4.1	.8	.018
Identity crystallization	3.7	1.0	4.0	.9	N.S.
Role assumption	3.7	.8	3.8	.8	N.S.

Competence in all personality functions except role assumption increased from early to middle adolescence. With maturity, adolescents showed an increased ability to maintain identity, to test reality regarding self and others, to communicate, to maintain identity in varied relationships and circumstances, and to demonstrate improved self-esteem. Although identity crystallization also tended to improve, this was less predictable. No increase in competence was noted in role assumption, which suggests that confidence and willingness to assume different behaviors in different situations remains problematic in accord with a developmental period that is filled with progressively changing social expectations and demands. There were no differences between boys and girls with respect to any particular personality function.

We were also interested in the consistency of individuals in personality functioning from early to middle adolescence. The subjects were found to be moderately consistent in their competence in personality functioning between the two ages, as measured by the total scores on the personality functions scale ($R[61] = 0.60$, $p < .0001$). Similarly, there was modest to moderate consistency on each of the individual personality functions. The greatest consistency was in relatedness and the least was in identity crystallization. These results are presented in table 5.

In order to provide a clearer picture of change or consistency in personality functioning between early and middle adolescence, the subjects were reclassified into three groups: (1) stable clear—those adolescents clear of disturbance at both ages; (2) stable disturbed—those adolescents rated as demonstrating some or marked disturbance at both ages; and (3) fluctuating—those adolescents who were clear of disturbance at one age but presented with some or marked disturbance

TABLE 5
CONSISTENCY IN PERSONALITY FUNCTIONS FROM EARLY
TO MIDDLE ADOLESCENCE

Variable	Pearson Product-Moment Correlation	Significance
Total scale score	.60	.0001
Relatedness..................................	.51	.0001
Role assumption	.47	.0001
Maintenance of identity	.44	.0001
Verbal communication	.40	.001
Self-esteem	.32	.006
Reality testing	.32	.007
Identity crystallization	.28	.015

at the other age. The results of this reclassification are presented in table 6.

This reclassification indicated that about half of the sample (47.5 percent) were stable clear, about one-quarter (24.6 percent) were stable disturbed, and about one-quarter (27.9 percent) fluctuated between presenting as disturbed and as clear. No significant differences were found between girls and boys in their tendency to be stable or to fluctuate.

Conclusions

The results reported above indicate that, when studied in cross-section, more than half of the adolescents appear clear of personality

TABLE 6
STABILITY OR CHANGE IN PERSONALITY
FUNCTIONING STATUS FROM AGE THIRTEEN
TO AGE SIXTEEN

	SEX		
GROUP	Male	Female	TOTAL
Stable clear	12	17	29 (47.5)
Fluctuating	8	9	17 (27.9)
Stable disturbed	11	4	15 (24.6)

NOTE.—Numbers in parentheses represent percentages.

disturbance at two developmental subphases—early (54 percent) and middle (67 percent). However, when studied longitudinally, more than half (52.5 percent) of the adolescents experience moderate to marked personality difficulties at some point in their development. Of this group, 24.6 percent demonstrate some or marked disturbance, which persists from age thirteen to age sixteen; 10 percent were consistently rated as markedly disturbed; and 27.9 percent demonstrate fluctuation, appearing clear of disturbance at one age and showing some or marked disturbance at another age. These data lend support to the position that while adolescent turmoil is not a universal phenomenon, it is widespread, influencing about one out of every four adolescents (Rutter, Graham, Chadwick, and Yule 1976).

The adolescents in our study demonstrated greater difficulties in personality functioning during their early adolescence than during middle adolescence. In middle adolescence, there was an increase in the number of adolescents assessed as clear of disturbance. In addition, for the sample as a whole, there was a significant increase in overall ratings of personality function competence. Individual functions also appeared less disturbed during middle adolescence. These findings suggest that early adolescence may represent a transitional phase of development accompanied by heightened stresses that affect personality organization in the vulnerable child. Middle adolescence may represent a period of calm and increased maturity.

In our population, potential stresses at early adolescence include the onset of puberty, the change from elementary to high school with the accompanying introduction to a different system of instruction, new friendships and new teachers, and the often sudden confrontation with significantly different "adolescent" role expectations.

Most interesting is the finding that 47.5 percent of the subjects remained clear of personality function disturbance from early to middle adolescence. To the best of our knowledge, these adolescents never experienced turmoil, did not demonstrate persistent or excessive anxiety or depression, were well related, had good role differentiation, and were secure in their established identity. This group seemed remarkably untroubled by their passage from middle childhood into middle adolescence. Two alternative explanations for this impressive course of development come to mind. These youngsters may represent a particularly "invulnerable" group capable of progressing with smooth personality development even within average expectable adverse environmental and family influences. Alternatively, this group may have

376

been "privileged" to an exceptionally growth-enhancing environment, unusually protected from significantly disturbing "life" events. An analysis of family data and life circumstances should help clarify this issue and will be the subject of a future report.

NOTE

This study was supported by a grant from the Ministry of Community and Social Services, Ontario, Canada. Dr. Harvey Golombek, principal investigator of the Toronto Adolescent Longitudinal Study, was supported by a Continuing Education Award from the Laidlaw Foundation, which allowed for his appointment as Visiting Scholar at the Maudsley Hospital, London, England (1985–1986); this appointment greatly facilitated the publication of this research. This work could not have been done without the continuing assistance of the Etobicoke Board of Education, Toronto, Ontario. We are also indebted to the adolescents and their families for their cooperation and interest and to Ms. S. Allon, social worker, and Mrs. M. Churchard, research assistant, for their invaluable contributions.

REFERENCES

Bowlby, J. 1982. Attachment and loss: retrospect and prospect. *American Journal of Ortho Psychiatry* 52(4): 664–678.

Cohen, J. 1960. A coefficient of agreement for nominal scales. *Educational and Psychological Measurement* 20:37–46.

Giovacchini, P., and Borowitz, G. 1974. An object relationships scale. *Adolescent Psychiatry* 3:186–195.

Golombek, H.; Marton, P.; Stein, B.; and Korenblum, M. 1986a. Personality dysfunction and behavioral disturbance in early adolescence. *Journal of the American Academy of Child Psychiatry* 25:697–703.

Golombek, H.; Marton, P.; Stein, B.; and Korenblum, M. 1986b. A study of disturbed and nondisturbed adolescents: The Toronto Adolescent Longitudinal Study. I. *Canadian Journal of Psychiatry* 31:532–535.

Rutter, M.; Graham, P.; Chadwick, O.; and Yule, W. 1976. Adolescent turmoil: fact or fiction? *Journal of Child Psychology and Psychiatry* 17:35–56.

Solnit, A. 1986. Object constancy and early triadic relationships. *Journal of the American Academy of Child Psychiatry* 25(1): 23–29.

377

24 PERSONALITY FUNCTIONING AND CHANGE IN CLINICAL PRESENTATION FROM EARLY TO MIDDLE ADOLESCENCE

BERNARD STEIN, HARVEY GOLOMBEK, PETER MARTON, AND MARSHALL KORENBLUM

The division of personality development in adolescence into early, middle, and late segments hypothesizes different tasks, stresses, conflicts, vulnerability, and presentation for each stage. Yet the sometimes subtle but significant distinguishing characteristics of each stage have not been clearly described or agreed upon (Douvan and Adelson 1966). The period of early adolescence has been described in psychoanalytic theory as an inevitably tumultuous period arising from the heightening of sexual and aggressive drives associated with pubescence. This is said to result in rebelliousness, regressive behavior associated with primitive defenses, and a deterioration of positive family relationships. At the same time, a mistrust of adults and a turning toward peers as a main source are described.

Middle adolescence has been labeled "adolescence proper," a time for consolidating the personality structures built up since childhood (Miller 1974) and searching for physical, social, sexual, and intellectual competence (Solnit 1983). There are differing opinions concerning the amount of inner turmoil and degree of resolution of the struggle for independence from parents during middle adolescence. Some (Esman 1984) see it as a period where there is some stabilization with less regressive potential, less rigid defenses, and a more secure sense of autonomy. Although there remains a deep involvement with peers, a revision of the intense, earlier, ambivalent attachment to parents takes place permitting the middle adolescent to be able to again turn to parents for support. Shifting moods and dysphoria are viewed as "normal" manifestations of growth, maturation, and object loss. Another view (Miller 1974) asserts that the middle adolescent still experiences much inner turmoil, which manifests itself in negativistic antisocial behavior, withdrawal, and uncommunicativeness toward parents. At the same time, cognition may be more analytical, objective, and reality oriented (Blos 1962).

Some investigators (Moriarity and Toussieng 1976) have found puberty to be followed by a brief rebellious period, usually over by age fifteen, and then succeeded by an emotionally serene period marked by the adolescent's turning toward the world and avoiding alienation from parents. The rebellious feeling and excessive mood swings so often associated with all of adolescence were found only in early adolescence, and the stabilization in mid adolescence was accomplished with the support of peers and a more refined coping style. Although some studies (Coleman 1980) have shown a shift to a greater interest in peers, others (Greenberg, Siegel, and Leitch 1983) have found that the quality of attachment to parents was significantly more powerful than that to peers in predicting good functioning throughout adolescence, and that these qualities of attachment did not shift significantly from early to middle adolescence.

Another way of examining the stability and consistency of personality features through adolescence has been through the investigation of specific aspects such as self-esteem and self-concept over time (Hauser, Jacobson, Noam, and Powers 1983). Again, there have been reports of both consistency and change. Some have found a relative stability of self-image (Engel 1959) from early to mid adolescence, while others (Piers and Harris 1964) found a drop in self-esteem in early adolescence compared to both latency and middle adolescence.

In an earlier paper (Stein, Golombek, Marton, and Korenblum 1986) describing the findings from psychiatric interviews of a nonclinical group of early adolescents, we reported that the majority demonstrated competent functioning with minimal dysphoria, positive attitudes that promote cooperation, self-awareness, and satisfaction in day-to-day living, the use of higher level defense mechanisms, and good involvement with peers and parental figures. This is in contrast with a minority who were more stereotypical of the concept of adolescent turmoil and demonstrated significantly more dysphoria, negative attitudes, more primitive defense mechanisms, and distant relationships with peers and parents.

The present study was undertaken to describe the clinical presentation and personality functioning in a sample of middle adolescents and to determine whether these observations are consistent over the period from early to middle adolescence.

Method

The procedure was the same as that reported in detail in Golombek, Marton, Stein, and Korenblum (1987). We employed a semistructured interview based on an object relations scale originally created by Giovacchini and Borowitz (1974) and modified for our purposes. This allowed for the subsequent rating of mental status phenomena (eight items), personality traits (ten items), mental mechanisms of defense (fourteen items), and personality functions (seven items). Degree of interest in significant others was also rated. Over the three-year period, only two of the sixty-three adolescents were lost from the sample, which therefore remained quite intact. The sex distribution also remained equal—thirty boys and thirty-one girls (see table 1).

Data Analysis

The ratings of clinical presentation on the personality functions scale at age thirteen and at age sixteen were examined. The method of analysis has been previously described (see Golombek et al. 1987). These analyses enabled us to determine the changes in the degree to which

TABLE 1
CHARACTERISTICS OF STUDY SAMPLE

	N
Gender:	
Male	31
Female	30
Socioeconomic status:	
Upper third	6
Middle third	18
Lower third	37

our sample, as a whole, displayed these personality functions at each of the two ages and also the degree to which the rating at one age predicted the rating obtained at the other.

Having identified the developmental changes that take place from early to middle adolescence for boys and girls, we examined next the features that distinguished the clinical presentation of those adolescents who throughout the period of early to middle adolescence were found to be clear of personality function disturbance, those who were found to manifest disturbance at both phases, and those who were found to manifest disturbance at only one phase. We then determined which of the items in the personality functions scale best differentiated among the three groups of adolescents using a discriminant functions analysis. This analysis combines the variables in a way that best differentiates among the groups and also indicates the relative contribution of each variable in differentiating among the groups. Thus, it is possible to identify those variables on which the groups can best be differentiated.

Closer examination of the early adolescents indicated that of those teenagers ($n = 27$) who manifested personality function disturbance at thirteen, a little over half ($n = 15$) continued to manifest disturbance in middle adolescence, while the remainder became clear of disturbance. We examined the data to determine which features of their clinical presentation at age thirteen would differentiate the two groups three years later in middle adolescence.

Results

As presented (see Golombek et al. 1987), teenagers during both early and middle adolescence can be differentiated into three groups according to competence or disturbance in personality functioning. At age thirteen, 54 percent were clear of personality disturbance, 21 percent demonstrated some disturbance, and 25 percent demonstrated marked disturbance in personality functioning.

At age sixteen, our sample presented as having more competent personality functioning overall, with 67 percent being clear of disturbance, 18 percent demonstrating some disturbance, and 15 percent demonstrating marked disturbance. This pattern of results was similar for boys and girls, and, as previously reported, the girls were not rated as demonstrating more or less competence in personality functioning.

GROUP CHANGES FROM EARLY TO
MIDDLE ADOLESCENCE

There were significant differences in mental status phenomena from early to middle adolescence ($F[1,48] = 6.08, p < .0001$).[1] The sixteen-year-olds were more verbally coherent, affectionate, and experienced more pleasure and less anxiety and depression. These results are presented in detail in table 2. For the most part, the subjects remained fairly constant in their personality traits, although the sixteen-year-olds were significantly more optimistic and introspective ($F[1,46] = 5.12$, $p < .0001$). These results are presented in table 3.

TABLE 2

CHANGE IN MENTAL STATUS PHENOMENA FROM EARLY
TO MIDDLE ADOLESCENCE

Variable	Age 13	Age 16	Significance*
Verbal coherence	3.3	3.7	.0001
	(.6)	(.5)	
Depression	2.2	1.7	.0001
	(.9)	(.9)	
Anxiety	3.3	2.8	.001
	(.7)	(.9)	
Affection	2.8	3.1	.001
	(.8)	(.7)	
Pleasure	3.0	3.2	.05
	(.6)	(1.6)	

NOTE.—Data in cols. 1 and 2 represent mean scale scores, with standard deviations in parentheses.
* Analysis of variance.

TABLE 3

CHANGE IN PERSONALITY TRAITS FROM EARLY
TO MIDDLE ADOLESCENCE

Variable	Age 13	Age 16	Significance*
Introspectiveness	2.0	2.6	.0001
	(.8)	(.6)	
Optimism	3.0	3.2	.006
	(.8)	(.7)	

NOTE.—Data in cols. 1 and 2 represent mean scale scores, with standard deviations in parentheses.
* Analysis of variance.

At age sixteen, the teenagers manifested an overall decrease in the use of a variety of defense mechanisms. Significantly less use was made of isolation, substitution, repression, somatization, projection, and denial. These results are presented in table 4. At age sixteen, the subjects were found to demonstrate a greater interest in significant others than at age thirteen ($F[1,37] = 2.48, p < .029$). Specifically, the middle adolescents were found to show greater interest in their mothers and also an increase in the greatest amount of interest shown toward any significant person in their lives. These results are presented in table 5.

TABLE 4

CHANGE IN MENTAL MECHANISMS OF DEFENSE FROM EARLY
TO MIDDLE ADOLESCENCE

Variable	Age 13	Age 16	Significance*
Isolation	2.4	1.4	.00001
	(1.1)	(.5)	
Substitution	3.4	2.8	.0001
	(.8)	(.9)	
Repression	3.5	3.1	.001
	(.7)	(.8)	
Somatization	1.3	1.0	.003
	(.7)	(.1)	
Projection	2.8	2.3	.007
	(1.3)	(1.1)	
Denial	3.3	3.0	.016
	(1.0)	(1.0)	

NOTE.—Data in cols. 1 and 2 represent mean scale scores, with standard deviations in parentheses.
* Analysis of variance.

TABLE 5

CHANGE IN INTEREST IN SIGNIFICANT OTHERS FROM EARLY
TO MIDDLE ADOLESCENCE

Variable	Age 13	Age 16	Significance*
Mother	3.2	3.5	.003
	(.5)	(.6)	
Highest interest in anyone	3.6	3.8	.029
	(.5)	(.5)	

NOTE.—Data in cols. 1 and 2 represent mean scale scores, with standard deviations in parentheses.
* Analysis of variance.

The findings presented thus far reflect changes associated with maturation and indicate that indeed the clinical presentation alters from early to middle adolescence.

CHANGES IN INDIVIDUALS FROM EARLY TO MIDDLE ADOLESCENCE

Having established that there are group developmental changes reflected in the average level of functioning of sixteen-year-olds as compared to thirteen-year-olds, we wished to describe the degree of change or consistency in the clinical presentation of individuals between the two ages. Examination of the correlation of the ratings obtained by individuals at the two ages on the four scales of the personality function scale indicated that there was a moderate amount of consistency such that it was possible to predict on the basis of presentation at age thirteen how an individual would present at sixteen. There was more consistency in mental status features and personality traits than in the degree of use of specific defense mechanisms or degree of interest in significant others. The specific correlation coefficients are presented in tables 6, 7, and 8.

TABLE 6
CONSISTENCY FROM AGE THIRTEEN TO AGE SIXTEEN

Variable	Correlation	Significance
Mental status phenomena	.47	.0001
Personality traits	.60	.0001

TABLE 7
CONSISTENCY IN DEFENSES FROM AGE THIRTEEN
TO AGE SIXTEEN

Variable	Correlation	Significance
Denial	.46	.0001
Withdrawal	.43	.0001
Projection	.43	.0001
Substitution	.33	.004
Rationalization	.29	.01

TABLE 8
CONSISTENCY IN INTEREST IN SIGNIFICANT OTHERS FROM AGE
THIRTEEN TO AGE SIXTEEN

Variable	Correlation	Significance
Sibling	.41	.001
Interviewer	.40	.001
Father	.36	.002

DIFFERENCES IN PERSONALITY FUNCTION COMPETENCE

In order to investigate further the relationship between competence in personality functioning and clinical presentation, we examined those characteristics that differentiate three groups of adolescents: those who were consistently clear of disturbance ($n = 29$), those who were consistently disturbed ($n = 15$), and those who experienced disturbance at only one developmental phase ($n = 17$). The three groups were found to differ in mental status phenomena ($F[2,96] = 6.06, p < .00001$). The consistently clear group presented as more competent than those who were consistently disturbed, while the fluctuating group fell in between. Differences were observed in the following areas: verbal quantity and coherence, anxiety, depression, pleasure, affection, and hate. These results are presented in table 9.

There was also a difference in personality traits among the three groups ($F[2,92] = 3.70, p < .0001$). The consistently clear group was found to be more cooperative, curious, approving, optimistic, and introspective. These results are presented in table 10.

The three groups differed in their use of defenses ($F[2,84] = 3.78, p < .0001$). The consistently clear group was found to use more identification and omnipotent idealization; the consistently disturbed group used more denial, projection, withdrawal, isolation, and masochistic surrender. These results are presented in table 11.

The three groups of adolescents were also found to differ in their interest in significant others ($F[2,74] = 2.19, p < .012$). The consistently clear group showed more interest in their mothers, fathers, peers, and the interviewer as well as having a higher average amount of interest in all significant others. These results are presented in table 12.

385

TABLE 9

MENTAL STATUS PHENOMENA ASSOCIATED WITH CHANGE IN PERSONALITY
FUNCTIONS FROM EARLY TO MIDDLE ADOLESCENCE

Variable	Stable Clear ($N=29$)	Stable Disturbed ($N=15$)	Unstable Fluctuating ($N=17$)	Significance*
Verbal coherence	3.7	3.1	3.4	.0001
	(.3)	(.4)	(.5)	
Depression	1.6	2.6	1.9	.0001
	(.7)	(.8)	(.9)	
Pleasure	3.3	2.7	3.1	.0001
	(.5)	(.5)	(.5)	
Affection	3.3	2.3	3.0	.0001
	(.6)	(.5)	(.7)	
Verbal quantity	3.2	2.6	3.4	.002
	(.6)	(.8)	(1.0)	
Anxiety	2.8	3.5	3.0	.002
	(.7)	(.6)	(.8)	
Hate	2.2	3.0	2.5	.002
	(.7)	(.8)	(.9)	

NOTE.—Data in cols. 1–3 represent mean scale scores, with standard deviations in parentheses.

* Analysis of variance.

TABLE 10

PERSONALITY TRAITS ASSOCIATED WITH CHANGE IN PERSONALITY
FUNCTIONS FROM EARLY TO MIDDLE ADOLESCENCE

Variable	Stable Clear ($N=29$)	Stable Disturbed ($N=15$)	Unstable Fluctuating ($N=17$)	Significance*
Cooperativeness	3.6	2.8	3.5	.0001
	(.5)	(.6)	(.6)	
Curiosity	3.2	2.3	3.1	.0001
	(.5)	(.6)	(.8)	
Approval	3.5	2.3	3.2	.0001
	(.6)	(.7)	(.7)	
Optimism	3.4	2.4	3.2	.0001
	(.6)	(.6)	(.7)	
Introspectiveness	2.6	1.7	2.2	.0001
	(.6)	(.5)	(.7)	

NOTE.—Data in cols. 1–3 represent mean scale scores, with standard deviations in parentheses.

* Analysis of variance.

386

TABLE 11
MENTAL MECHANISMS OF DEFENSE ASSOCIATED WITH CHANGE IN
PERSONALITY FUNCTIONS FROM EARLY TO MIDDLE ADOLESCENCE

Variable	Stable Clear $(N=29)$	Stable Disturbed $(N=15)$	Unstable Fluctuating $(N=17)$	Significance*
Withdrawal	2.2	3.7	2.6	.0001
	(.8)	(1.1)	(1.1)	
Projection	2.1	3.4	2.6	.0001
	(1.0)	(1.1)	(1.3)	
Denial	2.6	3.9	3.4	.0001
	(1.0)	(.6)	(.8)	
Isolation	1.7	2.4	1.7	.002
	(.7)	(.8)	(.8)	
Identification	3.6	3.1	3.6	.005
	(.6)	(.7)	(.6)	
Omnipotent idealization	2.4	1.7	2.0	.009
	(1.0)	(.8)	(1.0)	
Masochistic surrender	1.9	2.4	2.1	.014
	(.8)	(.8)	(.9)	

NOTE.—Data in cols. 1–3 represent mean scale scores, with standard deviations in parentheses.
* Analysis of variance.

TABLE 12
INTEREST IN SIGNIFICANT OTHERS ASSOCIATED WITH CHANGE IN
PERSONALITY FUNCTIONS FROM EARLY TO MIDDLE ADOLESCENCE

Variable	Stable Clear $(N=29)$	Stable Disturbed $(N=15)$	Unstable Fluctuating $(N=17)$	Significance*
Mother	3.5	3.0	3.4	.0001
	(.5)	(.5)	(.6)	
Father	3.1	2.4	3.1	.0001
	(.7)	(.7)	(.8)	
Interviewer	3.1	2.2	3.0	.0001
	(.4)	(.5)	(.9)	
Average interest	3.0	2.6	3.1	.001
	(.3)	(.3)	(.4)	
Peers	3.4	2.7	3.5	.003
	(.7)	(.8)	(.6)	

NOTE.—Data in cols. 1–3 represent mean scale scores, with standard deviations in parentheses.
* Analysis of variance.

The same difference between the three groups was found at both ages thirteen and sixteen, with the single exception that in the consistently disturbed group, younger adolescents were more domineering than older adolescents. Girls and boys were found to show the same pattern of results.

The discriminant function analysis of personality variables revealed that at age thirteen the following variables best differentiated the three groups: the qualities of introspectiveness, approval, interest in peers, interest in mother, and pleasure, which are associated with competent personality functioning, and hate, denial, and projection, which are associated with personality disturbance. At age sixteen, the three groups were best differentiated by the qualities of verbal coherence, interest in the interviewer, introspectiveness, pleasure, and optimism, which are associated with competent personality functioning, and verbal quantity, hate, isolation, and pessimism, which are associated with personality disturbance.

Having established that there were differences in clinical presentation associated with personality competence, we wished to identify those characteristics that would be associated with the development of more competent functioning over time. We determined which aspects of clinical presentation of disturbed adolescents at age thirteen would differentiate those subjects who would continue to be disturbed at age sixteen ($n = 15$) from those who would develop competent functioning ($n = 12$). These results are presented in table 13.

The comparison indicated that among the mental status phenomena, the one differentiating factor was that the consistently disturbed adolescents were more depressed at age thirteen. Also, those adolescents who would develop more competent functioning in middle adolescence differed in personality traits assessed at age thirteen; they were more affectionate, cooperative, approving of others, optimistic, and intellectually curious. The consistently disturbed adolescents were found to use more denial and projection as defense mechanisms. The only difference observed in their interest in significant others was that the adolescents who became more competent were more interested in their peers. We also examined whether the two groups differed in any of the specific personality functions. The only difference was that those who became more competent had better relatedness—the ability to establish satisfying intimate relationships with others.

TABLE 13
CHARACTERISTICS DIFFERENTIATING EARLY ADOLESCENTS WHO STAY
DISTURBED FROM THOSE WHO IMPROVE IN MIDDLE ADOLESCENCE

Variable	Improve ($N = 12$)	Stay Disturbed ($N = 15$)	Significance*
Affection	2.9	2.1	.002
	(.8)	(.5)	
Depression	2.3	3.0	.03
	(1.1)	(.7)	
Cooperativeness	3.5	2.8	.007
	(.7)	(.6)	
Approval	3.1	2.3	.011
	(.8)	(.6)	
Optimism	2.9	2.3	.033
	(.9)	(.6)	
Curiosity	2.9	2.2	.046
	(1.2)	(.6)	
Denial	3.7	4.1	.048
	(.7)	(.5)	
Projection	2.8	3.9	.059
	(1.6)	(1.1)	
Peers	3.2	2.7	.041
	(.6)	(.6)	
Relatedness	3.4	2.9	.016
	(.5)	(.5)	

NOTE.—Data in cols. 1 and 2 represent mean scale scores, with standard deviations in parentheses.
* Analysis of variance.

Discussion

Over the three-year period from early to mid adolescence, the proportion of teenagers clear of personality disturbance rose from 54 percent to 67 percent, and the proportion of those with marked disturbance fell from 25 percent to 15 percent, indicating greater overall competence for middle adolescents as a group. These subjects appeared to improve in their mood and communication pattern rather than experience more difficulties. These findings support the views of others (Esman 1984; Moriarity and Toussieng 1976) who have found middle adolescence to be a period of stabilization with less dysphoria and less disturbance.

Along with the changes in mental status phenomena, the changes in defense mechanisms suggest an overall decrease in the need to defend

389

against unacceptable drives and feelings. Middle adolescents are better able to cope and have a defensive style that is more adaptive and reality oriented.

Certain aspects, however, remain more consistent over time than others. Overall personality traits and attitudes are fairly consistent over time, with the exception that, again, middle adolescents improve in their adaptation; they are more optimistic and introspective than younger adolescents. Therefore, the changes that occur over time are in the direction of better coping.

The consistency in relatedness to peers, fathers, siblings, and the interviewer suggests a stability in these relationships over time. Peers have become important to early adolescents and remain so three years later. Closeness or distance to fathers does not need to change because this relationship has not been as intense as that with the mother. Therefore, adolescents do not appear to have to reconsider this relationship in terms of closeness or internal significance. The change in relatedness to mothers supports the hypothesis of a rapprochement and a resolution of that earlier ambivalent attitude. Middle adolescents no longer have to fight for a fragile sense of autonomy and can acknowledge affection for and closeness with their mothers. This appears to be the case for both boys and girls in our sample.

The period of middle adolescence, therefore, can be viewed as a period when teenagers regain a sense of being comfortable with both themselves and others; along with maturation comes a greater facility for coping and adaptation.

It is of interest that an individual adolescent will be more consistent in his phenomenological appearance and manifest attitudes over time than in his use of defenses or interest in others. The younger adolescent who is anxious, depressed, and angry, with little affection, is likely to be similar three years later, when he or she is through pubescence. Also, a domineering, disapproving, pessimistic attitude is likely to be present three years later, contributing to dysfunctional interactions. On the other hand, a positive appearance and attitude adopted in early adolescence usually continues into middle adolescence.

One characteristic in early adolescence that seems most clearly to distinguish competent from disturbed functioning is a higher degree of interest in both peers and mother. Competent adolescents do not feel the need to abandon one in favor of the other as do disturbed adolescents who have problems with separation and individuation. Also, at this age, we see the effects of more primitive defense mechanisms as powerful discriminating factors. In middle adolescence, verbal presentation emerges as an important factor differentiating personality functioning. Competent adolescents are able to communicate clearly and coherently, while disturbed adolescents use a lot of verbiage that often clouds and distorts information defensively. It is of interest that introspectiveness, optimism, and pessimism are significant features that distinguish between competent and disturbed personality functioning in middle adolescents. This suggests that teenagers who are aware of themselves and their competence in personality functioning are realistically hopeful about their future, whereas those who are functioning less competently are less hopeful without understanding why.

Adolescents who are consistently competent in their personality functioning from age thirteen to sixteen are different from those who consistently show disturbance in a large number of areas in mental status, personality traits, defenses, and interest in significant others. This clearly illustrates the differences in clinical presentation of adolescents in relation to personality functioning and how competence or disturbance remains stable over time. However, the minority (28 percent) who shift in personality functioning present a challenge for the understanding of personality development in adolescence. This fluctuating or unstable group generally was rated intermediate between the stable clear group and the stable disturbed group. When there are subtle signs of personality disturbance, it is not easy to determine whether, over time, these will progress toward better or worse functioning. Obviously, there are other factors, both maturational and environmental, that may influence the direction of that growth.

The question of which adolescent manifesting personality disturbance at age thirteen continues to show disturbance at age sixteen and which goes on to more competent functioning is an important one. It is notable that the only mental status phenomenon that differentiates stably disturbed young adolescents from those who improve is the amount of depression. This affect may be the important criterion that is enduring and indicative of personality disturbance, in contrast to the other phenomena—such as anxiety, anger, and communication difficulty—that may be more related to the turmoil and change of early adolescence. The presence of depressive symptoms in nonclinical adolescents has recently been shown to be a significant predictor of depression and social problems in young adults (Kandel and Davies

391

1986). On the other hand, there are protecting factors that may point to an improvement in time—positive attitudes, few primitive defenses, and better peer relationships. The latter finding suggests that when there are personality problems in early adolescence, the presence of good peer relationships is a good prognostic indicator. This contrasts with other studies (Greenberg, Siegel, and Leitch 1983) that stress positive family relationships as a predictor of good functioning throughout adolescence.

Conclusions

These clinical interviews have demonstrated that there is both consistency and change between early and middle adolescence. As a group, there is better overall personality functioning in middle compared to early adolescence. Changes in mental status and defense mechanisms are in the direction of better functioning over time. Relationships generally remain stable, but middle adolescents are better able to be close to their mothers. The findings also suggest that a minority (20 percent) of adolescents manifest personality disturbance at age thirteen but not at age sixteen and may therefore represent that group labeled "early adolescent turmoil." Future reports will demonstrate to what degree there is further change or consistency in personality functioning as this nonclinical sample is studied during late adolescence.

NOTES

This study was supported by a grant from the Ministry of Community and Social Services, Ontario, Canada. This work could not have been done without the continuing assistance of the Etobicoke Board of Education, Toronto, Ontario. We are also indebted to the adolescents and their families for their cooperation and interest and to Ms. S. Allon, social worker, and Mrs. M. Churchard, research assistant, for their invaluable contribution.

1. The multivariate statistics are presented in the text, while the univariate significance levels are presented in the tables.

REFERENCES

Blos, P. 1962. *On Adolescence*. New York: Free Press.
Coleman, J. C. 1980. *The Nature of Adolescence*. New York: Methuen.

Douvan, E., and Adelson, J. 1966. *The Adolescent Experience*. New York: Wiley.

Engel, M. 1959. The stability of the self-concept in adolescence. *Journal of Abnormal Social Psychology* 58:74–83.

Esman, A. H. 1984. A developmental approach to the psychotherapy of adolescents. *Adolescent Psychiatry* 12:119–133.

Giovacchini, P. L., and Borowitz, G. H. 1974. An object relationship scale. *Adolescent Psychiatry* 3:186–212.

Golombek, H.; Marton, P.; Stein, B.; and Korenblum, M. 1987. Personality functioning status during early and middle adolescence. *Adolescent Psychiatry* (in this volume).

Greenberg, M. T.; Siegel, M. S.; and Leitch, C. J. 1983. The nature and importance of attachment relationships to parents and peers during adolescence. *Journal of Youth and Adolescence* 12(5): 373–386.

Hauser, S. T.; Jacobson, A. M.; Noam, G.; and Powers, S. 1983. Ego development and self-image complexity in early adolescence. *Archives of General Psychiatry* 40:325–332.

Kandel, D. B., and Davies, M. 1986. Adult sequelae of adolescent depressive symptoms. *Archives of General Psychiatry* 43:255–262.

Miller, D. 1974. *Adolescence: Psychology, Psychopathology and Psychotherapy*. New York: Jason Aaronson.

Moriarity, A. E., and Toussieng, P. W. 1976. *Adolescent Coping*. New York: Grune & Stratten.

Piers, E. V., and Harris, D. B. 1964. Age and other correlates of self-concept in children. *Journal of Education Psychology* 55:91–95.

Solnit, A. J. 1983. Obstacles and pathways in the journey from adolescence to parenthood. *Adolescent Psychiatry* 11:14–26.

Stein, B.; Golombek, H.; Marton, P.; and Korenblum, M. 1986. Personality functioning and clinical presentation in early adolescence. *Canadian Journal of Psychiatry* 31:536–541.

393

25 BEHAVIOR DISTURBANCE AND CHANGES IN PERSONALITY DYSFUNCTION FROM EARLY TO MIDDLE ADOLESCENCE

PETER MARTON, HARVEY GOLOMBEK, BERNARD STEIN,
AND MARSHALL KORENBLUM

Many of our models of psychopathology tend toward broad conceptualization and oversimplification. This is particularly true for child and adolescent psychological disturbance. The challenge for research is to account for the psychological complexity of children and adolescents as well as the dramatic changes that take place as individuals develop.

One limitation in this effort is that workers from different theoretical schools and different disciplines tend to ignore the models and findings in other areas. The reasons for this are obvious—the difficulties in bridging the boundaries are great. However, in order to begin to understand adolescent development it will be necessary to link different conceptual models and different methods of investigation.

In a modest attempt to meet this challenge, we have begun to examine the relation between dysfunction in personality and disturbance in behavior.

In a previous paper (Golombek, Marton, Stein, and Korenblum 1986a), we found that at age thirteen adolescents who were disturbed in personality functioning also had more behavior problems at home and in school. These behavior problems were indicative of immaturity, poor interpersonal relations, and ineffectiveness in task accomplishment. When examined cross-sectionally, adolescents with marked personality disturbance did not differ from adolescents with moderate disturbance or those clear of disturbance in behavior problems associated with conduct problems or hyperactivity. As we have continued to follow this cohort of adolescents from early to middle adolescence, we have become interested in tracing changes in behavior as a function of adolescent development. In addition, we are also interested in differentiating behavior patterns associated with disturbed and nondisturbed personality functioning.

Method

SUBJECTS

SAMPLE SELECTION

The study sample has been described in detail in a previous paper (Golombek, Marton, Stein, and Korenblum 1986b). In this chapter, we present data on the behavior of the sixty-one adolescents who were assessed at both ages thirteen and sixteen. It is useful to keep in mind that they were selected to be representative of the full range of behavioral disturbance presented by students enrolled in the regular education system.

PROTOCOL

In addition to the semistructured interviews that each adolescent underwent to assess their personality functioning, the mothers and teachers also completed behavior ratings of the adolescent each year. When the adolescents were age thirteen and sixteen, the mothers completed a seventy-six-item behavior checklist (Arnold and Smeltzer 1974). This scale assesses behavior problems organized around seven factors: unsocialized aggression, inattentive-unproductiveness, sociopathy, hyperactivity, withdrawal depression, somatic neuroticism, and sleep disturbance. As a more comprehensive checklist became available, we incorporated into the study the Achenbach Child Behavior Checklist (Achenbach and Edelbrock 1981), which the parents completed when their children were ages fourteen and sixteen. The Child Behavior Checklist assesses competence in activities, interpersonal relations, and school performance. In addition, it surveys by means of 118 items behavior problems organized into two major areas of functioning: internalizing problems (problems within the self) and externalizing prob-

395

lems (problems with others). The scale also taps a number of more specific areas, which are called narrow band factors. These factors are different for boys and girls.

At ages thirteen and sixteen, the teachers completed the thirty-nine-item Conners Behavior Rating Scale (Conners 1969). This scale enables the teacher to report on four areas of behavior problems: conduct problems, inattentiveness-passivity, tension-anxiety, and hyperactivity.

DATA ANALYSIS

The data were analyzed to answer three principal questions. (1) What changes take place from early to middle adolescence in the level and extent of behavior problems? (2) What types of behavior problems differentiate adolescents who are consistently clear of personality disturbance, those who are consistently disturbed, and those whose disturbance is transitory? (3) Of those adolescents who experience personality disturbance in early adolescence, what aspects of behavior differentiate those whose disturbance is transitory from those whose disturbance is long lasting?

The adolescents in the sample were divided into three groups on the basis of their personality functioning: adolescents who were consistently clear, adolescents who were consistently disturbed, and those who experienced disturbance at only one of the two ages. In order to examine changes over time between early and middle adolescence as well as to determine whether the three groups differed in behavior, multivariate analyses of variance with repeated measures (group × sex × time) followed by univariate analyses of variance with repeated measures (group × sex × time) were carried out on each of the teacher and parent behavior rating scales. Multiple stepwise discriminant function analyses were used to determine which of the variables, on which there were significant differences between the groups, best differentiated among the three groups of adolescents at age thirteen and again at age sixteen. In order to examine differences between those adolescents who were disturbed in early adolescence but who improved to become clear in middle adolescence and those who were disturbed in early adolescence and who remained disturbed in middle adolescence, multivariate analyses of variance followed by univariate analyses of variance were carried out. For all analyses of variance, post hoc comparisons using the Scheffé test were used to examine differences between specific groups.

In order to assess consistency among individuals over time on the various behavioral scales, Pearson product-moment correlations were derived.

Results[1]

ADOLESCENT DEVELOPMENT AND CHANGES IN BEHAVIOR

Examination of changes in behavior of the students from ages thirteen to sixteen indicated that the middle adolescents were rated by both parents and teachers as being less disturbing than the thirteen-year-olds. The teachers reported that they observed fewer conduct problems. The parents reported on the Arnold and Smeltzer checklist that they observed fewer behavior problems in total and also on five of the seven factors in middle adolescence than during early adolescence. In middle adolescence the teenagers exhibited less unsocialized aggression, less antisocial behavior, they were less inattentive and unproductive, less hyperactive, and were less likely to make somatic complaints. These results are presented in table 1.

On the Achenbach Child Behavior Checklist, the sixteen-year-olds were rated by their mothers as having fewer problems in total, fewer

TABLE 1
CHANGES IN BEHAVIOR FROM EARLY
TO MIDDLE ADOLESCENCE

Conners Teacher's Behavior Rating Scale:
   Conduct problems

Arnold and Smeltzer Parent Behavior Checklist:
   Total score
   Unsocialized aggression
   Inattentive-unproductiveness
   Sociopathy
   Hyperactivity
   Somatic complaints

Achenbach Child Behavior Checklist:
   Total competence score
   Social competence score
   Total problems score
   Internalizing factor
   Externalizing factor

externalizing problems (problems with others), and fewer internalizing problems (problems within the self). Hence parents and teachers report that as adolescents mature from age thirteen to sixteen, they exhibit fewer behavior problems.

When we examined how consistent individual adolescents were from early to middle adolescence, we found that the parents reported a moderate amount of consistency in individuals over the two ages. However, the teachers' ratings indicated little consistency in classroom behavior. This suggests that the consistency in behavior problems can be attributed largely to consistency in the parent and the home situation. At school, the teacher, the classmates, and the environment change a great deal. These results are presented in table 2.

BEHAVIOR PROBLEMS ASSOCIATED WITH PERSONALITY DYSFUNCTION

We next examined whether behavior problems were associated with disturbance in personality functioning.

TABLE 2
CONSISTENCY OF BEHAVIOR FROM AGE THIRTEEN
TO SIXTEEN

Variable	Correlation
Conners Teacher's Behavior Rating Scale:	
Inattentive-passive	.33
Arnold and Smeltzer Parent Behavior Checklist:	
Unsocialized aggression	.83
Total score	.64
Sociopathy	.64
Somatic complaints	.60
Hyperactivity	.56
Inattentive-unproductiveness	.51
Achenbach Child Behavior Checklist:	
Total problems score	.80
Externalizing factor	.80
Internalizing factor	.75
Other problems	.53
Total competence score	.50
Activities....s18.	.31

BEHAVIOR AT SCHOOL

The teachers indicated differences in behavior problems among the three groups of adolescents—those who were consistently clear, those who were consistently disturbed, and those who fluctuated. Teachers identified the stable disturbed group as having the most behavior problems as well as exhibiting the most behaviors indicative of being inattentive or passive, having conduct problems, or experiencing tension or anxiety. These results are presented in table 3.

The teachers also differentiated the three groups of adolescents on a number of specific items. Again, the stable disturbed group was found to exhibit most problems on the items listed in table 4. The teachers

TABLE 3
BEHAVIOR ASSOCIATED WITH PERSONALITY
FUNCTIONS DISTURBANCE
IN EARLY AND MIDDLE ADOLESCENCE

Conners Teacher's Behavior Rating Scale:
   Total score
   Inattentive-passive
   Conduct problems
   Tension-anxiety

Arnold and Smeltzer Parent Behavior Checklist:
   Total score
   Inattentive-unproductiveness
   Unsocialized aggression
   Sociopathy

Achenbach Child Behavior Checklist:
   Total competence score
   Total problems score
   Externalizing factor
   Internalizing factor

Females:
   Immature-hyperactive
   Delinquent

Males:
   Hyperactive
   Uncommunicative
   Hostile-withdrawn
   Immature
   Somatic complaints

TABLE 4

ITEMS ON THE CONNERS TEACHER'S
SCALE ASSOCIATED WITH PERSONALITY
FUNCTIONS DISTURBANCE

Submissive
Sullen or sulky
Stubborn
Uncooperative
No sense of fair play

Poor coordination
Appears to lack leadership
Fails to finish things he starts
Daydreams

Serious or sad
Isolates himself from other children
Does not get along with same sex
Demands must be met immediately
Appears to be unaccepted in a group
Does not get along with opposite sex
No sense of fair play

appear to have differentiated the adolescents on the basis of difficulties in getting along with others and their competence in task accomplishment.

BEHAVIOR AT HOME

The parents also described the three groups of adolescents as being different in their behavior at home. On the Parent Behavior Checklist (Arnold and Smeltzer 1974), parents' ratings indicated that the three groups of adolescents differed in the total number of behavior problems. They also differed in ratings of the following factors: inattentive-unproductiveness, unsocialized aggression, and sociopathy. As expected, the adolescents who were stable disturbed were described as having greater problems in each area.

Examination of the specific items on which the three groups were found to differ indicated that the adolescents who were stable disturbed were described by parents as exhibiting most problems with behaviors indicative of delinquency as well as difficulty in getting along with others. These results are presented in table 5.

TABLE 5
ITEMS ON THE PARENT BEHAVIOR CHECKLIST
(Arnold and Smeltzer) ASSOCIATED
WITH PERSONALITY FUNCTIONS DISTURBANCE

Rude to grown-ups
Misbehaves even after warning
Refuses to obey parents
Refuses to admit he is wrong
Uses people to get what he wants
Shows temper in an extreme way

Fails to learn by mistakes
Dislikes going to school

Undependable
Denies having done wrong
Has had trouble with police

Things must be done the same way every time

Gets confused in his thinking
Has to have his own way right now
Hard to know what he is trying to tell you
Bad judgment
Bragging or boasting
Mood changes quickly and goes to extremes

On the Achenbach Child Behavior Checklist, parents indicated that the three groups differed in their total competence and the total number of behavior problems observed as well as in externalizing and internalizing behaviors. This scale assesses different factors for boys and girls. The boys differed in being hyperactive, uncommunicative, hostile-withdrawn, and immature and in expressing somatic complaints. The girls differed in being immature-hyperactive and delinquent.

We next attempted to determine which of these components of disturbing behavior best differentiated the three groups of adolescents at age thirteen and at age sixteen. During early adolescence, overall competence, being inattentive or unproductive, and exhibiting tension or anxiety at home, together with conduct problems at school, best differentiated the three groups. During middle adolescence, overall competence, being inattentive or unproductive, and demonstrating unsocialized aggression at home best differentiated the three groups. Thus, a similar pattern of behavior characterizes the three groups at both ages. Consistently healthy adolescents are more competent, more attentive and productive, and are less aggressive. Adolescents who are consistently disturbed display a pattern of behavior that combines neurotic and antisocial features.

BEHAVIOR IN EARLY ADOLESCENCE DIFFERENTIATING ADOLESCENTS WHO REMAIN DISTURBED FROM THOSE WHO IMPROVE IN MIDDLE ADOLESCENCE

Closer examination of the early adolescents indicated that of the twenty-seven youngsters who manifested personality functions disturbance at age thirteen, fifteen continued to manifest disturbance in middle adolescence while the remainder became clear of disturbance. A comparison was made of their behavior at age thirteen to determine whether teenagers who improve in middle adolescence differ from their peers who remain disturbed. It was thought that examination of the characteristics of those adolescents whose personality functioning improves might give some clues regarding behavior patterns that are associated with change. The teachers were able to differentiate the two groups, reporting that the adolescents who improved manifested less behavior problems indicative of inattentiveness, passivity, and tension or anxiety.

The specific behaviors that differentiated the two groups were the following: poor coordination, submissiveness, being easily led, lacking leadership, and failing to finish things. These results are presented in table 6.

TABLE 6
VARIABLES ON THE CONNERS TEACHER'S
SCALE DIFFERENTIATING ADOLESCENTS AT
THIRTEEN WHO CONTINUE TO BE
DISTURBED FROM THOSE WHO IMPROVE

Factors:
Inattentive-passive
Tension-anxiety

Items:
Coordination poor
Submissive
Easily lead
Lacks leadership
Fails to finish things he starts

Thus, it is less competent behavior that primarily differentiates those adolescents who remain disturbed from those whose personality functioning improves. It is interesting that the parents did not differentiate between the two groups. Hence, teachers appear more capable of assessing characteristics of adolescents that are indicators of longer-term disturbance.

Discussion

Our findings indicate that the transition from early to middle adolescence is accompanied by a general decrease in the amount of disturbing behavior exhibited by adolescents in the classroom and at home. This trend supports the findings reported by Golombek, Marton, Stein, and Korenblum (1987) that in middle adolescence there is a diminution of the prevalence of disturbance in personality functions and by Stein, Golombek, Marton, and Korenblum (1987) that there is a shift toward healthier clinical presentation.

The adolescents who were consistently clear of personality functions disturbance, those who were consistently disturbed, and those who fluctuated were found to differ in their general level of competence and in the presence of behavior problems. Their behavior problems included both neurotic (internalizing) and antisocial (externalizing) characteristics. They were described as having difficulties in getting along with others and in being able to accomplish tasks.

Of those young adolescents who at age thirteen demonstrated disturbed personality functioning, about half remained disturbed in middle adolescence and half became clear of disturbance. We found that these young adolescents were described by their teachers differently at age thirteen. Primarily, the adolescents who remained disturbed were less competent, more passive and submissive, and were described as being less able to direct themselves and to accomplish tasks. Thus, adolescents who are more engaged with others and more responsive to external expectations are more likely to improve than peers who are less engaged and less responsive to their social environment.

Although there are some indications in the literature (Rutter, Graham, Chadwick, and Yule 1976) of a small increase in the prevalence of psychiatric disorder from childhood to adolescence, our findings indicate that during adolescence itself there is a gradual reduction in disturbing behavior and in personality disturbance from early to middle adolescence. Such a trend is in keeping with a general reduction in

403

behavior problems over the entire span of childhood. Early adolescence is a stressful developmental phase, and the heightened disturbances are most likely attributed to the biological and psychosocial changes associated with the transition from childhood to adolescence.

A cross-sectional examination of personality disturbance at any particular age demonstrates that those adolescents who are disturbed demonstrate behavior primarily characteristic of neuroticism or internalizing problems. However, those adolescents who remain consistently disturbed during early and middle adolescence are characterized by a combination of both neurotic-internalizing problems and antisocial-externalizing problems. This finding is consistent with reports from the Isle of Wight study (Rutter et al. 1976) that indicate that antisocial behavior problems are more stable than neurotic behavior problems from age ten to fifteen. Thus, disturbed personality development during adolescence is associated with behavior that is less competent and more antisocial and neurotic.

Interestingly, what differentiates those early adolescents who remain disturbed in middle adolescence from those who become clear of disturbance is greater engagement with others and more active involvement with their environment. Thus, although at thirteen both groups were seen as being similarly antisocial, the less engaged and less active individuals maintain their antisocial behavior and personality disturbance, whereas the more engaged and more active adolescents attain more healthy personality functioning and manifest less antisocial behavior. This suggests that it is the interplay of personality characteristics and social interaction that influences further personality development.

Conclusions

Our data indicate that during early and middle adolescence about half of the adolescent population can be expected to demonstrate steady development free from disturbance, about one-quarter can be expected to exhibit disturbed development suggestive of psychiatric disturbance, and another quarter experience adolescent turmoil. Adolescents whose personality development reflects these different developmental lines exhibit different behavior both at home and at school. The adolescent who is consistently disturbed exhibits more conduct problems combined with neurotic behavior. Furthermore, he differs from the adolescent whose disturbance is characteristic of adolescent turmoil in that he is less engaged with his environment.

NOTES

This study was supported by a grant from the Ministry of Community and Social Services, Ontario, Canada. This work could not be done without the continuing assistance of the Etobicoke Board of Education, Toronto, Ontario. We are also indebted to the adolescents and their families for their cooperation and interest and to Ms. S. Allon, social worker, and Mrs. M. Churchard, research assistant, for their invaluable contributions.

1. The results reported represent findings that met conventional levels of statistical significance. In order to simplify the presentation, the specific scale and item scores, the values of each statistic, and exact significance levels have been omitted. These may be obtained on request from the senior author.

REFERENCES

Achenbach, T., and Edelbrock, C. 1981. Behavioral problems and competencies reported by parents of normal and disturbed children aged 4 through 16. *Monographs of the Society for Research in Child Development*, vol. 46, no. 188.

Arnold, L., and Smeltzer, M. 1974. Behavior checklist factor analysis for children and adolescents. *Archives of General Psychiatry* 30:799–804.

Conners, C. 1969. A teacher rating scale for use in drug studies with children. *American Journal of Psychiatry* 126:152–155.

Golombek, H.; Marton, P.; Stein, B.; and Korenblum, M. 1986a. Personality dysfunction and behavior disturbance in early adolescence. *Journal of the American Academy of Child Psychiatry* 25:697–703.

Golombek, H.; Marton, P.; Stein, B.; and Korenblum, M. 1986b. A study of disturbed and non-disturbed adolescents: the Toronto adolescent longitudinal study. *Canadian Journal of Psychiatry* 31:532–535.

Golombek, H.; Marton, P.; Stein, B.; and Korenblum, M. 1987. Personality functioning status during early and middle adolescence. *Adolescent Psychiatry* (in this volume).

Rutter, M.; Graham, P.; Chadwick, O.; and Yule, W. 1976. Adolescent turmoil: fact or fiction? *Journal of Child Psychology, Psychiatry and Allied Disciplines* 17:35–56.

Stein, B.; Golombek, H.; Marton, P.; and Korenblum, M. 1987. Personality functioning and change in clinical presentation from early to middle adolescence. *Adolescent Psychiatry* (in this volume).

26 DISTURBED PERSONALITY FUNCTIONING: PATTERNS OF CHANGE FROM EARLY TO MIDDLE ADOLESCENCE

MARSHALL KORENBLUM, PETER MARTON, HARVEY GOLOMBEK, AND BERNARD STEIN

Controversy surrounding the existence of disturbed personality functioning in adolescence dates at least as far back as the beginning of the twentieth century. Hall (1904) characterized adolescence as a phase of inevitable "*Sturm und Drang*." He based his theory of adolescence on the principle of recapitulation, which had enjoyed a long history in the biological sciences. This principle postulates that the child passes through or retraces in its development the course already taken by the human race. Hall speculated that adolescence corresponded to a period in prehistory marked by large-scale migration. For both the race and the individual, it was a time of upheaval. This viewpoint readily harmonized with the evolutionary orientation of American psychology, itself heavily influenced by Charles Darwin.

The notion of discontinuity of development prevailed through psychoanalytic writings on adolescence during the period 1930–1960. It was asserted that adolescents normatively display varying degrees and kinds of character pathology that resemble but do not constitute true psychiatric illness (Freud 1958). Those who espoused this view suggested that psychiatric symptoms were common, transient, fluctuating, and essentially benign in most adolescents. In addition, it was thought that the prognosis of adolescent symptomatology was difficult if not impossible to determine.

The research methodology of the 1960s and 1970s challenged this traditional view of the disruptive nature of adolescent development. Studies such as those of Offer (1969), Masterson (1967), and Rutter, Graham, Chadwick, and Yule (1976) suggest that adolescent development is marked by relative continuity from childhood. According to these authors, adolescents normatively maintain psychic equilibrium as they struggle with developmental tasks. When symptom patterns and personality disorders do appear, they tend to persist and become better differentiated over time.

With the increasing acceptance of these empirically based conceptualizations of adolescent development, attention turned to the classification of adolescent psychopathology and the question of constancy and change over time.

Numerous authors (King and Pittman 1969; Masterson 1967; Weiner and Del Gaudio 1976) have reported a high degree of persistence of symptomatology and characterologic maladaptation over time in clinical populations. Fard, Hudgens, and Welner (1978) concluded that "a confused clinical picture became more typical as the subjects grew from adolescence into adulthood. The psychiatric disorders of teenagers are not a breed apart. They are the same syndromes we see in adults. It is just that some patients must become adults before their illnesses have a familiar look." The present chapter examines whether this same trend exists in a nonclinical population.

Purpose

In previous papers (Golombek, Marton, Stein, and Korenblum 1986; Stein, Golombek, Marton, and Korenblum 1986), we reported that 46 percent of a representative nonclinical sample of urban Canadian thirteen-year-olds displayed some degree of personality dysfunction. This cross-sectional snapshot of early adolescence raised the question of whether such disturbance is transient or persists over time. We therefore followed our nonclinical subjects into middle adolescence in order to study the types of disturbed personality functioning that they displayed and the degree of consistency or change of their personality dysfunction. The purposes of this chapter are twofold: (1) to describe the types of personality psychopathology present in adolescents at ages thirteen and sixteen and (2) to determine the stability of such psychopathology over time.

Method

SUBJECTS

This chapter presents data on the subgroup of adolescents who displayed characterologic psychopathology. The sample as a whole has been described in detail in a previous chapter (Golombek, Marton, Stein, and Korenblum 1987).

At age thirteen, twenty-seven of the sixty-three adolescents were found to have some degree of disturbed personality functioning. In 1982, at age sixteen, twenty out of sixty-one adolescents fell into this category, representing approximately 33 percent of the entire sample.

Procedure

Each adolescent underwent a one-hour, semistructured interview that focused on interpersonal relationships. This interview was videotaped and then rated according to a modified object relations scale. The presence of disturbed personality functioning was determined on the basis of the ratings.

Subsequently, two clinicians using Axis II categories of DSM-III independently classified the type of disturbed personality functioning demonstrated by these adolescents at ages thirteen and sixteen. This was not an attempt at diagnosis per se. Rather, the raters used clinical judgment to decide how similar the adolescents' global presentation was to the descriptions outlined in Axis II. Disagreements were resolved by invoking a third rater. Each psychiatrist was blind to the other's classification.

Because the group of disturbed adolescents was heterogeneous and somewhat small in number, the categories were clustered. Table 1 illustrates how Axis II categories of DSM-III naturally fall into five

TABLE 1
CLUSTERS OF PERSONALITY DISORDERS
(DSM-III, AXIS II)

A. Paranoid, schizoid, schizotypal
B. Histrionic, borderline, narcissistic
C. Antisocial
D. Avoidant, dependent, compulsive, passive-aggressive
E. Atypical, mixed, other

clusters (DSM-III 1980). The first cluster consists of categories that apply to individuals who appear odd or eccentric. Individuals in the second cluster appear to be dramatic, emotional, or erratic. The third category was designated as a separate entity because of the hypothesis that subjects in this group would be sufficiently homogeneous to warrant such separation and because it was thought that adolescents meeting this description did not fit into the second cluster (which is where DSM-III would have otherwise placed them). Individuals with disorders in the fourth cluster appear anxious or fearful, and the final cluster is a residual one for individuals who do not meet requirements for any specific disorder.

Classification hinges on reliability, and we ensured that this was adequate before proceeding. In 1979 (when the subjects were age thirteen), there was 77 percent agreement about cluster assignment. In 1982 (when the subjects were age sixteen), the agreement was 75 percent. These levels of reliability were thought to be satisfactory.

In addition to classifying the subjects according to DSM-III clusters, we also divided the sample into two different subgroups to reflect the change or stability in the presence of disturbance at ages thirteen and sixteen. (1) Stable disturbed: these adolescents were rated as demonstrating some degree of disturbance at both ages. (2) Fluctuating: these adolescents were clear of disturbance at one age but presented with some degree of disturbance at the other age.

Results

In both 1979 and 1982, the subjects with some degree of personality dysfunction were classified according to the five clusters outlined above. The results for age thirteen are presented in figure 1. Fifty-five percent of the disturbed adolescents fell into cluster D, 30 percent fell into cluster C, 7 percent were in each of clusters A and E, and there were no individuals in cluster B. The adolescents were essentially divided into two groups—a large number who were anxious or fearful and a smaller number of antisocial individuals. All of the cluster A and practically all of the cluster C subjects were in the stable disturbed subgroup. On the other hand, all of the cluster E and 60 percent of the cluster D subjects were in the fluctuating subgroup.

In 1982, when the subjects were age sixteen, the distribution of the type of dysfunction was quite different. As figure 2 demonstrates, 35

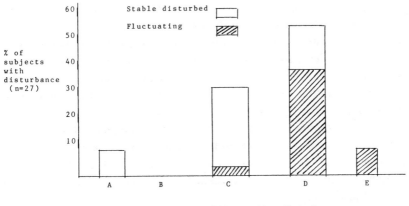

FIG. 1.—Distribution of subjects with personality dysfunction at age thirteen

percent of the sample fell into each of clusters C and E, while 10 percent fell into clusters A, B, and D. All of the subjects in clusters A and D were from the stable disturbed subgroup, and 86 percent of the cluster C subjects were also stable disturbed. On the other hand, half of the cluster B and over 40 percent of the cluster E subjects were from the fluctuating subgroup.

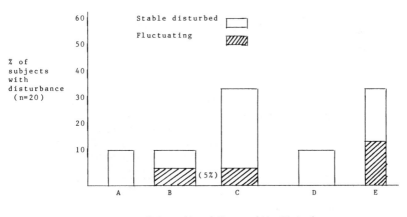

FIG. 2.—Distribution of subjects with personality dysfunction at age sixteen

411

Table 2 emphasizes the stability or change in clusters from 1979 to 1982. The most noticeable shifts are a decrease in cluster D and an increase in cluster E. Table 3 presents the consistency of pathology in individual subjects from age thirteen to sixteen. The greatest consistency was in cluster A and cluster C subjects, while very few of the cluster D and none of the cluster E subjects retained the same type of disturbance.

It should be noted that three-quarters of the subjects who fluctuated from disturbance at age thirteen to no disturbance at age sixteen came from cluster D. Sixty percent of the subjects who fluctuated from no disturbance at age thirteen to disturbance at age sixteen were categorized in cluster E.

In total, fifteen subjects were stable disturbed, while seventeen were in the fluctuating group. Of this fluctuating group, five went from no disturbance to disturbance, while twelve went from disturbance to no disturbance.

TABLE 2
DISTRIBUTION OF TYPES OF PERSONALITY DYSFUNCTION
AT AGES THIRTEEN AND SIXTEEN

	A	B	C	D	E
Age thirteen (%)	7	0	30	55	7
Age sixteen (%)	10	10	35	10	35

TABLE 3
CONSISTENCY OF THE TYPE OF PERSONALITY
DYSFUNCTION FROM AGES THIRTEEN TO SIXTEEN

Cluster	Percentage Who Remained in the Same Cluster
A	100
B	. . .
C	71
D	33
E	0

Discussion

The results of this study indicate that it is possible to identify reliably teenagers who have some degree of disturbed personality functioning in early and middle adolescence. At age thirteen, such adolescents tend to distribute themselves into two major groups—the majority appear to be anxious or fearful, while a smaller segment are characterized by antisocial tendencies. At age sixteen, they distribute themselves quite differently—roughly one-third are antisocial, another third fall into a mixed group of atypical and/or immature types, and there are smaller segments of odd, erratic, and anxious types. Overall, there is a decrease in the prevalence of personality dysfunction from early to middle adolescence. In addition, the form of this disturbance changes to a somewhat more diffuse, less well defined pattern.

For the antisocial cluster, there was both group and individual stability over time. This is consistent with the many studies that have shown the enduring nature of antisocial predilection in children and adolescents. Glueck and Glueck (1968) found that among 500 delinquent children, 70 percent had multiple convictions by the time they had reached age seventeen to twenty-five. Robins, in her longitudinal cohort studies (1966, 1978), found that 90 percent of adult sociopaths had been antisocial as children.

For cluster A, there was also a high degree of group and individual stability over time. This is again consistent with studies that have shown that shy and withdrawn children are, as a group, quiet and retiring in adult life (Morris, Soroker, and Burrus 1954). One study showed that over 90 percent of boys diagnosed as schizoid at age ten were given the same diagnosis by an independent psychiatrist ten years later (Wolff and Chick 1980).

On the other hand, avoidant, dependent, compulsive, and passive-aggressive adolescents, who may be conceptualized as approximating the more neurotic end of the spectrum, do seem to "grow out of" their dysfunction. Fully three-quarters of the group of adolescents that fluctuated from disturbance to nondisturbance came from cluster D. In the stable disturbed group, only one-third of subjects from cluster D stayed in that cluster. The majority later displayed some other type of dysfunction. The implication of these findings is that early adolescents displaying this type of disturbance may have a better prognosis and a more benign course than those who seem schizoid or antisocial.

413

The group fluctuating from normalcy at thirteen into disturbance at sixteen were classified largely as mixed, atypical, or other disorder. This may mean that a subsegment of the population drifts into dysfunction in middle adolescence, but it is extremely hard to define the precise nature of this dysfunction. This could represent a midadolescent "turmoil" group.

Our findings support Rutter's Isle of Wight data (Rutter et al. 1976) on adolescent turmoil. He found that conditions arising for the first time during adolescence differ from those that have persisted from earlier time periods. There was a tendency for the most severe disorders to be found in his persistent group. This parallels our data that clusters A and C were composed primarily of adolescents who were disturbed at both ages thirteen and sixteen.

The trajectories that our adolescents seem to be following are consistent with longitudinal principles that have recently been outlined by Strauss, Hafez, Lieberman, and Harding (1985). They point out that most disturbances follow a nonlinear course and that there are identifiable phases to certain disorders. In particular, they describe so-called moratoriums during which subjects experience stability. The middle adolescence of most of our subjects seems to represent such a phase. He also describes change points that involve considerable shifts in functioning. This corresponds to our fluctuating subgroups. Whether these patterns are simply reflective of developmental thrusts or are inherent to deviant patterns of growth is a moot point and cannot yet be determined from our data. We have, however, followed all of the adolescents to their eighteenth birthday. Each year they received the same object relations interview. When they entered late adolescence we added a structured interview, which has enabled us to assess personality dysfunctioning according to formal Axis II, DSM-III criteria. We look forward to sharing the results of these measures insofar as they may shed further light on the question of continuity versus change in personality function disturbance.

Conclusions

(1) There is a decrease in the prevalence of personality dysfunction from early to middle adolescence in this nonclinical sample (46 percent to 33 percent). (2) The form of this disturbance changes from a bimodal distribution of anxious-fearful and antisocial types in early adolescence

to a more diffuse, less well defined pattern in middle adolescence. (3) There is both group and individual stability over time among the antisocial and eccentric-withdrawn adolescents. The anxious-fearful adolescents are more likely to "grow out of" their difficulties. (4) One-quarter of the sample as a whole (fifteen out of sixty-one) manifested disturbance in both early and middle adolescence. A further 28 percent (seventeen out of sixty-one) fluctuated from some personality dysfunction at one age to essentially no disturbance at the other age. There was movement in both directions in the latter group, but the large majority developed toward health.

NOTE

This study was supported by a grant from the Ministry of Community and Social Services, Ontario, Canada. This work could not have been done without the continuing assistance of the Etobicoke Board of Education, Toronto, Ontario. We are also indebted to the adolescents and their families for their cooperation and interest and to Ms. S. Allon, social worker, and Mrs. M. Churchard, research assistant, for their invaluable contributions.

REFERENCES

Diagnostic and Statistical Manual of Mental Disorders (DSM-III). 1980. 3d ed. Washington, D.C.: American Psychiatric Press.

Fard, K.; Hudgens, R. W.; and Welner, A. 1978. Undiagnosed psychiatric illness in adolescents: a prospective study and seven-year follow-up. *Archives of General Psychiatry* 35:279–282.

Freud, A. 1958. Adolescence. *Psychoanalytic Study of the Child* 13:255–273.

Glueck, S., and Glueck, E. 1968. *Delinquents and Non-delinquents in Perspective*. Cambridge, Mass.: Harvard University Press.

Golombek, H.; Marton, P.; Stein, B.; and Korenblum, M. 1986. A study of disturbed and non-disturbed adolescents: the Toronto adolescent longitudinal study. I. *Canadian Journal of Psychiatry* 31(6): 532–535.

Golombek, H.; Marton, P.; Stein, B.; and Korenblum, M. 1987. Personality functioning status during early and middle adolescence. *Adolescent Psychiatry* (in this volume).

Hall, G. S. 1904. *Adolescence: Its Psychology and Its Relations to Anthropology, Sociobiology, Sex, Crime, Religion, and Education.* Vols. 1, 2. New York: Appleton.

King, L. J., and Pittman, G. D. 1969. A six-year follow-up study of 65 adolescent patients: predictive value of presenting clinical picture. *British Journal of Psychiatry* 115:1437–1441.

Masterson, J. F. 1967. *The Psychiatric Dilemma of Adolescence.* Boston: Little, Brown.

Morris, D. P.; Soroker, E.; and Burrus, G. 1954. Follow-up study of shy and withdrawn children. I. Evaluation of later adjustment. *American Journal of Orthopsychiatry* 24:743–754.

Offer, D. 1969. *The Psychological World of the Teenager.* New York: Basic.

Robins, L. 1966. *Deviant Children Grown Up.* Baltimore: Williams & Wilkins.

Robins, L. N. 1978. Sturdy childhood predictors of adult antisocial behavior: replications from longitudinal studies. *Psychological Medicine* 8:611–622.

Rutter, M.; Graham, P.; Chadwick, O.; and Yule, W. 1976. Adolescent turmoil: fact or fiction? *Journal of Child Psychology and Psychiatry* 17:35–56.

Stein, B.; Golombek, H.; Marton, P.; and Korenblum, M. 1986. Personality functioning and clinical presentation in early adolescence. II. *Canadian Journal of Psychiatry* 31(6): 536–541.

Strauss, J. S.; Hafez, H.; Lieberman, P.; and Harding, C. M. 1985. The course of psychiatric disorder. III. Longitudinal principles. *American Journal of Psychiatry* 142:289–296.

Weiner, I. B., and Del Gaudio, A. C. 1976. Psychopathology in adolescence: an epidemiological study. *Archives of General Psychiatry* 33:187–193.

Wolff, S., and Chick, J. 1980. Schizoid personality in childhood: a controlled follow-up study. *Psychological Medicine* 10:85–100.

PSYCHIC DISCONTINUITY DURING

ADOLESCENCE: DISCUSSION OF PANEL

PRESENTATIONS, AMERICAN SOCIETY FOR

ADOLESCENT PSYCHIATRY, MAY 1986

PETER L. GIOVACCHINI

In my opinion, the conclusions reached by the presentations of this panel are useful from several viewpoints. As a clinician, I am offered certain guidelines and orientations that will help me understand my adolescent patients so that I will be able to treat them more effectively. There are also some implications that can be derived from the investigators' data that can be helpful for the understanding of all patients. I am referring specifically to the interaction of physiological and psychological elements and generally to the effects of particular stresses on personality functioning, but I shall return to these topics later.

Another viewpoint that is clarified by this research refers to popular and impressionistic notions about adolescent emotional development and motivation. In the past, we have heard that adolescence is a period of turmoil. We have also heard the opposite opinion that we need not assume that there will be any undue stress during the passage from childhood to adulthood. In the samples studied by the participants of this panel, we learn that there are characteristic patterns of functioning—at times psychopathological functioning—that are typical (at least from a statistical perspective) of early and middle adolescence. The investigative approach pursued by the panelists leads to objective evaluations about the phenomenology of adolescence, a subject that is, in spite of our increasing sophistication and continued interest, still predominantly shrouded by impressionistic notions and speculative formulations. Their precision in locating functional competency and the dominant use of certain defense mechanisms such as projection and denial during early adolescence should help us in our efforts to define the adolescent process in terms of its relevance to emotional development and psychopathology. These goals are equally important for both the clinician and the academician.

I wish quickly to set aside the issue of cultural relativism, a topic that has more often confused than clarified our attempts to study the adolescent process. True, in some societies both present and past, there may have been no such thing as an adolescent from the perspective of a unique psychic configuration. The passage from childhood to adulthood may have progressed on a smooth, unbroken continuum. This is, however, not true in the United States, as many studies indicate, and apparently not so in Canada as our colleagues here today emphasize. They have convincingly demonstrated that there are characterological patterns and sequences that are found in a statistically significant number of teenagers.

Our colleagues also point to the relevance of an ego-psychological frame of reference. The seven variables they use as indexes of measurement—identity crystallization, maintenance of identity, role assumption, communication with self and others, reality testing, and self-esteem—all refer to ego functions and ego subsystems. The main ego functions refer to object relationships, and from a structural frame the self-representation is in the forefront.

These variables cannot be equally weighted. In some instances one variable is a subcategory of a more general one. For example, maintenance of identity would involve the psyche's capacity to assume a particular role. The crystallization of the identity sense would be important in the production of or loss of self-esteem. I am referring to this methodological issue to make explicit what the authors know but did not need to emphasize because of their research goal of exploring the functional capacities of specific chronological periods of adolescence. Still, I believe this point is important for future endeavors aimed at studying the continuity of character development and its relationship to both the developmental process and psychopathology.

The panelists traced, from a phenomenological perspective, the passage from early to middle adolescence. They noted that quantitative and qualitative aspects of emotional equilibrium at the age of thirteen led to certain adjustive patterns at sixteen. They observed a certain amount of homogeneity, although from what I understood they cannot as yet establish specificity. I am inclined to believe that as they pursue their studies they will be able to discover *clusters of developmental movement* that are the outcome of particular environmental configurations. To put it more simply, I hope they will define sequences of character formation that are typically associated with specific family orientations. The latter would, of course, emphasize the maternal relationship and nurturing and soothing interactions as they determine emotional stability and the acquisition of psychic structure. This is an area that currently belongs to neonatologists.

In a similar vein, research regarding psychic development during adolescence, a natural extension of the phenomena studied by neonatologists, will also lead to insights about character formation and psychopathological vicissitudes. I believe that the chapters just presented point to both the continuities and discontinuities of structural development and give us the opportunity to make some inferences about the impact of both internal (physiological) stimuli and external influences. The latter involve significant object relationships and the expectations of the milieu as they are related to changing demands on role assumption, necessitating a reconstruction of the self-representation and the identity sense.

The conclusions reached about what we might refer to as the *vulnerability* of early adolescence are highly plausible. No matter how supportive the environment might be, puberty represents a monumental change and leads to tremendous shifts in psychic equilibrium. There is a devastating transformation in the body configuration, and the repertoire of feelings is drastically expanded as sexuality joins the ranks of desires. The child, so to speak, has adult needs, but he has adaptations—that is, ego executive techniques—that are appropriate only to childhood inpulses. The early adolescent suffers from a lag between instinctual needs, created by the hormonal upheaval of puberty, and a consolidation of the identity sense. The somatic elements of the self-representation stand out in bold relief when there is a lack of synchrony between the psyche and the soma, and this seems to be what happens at puberty. It occurs independent of psychopathology, although psychopathology would, of course, intensify the difficulties the early adolescent will experience.

The modern clinician is faced with patients who can best be explained in terms of defects in psychic structure. This forces us to look at early developmental processes, and since adolescence is the period when the adult personality is formed—that is, the period of character consolidation—the sequence of development during the postpuberty years acquires increasing significance. Whether there is a smooth continuity between the various phases of adolescence is clinically most meaningful, because inasmuch as some forms of psychopathology are based on exaggerations or distortions of ordinary development, the lack of developmental continuity can be reflected in the production of clinical syndromes during both adolescence and adulthood.

This lack of developmental continuity—besides creating clinical syndromes—is also reflected in character traits that have been considered to be typically adolescent. For example, we are all familiar with the taciturn and what at times appears to be the shy and awkward teenager. In treatment, this can be a frustrating experience since the therapist feels forced to intrude during the process of gathering information. Our efforts are constantly thwarted as they parry our questions with either silence or monosyllabic, noninformative answers. Our psychotherapeutic purpose is threatened by the patient's lack of spontaneity and absence of psychological mindedness. I refer to this common enough but far from universal situation with adolescents to point out what seems to be a lack of connection, a discontinuity, between inner feelings and the higher levels of the psyche that are involved in communication.

Heretofore, we have explained such phenomena as the outcome of repression, a purposeful but unconscious shutting out of feelings and urges that would be conflictful, anxiety producing, and painful if allowed access to consciousness. In many instances, this is the case. I believe, however, that more frequently we are confronted with a character trait rather than an attempt by the psyche to maintain psychodynamic equilibrium, a character trait that is related to what I call *structural discontinuity* and which is especially prominent during adolescence, when there is a relative lack of characterological consolidation.

For example, a nineteen-year-old college student began most of his sessions by announcing that he had nothing to say. He did not seem anxious or otherwise uncomfortable. He would just sit on my couch, remaining silent and appearing calm. Ordinarily I am not disturbed by a patient not talking, but with this young man I had the feeling that this lack of verbal interaction would continue forever if I did not intervene in some way. I was thinking in terms of resistance and repression, seeing a purpose in the patient's behavior.

The patient, however, did not agree with my assessment that there was some purpose to his behavior. He simply stated that he did not say anything because he had nothing to say. That is all there was to it, and I was trying "to find a meaning for something that had no meaning." He accused me of "making something out of nothing." On occasion I had the feeling that he felt sorry for me because of my fruitless efforts, and I believed that he ruefully shook his head at my obtuseness as I was pursuing the principle of psychic determinism. He seemed to have tolerantly accepted the possibility that I would never learn.

I was grateful for even this limited exchange as I puzzled over the possibility that perhaps he really did not have anything to say. I was reminded of the fact that he claimed that he never dreamed, since in my efforts to gather "material" I had inquired about dreams. His descriptions of events when I asked him pointed questions were extremely concrete, a factual report without any elaboration or reference to feelings or emotional states.

After several months of almost total silence, we discussed a fantasy. At this moment, I do not recall whether it was his fantasy or mine, but in any case, it proved to be most instructive. In this fantasy the patient and I were both in a totally dark room. Since neither one of us could see, we were completely unaware of each other's presence. From my perspective, I was alone in this room, and he felt the same way. We did not exist for each other. For a while, this was all there was in this mental image, simply a state of isolated being and no action or feelings. Then the patient moves his hand in the dark and touches an overhanging string. He pulls it and turns on a light. Suddenly we both exist. He can see me and I can see him, and by turning on the light we have created each other. The patient then wondered if I now understood that he really meant it when he stated that he had nothing to say.

The patient could not free associate, but I could. I treated the fantasy as if it were my own, especially since I found it a most apt description of our relationship. I viewed the darkness as a state of nonexistence and equated it with his contention of having nothing to say. The light represented a source of energy—in metapsychological terms, a method of cathecting psychic structure and external objects. From his viewpoint, I did not exist unless he could energize parts of his psychic apparatus. In a similar fashion, he usually could not cathect his unconscious and the outer world, so he could not get in touch with the deeper levels of his psyche. To be able to communicate id elements, he had to be able to form a mental representation of me—something he was usually unable to do. The surface of his mind that contains the perceptual apparatus in a sense was isolated from the deeper recesses of the unconscious.

From the viewpoint of psychic structure, there does not seem to be a smooth continuum, a hierarchal spectrum between id primary process elements and higher-level, reality-directed secondary process operations. This characterological configuration has to be distinguished from repression, an intrapsychic defensive interaction, as well as the more familiar structural changes that accompany splitting or dissociative mechanisms. Obviously, what I am describing is a structural deficit that involves continuity between deeper and surface psychic elements rather than a psychic force pushing unacceptable impulses and feelings out of conscious awareness. Splitting refers to separation of psychic elements, but this occurs at the same ego level and involves a splitting of the self-representation, usually into good and bad. My patient did not have access to both his id and the outer world. The separation here involved different strata of the psyche rather than the same level.

I believe this type of structural deficit is typical of adolescence and probably begins with the changes of puberty during early adolescence. This configuration, however, will contribute to the psychopathological distortions of the final character structure of adulthood. Freud has taught us that behind every adult neurosis we will find a childhood or infantile neurosis. The emotional disturbances of adulthood can be traced to disturbances of the early years of life. We can draw a parallel with the psychopathology so frequently encountered currently that involves defects in character structure, as seen in the numerous patients suffering from character disorders and borderline states. The events and psychic processes of early adolescence are the etiological precursors of later characterological disturbances in the same way that infantile trauma determines the adult neurosis. It is my opinion that the research that is reported in this section supports this thesis.

PART VI

EDUCATIONAL ISSUES IN ADOLESCENT PSYCHIATRY

EDITORS' INTRODUCTION

Becoming educated in the institutions that are called "schools" in our society should be an organizing experience. The vast majority of children find school a positive aspect of their lives, but a substantial proportion (depending on socioeconomic factors) struggle with learning. Learning theory hardly deals with the loss aspect of acquiring knowledge, but it is the struggle with loss that leads to emotional stress and eventual breakdown. This part is devoted to educational issues in adolescent psychiatry and features chapters on underachievement by Max Sugar and Howard S. Baker and a special section, edited by Irving H. Berkovitz, on therapeutic potentials in school programs.

Max Sugar considers the diagnostic aspects of school underachievement in adolescents. He focuses on factors that affect optimal achievement and discusses heredity, prenatal complications, neurological findings, cognitive issues (minimal brain dysfunction, developmental output failure, interference in the sensorimotor period, and formal operations), and emotional factors (developmental and familial). Sugar believes a large number of underachievers exist and require early detection, proper placement, and remedial efforts.

Howard S. Baker examines the sources of psychopathology that lead to underachievement and failure in college students; childhood trauma, oedipal conflicts, biology, family interactions, and social relations from the viewpoint of self psychology. He thus views psychopathology as resulting from deficits in internal structures rather than from unresolved conflicts, and discusses problems of maintaining self-esteem and disruptions in selfobject relationships. Baker reviews self psychology theory and concludes that self psychology can provide a basis for interventions that range from psychoanalytic to cognitive psychotherapy.

Carl Feinstein and Richard Lytle conclude that deaf teenagers are more vulnerable to problems of adjustment than are hearing youngsters. This increased vulnerability is due not to a characteristic "deaf personality" but rather to the greater stress from the special minority experience of being deaf and isolated.

426

MAX SUGAR

The designation underachievement usually begins when parents learn from the school report card that their youngster has not done as well as hoped. The report usually contains remarks from the teacher such as "not participating" or "not paying attention." Academic underachievement is the single most frequent symptom leading young people to psychiatric evaluation. Doing poorly in school is usually thought of as equivalent to being "bad." This is often reinforced by the parental statement, "you could do better," which reflects the teacher's comments on report cards. The youngster often feels embarrassed or guilty about not having done better work and is loathe to tell his parents about his failures at school. He may even go so far as to forge better grades on his school work and/or report cards.

Contributing Factors

This chapter focuses on the broad spectrum of underachievement and some particular factors that affect optimal achievement. Most underachievement is not of emotional origin (Blanchard 1946). A recent underachievement survey (Cartwright, Rosin, and Price 1980) reaffirmed this with percentages of causes as follows: IQ—retardation or borderline, 38 percent; social and emotional problems, 25 percent; speech and hearing disorders, 10 percent; developmental problems, 8 percent; and learning difficulties, 17 percent. As table 1 shows, there are multiple causes of underachievement.

TABLE 1

CAUSES OF UNDERACHIEVEMENT

1. Hereditary—e.g., sickle cell anemia, temperament
2. Congenital—e.g., sensory defects (rubella)
3. Developmental—e.g., intracranial hemorrhage, learning disabilities, prematurity
4. Infections—e.g., encephalitis
5. Metabolic and hormonal—e.g., cretinism, phenylketonuria, iron deficiency anemia
6. Toxins—e.g., pica, substance abuse
7. Trauma—e.g., concussion
8. Tumors—e.g., CNS tumors, blood dyscrasias, leukemia
9. Neurological—e.g., epilepsy
10. Nutritional deficiencies
11. Cognitive—e.g., dyslexia, absence of abstract thinking
12. Emotional—e.g., psychosis, neurosis, situational, post-trauma
13. Family
14. Educational system

1. HEREDITY

Some children underachieve because of their temperaments—being reflective and quiet is more rewarded and rewarding in academic tasks than being impulsive and action oriented. A youth with the latter characteristics will have a greater likelihood of underachieving than the reflective one, even if all other factors—such as family, socioeconomic status, and IQ—are similar.

Genetic studies have found evidence for an autosomal recessive transmission of dyslexia (Finucci and Childs 1983).

2. PRENATAL FACTORS

Recent research has shown that many events in pregnancy may contribute to learning disabilities. Among these are poor maternal nutrition; small for gestational age due to fetal malnourishment; congenital infection from cytomegalovirus; oxytocin exposure; scopolamine exposure; lead exposure; cadmium exposure; manganese exposure; lithium exposure; phenobarbitol exposure; cigarette smoking causing low birth weight; alcohol abuse leading to fetal alcohol syndrome; inhalation anesthetics; complications of labor and delivery; and cesarean section. The placenta, once thought to be an impenetrable barrier, is clearly not impervious to the listed metals, drugs, viruses, and toxins.

428

3. NEUROLOGICAL FACTORS

Neurological difficulties—such as seizure disorders, postinflammatory sources (e.g., post encephalitis or post concussion), brain tumors, and hemorrhage—may be the cause of underachievement.

Among youngsters with epilepsy, those with major epilepsy are more likely to fail than those with petit mal (Holdsworth and Whitmore 1974). Baird, John, Ahn, and Maisel (1980) believe that the presence of epileptiform activity in children is an indication of possible learning problems. Estimates of the percentage of epileptic children who have educational difficulties range from 33 to 70 percent. Even epileptics with normal IQs have specific learning disabilities. Baird et al. question whether medication controls all seizure activity and note that subclinical paroxysms may be present in the absence of overt signs of epilepsy. This would be a cause for the youngster's difficulties in attention and thus in learning.

4. COGNITIVE FACTORS

MINIMAL BRAIN DYSFUNCTION (MBD)

Statistics show that 10 to 20 percent of youngsters have MBD, with a male to female ratio of 4:1. Early in the study of MBD, youngsters were believed to outgrow the disorder in early adolescence. Then evidence accumulated that this was not the case; in fact, the disability remained for a lifetime, and adult attention deficit disorder is now a diagnostic entity. More recently it was reported that the condition has three different courses and possibilities for duration: one group of children seem to mature out of their disabilities by about age eight; another group achieves this by age twelve; and a third group has the dysfunction permanently (Silver 1983).

We are now seeing more of the following cases clinically.

Case Example 1

When a fifteen-year-old girl was evaluated for severe depression and suicidal behavior, it was learned that she was barely getting by in school. Her chronic low self-esteem and impulsivity were problems of long duration. Between ages eight and eleven she had received remediation for her learning disability along with physiotherapy and special education. On clinical examination her intelligence appeared to be average, and she had no evidence of a hyperactive syndrome or attention deficit disorder. Psychological testing confirmed the above findings and showed no evidence of visual or auditory perceptual difficulty, organicity, or residuals thereof. It is now impossible to establish whether she ever had a learning disability with visual or auditory perceptual deficits. She had for years, however, thought herself to be dumb, helpless, and incompetent. Whether these feelings followed or preceded the learning disability diagnosis could not be discerned.

In other cases the psychological testing has clearly recognized the residual of a learning disability that has been overcome by maturation. Perhaps the cited case was one of diagnostic error, halo effect, or maturational improvement. Nonetheless, the suggestion follows that once a diagnosis of MBD is made, it behooves us to repeat the evaluation by age eight or nine and again in early adolescence.

Levine, Oberklaid, and Meltzer (1981) noted a subgroup of youngsters with low academic achievement in late elementary and junior high school who had underlying subtle handicaps that resulted in reduced productivity and chronic underachievement. They characterized these as developmental output failure. The group showed problems with expressive language, fine motor tasks, finger-agnosia, attention, and retrieval memory. This group of youngsters is much more difficult to discern than those with the visual-perceptual or auditory-perceptual problems in MBD.

An interesting connection has been proposed between sex chromosome aberrations and learning disability, but Hier, Atkins, and Perlo (1980) detected no sex chromosome aberrations in their prospective study of twenty adult dyslexic men. In a retrospective study, however, twenty of eighty subjects with known chromosome abnormalities were found to be mentally retarded.

Zinkus, Gottlieb, and Zinkus (1979) raised the question of juvenile delinquents being learning disabled and suggested that juvenile delinquents' disabilities can be dealt with by early intervention to help the perceptually handicapped youngsters.

Youngsters with MBD think they are retarded because they cannot catch on and do things like other youngsters. Frequently their sense of worthlessness leads them to attach themselves to anyone who

430

praises them. They may then be exploited or recruited for delinquent behavior.

As McKay and Brumback (1980) noted, MBD youngsters may have difficulty in learning in the regular classroom despite aptitudes in various performance areas. However, classroom performance skills are not stressed and there is no success gradient for such endeavors. One of the problems in regular high school for such youngsters is that they are forced to do tasks that are difficult for them while they are deprived of areas of experience in performance where they might excel. Some MBD youngsters may do particularly well with subjects such as carpentry, brickwork, plumbing, or auto mechanics, but few schools offer such courses for credit in a regular high school curriculum.

INTERFERENCE IN THE SENSORIMOTOR PERIOD

Interference with, or deprivation of, suitable environmental stimulation at age four to eight months during Piaget's (1952) third stage of the sensorimotor period may lead to disruption of beginning intentionality. This might also delay or interfere with proper development of stage four, that is, genuine intentionality. That stigma might hamper optimal educational achievement, both in childhood and throughout life. The initial interference ''might be trauma, disturbed or disassociated feeding-hunger contrasts, maternal separation, an uninvolved mother with a blind or deaf infant, or a premature who is 'prop-fed' '' (Sugar 1982).

FORMAL OPERATIONS

Forty percent of college freshmen have not achieved formal operations and therefore will be deficient academically on those subjects requiring abstract thinking. They may have gotten by in high school without this ability, but in college this lack becomes a major barrier to further academic progress.

5. EMOTIONAL FACTORS

Freud (1905) wrote that from age three to five the impulse for knowledge and investigation sets in. Causes of an interference with a healthy sublimation of these impulses are of special interest.

The normative questions of adolescents to themselves—such as how tall will I be? or how attractive am I? or what career will I choose? or does masturbation melt the brain?—are not likely to be pervasive or interfere continually with concentration in school work. The temporary slump in seventh and eighth grades may be related to these items as well as to the giving up of infantile objects (Sugar 1968).

The girl who is pregnant may be dwelling on the alternatives to delivery and fear of parental response. This state would lead her to focus less on grades and more on major decision making about her options, with the potential to become a dropout. The boy who may become the legal father, depending on the girl's decision, is involved in guilt and burdens of responsibility that he might need to assume instead of school achievement. Adoptees have been found to have a higher percentage of emotional problems and, thereby, a greater than average potential for resultant learning disabilities.

Case Example 2

A thirteen-year-old adopted boy with above-average learning potential failed in all his subjects in his first year in high school. In the primary school he previously attended, where he knew everybody, he felt he belonged. In the huge high school he felt he "belonged to nobody, while all the other students belonged." He then regressed to living in fantasy, which engaged him all day. His fantasies involved finding his biological mother and being rejected by her; looking for students who had a complexion, eye, or hair color similar to his, with whom he fantasized a sibship or kinship; making the junior football team as quarterback; throwing passes of fifty yards and catching them; and partying with lots of girls in a hotel room he would rent for the weekend of the school dance.

The oppositional child behaves with parents, teachers, and peers in a most trying fashion. He is opposed to taking anything given to him and cannot easily assimilate material in the classroom, even though his intelligence may be quite high. The obsessive has to check everything, ruminates, and is unable to go along with the regular pace of working in the classroom or in homework. He thus becomes fatigued and everything is too much of a burden as he procrastinates, with never enough time to finish the work. Anxiety reactions will certainly affect the youngster's ability to concentrate, look, explore, and learn due to intense inhibition and castration anxiety. The depressed youngster will be essentially withdrawn from activities and unable to focus and concentrate as well as he might otherwise.

The teenager who wants to do better and hungers for an all-"A" report card may be unable to improve his grades because of average or low IQ, and his problem is not underachieving but an unrealistic compulsive need to overachieve.

Youngsters with a psychosis may not be readily recognized by the teacher and the pediatrician. They have disordered thinking along with difficulty in concentrating and comprehending. Psychosis may lead to lowered IQ on testing, and the youngster's poor grades may be diagnosed as due to borderline retardation if the proper diagnosis is overlooked. The IQ of some youngsters may be in the genius range, but because they are schizophrenic, they cannot comprehend ordinary classroom work even at a very low primary-grade level.

In the case of separation anxiety, the youngster may have a high rate of absenteeism which leaves a gap in his information and classroom experience. In this situation, the family as well as the teenager needs to deal with the issue of separation and not treat it as a reaction to something dangerous in school.

Grades often drop in the senior year of high school, most notably when vocational goals are unclear. There could be fears of the demands of college with feelings of inadequacy. There may be marked separation anxiety on leaving the familiar turf of school, home, and friends. The same may occur in the first and second semesters of college, especially when the student is away from home. There is also competition anxiety to consider as well as stranger anxiety (reactivations). As often happens when any change is made, separation problems may emerge.

Children with superior or higher IQ often become bored in an average classroom (unless offered extra challenging work) and may engage in fantasy and miss the instructions given. Borderline IQ and retarded youngsters may also underachieve because of emotional problems and situational difficulties. Just as happens to higher IQ youngsters, retardates may also have exam anxiety and underachieve on tests.

With the epidemic of substance and alcohol abuse in youngsters, toxic effects may lead to decreased attention and concentration, with resultant underachievement and reduced attendance.

After the death of a loved one, a youngster has an intense period of mourning, depending on his age and understanding of death. He may

433

see the loss as temporary or permanent. He may feel guilty in some way about the loss, believing that he contributed through some death wishes during an argument with the parent who died.

In the United States, about fifty percent of marriages end in divorce. Youngsters in a divorced family frequently have problems in concentration that interfere with learning because of a reactive depression. Children of divorce, of whatever age, are involved with a mourning reaction, conflicts of loyalties, feelings of guilt, and feelings that they may have caused the divorce or that they are the cause of the loss of a parent (Sugar 1970). With their minds focused and drained every day with constant guilt and self-deprecatory feelings, they have difficulty in concentrating, attending in class, or doing homework.

Case Example 3

A bright, early-adolescent boy with an engaging personality was developing suitably until his parents divorced. He remained with his mother, and he seemed to be doing well despite the divorce until she remarried and became more involved in an active social life with frequent excessive alcohol intake.

The youngster now experienced a double loss—his mother's inebriation and absence as well as loss of his original family. He felt neglected, angry, and rejected. He fantasized a great deal, imagining the parents reunited, happy, and living together once more with him. He shared none of his thoughts with his scattered older siblings, who were also going through their own turmoil and difficulties. The ordinary support system that otherwise would have been available was gone. He could not turn to his parents or siblings for support or any discussion of his troubled feelings. He was failing in school at the time he was seen for consultation.

During his six months of therapy, his feelings were clarified and dealt with. He was given additional support along with having his parents understand some of the features of his difficulty. He began to show more interest in school, his grades improved, his symptoms decreased, and underachievement was no longer a problem.

Vulnerabilities to learning come from such sources in the family as low socioeconomic status and nutritional deficiencies. The link between nutritional deficits (especially protein) and increased difficulties in learning has been understood for the past forty years (Blanchard 1946;

Cravioto 1973). This finding has recently been substantiated again in an extensive study by Galler, Ramsey, Solomano, Lowell, and Mason (1983a, 1983b) in which learning disabilities and attention deficit disorders were related to malnutrition.

Youngsters who have abusing or battering parents generally have a lower achievement than their potential. Although Pavenstedt (1967) found a pseudoprecocity in children of disorganized families, these children were handicapped emotionally and intellectually by nursery-school age. Despite "street" knowledge, they were delayed in perceptual and cognitive development, and by the time they arrived at adolescence, they were further handicapped.

Parental ambitiousness may be a factor for an underachieving child who is of average IQ and/or lacks burning ambitiousness. If the parents cannot accept the youngster as he or she is, and they chastise or punish the youngster for not fulfilling their wish, he or she may simply give up and do even worse academically. Professional people, doctors included, are prone to push their offspring for greater achievements.

Extremely wealthy, powerful, or successful people, who give their adolescents the idea that they will never have to work because the business or inheritance is theirs, rob the youngsters of the drive and motivation to learn and the desire to make something of, and for, themselves.

Immigrant families with a marked conflict in cultural values between the generations (the old adhering to the source culture and the young generation assimilating the conflict ridden and alien new) may be beset with the further problems of underachieving adolescents due to the family conflict. Displaced negative feelings from the parents to the teacher or vice versa may lead to decreased involvement in the learning effort by the student.

Youngsters who are achieving well academically often have a drop in grades when there is destabilization of the family through some major crisis (i.e., illness, a move, or alcoholism) in the parents. When this occurs, the youngster turns to peers (often unstable ones) for support and approval, disparages education and the parents, and views making good grades as being a traitor to the peer groups.

In families that disparage education, attending school and making good grades becomes a conflicted activity. Loyalty to family values may be in the ascendancy; the youngster remains in school solely to fulfill the law and quits as soon as possible, with or without a job. The same is often the case when youngsters hew to the ideals of their adolescent peers. Boys often view learning as feminine, when it is promoted only by mothers. This may be especially so in families with absent fathers; the males try to escape it since it is perceived as threatening to their masculinity.

The amount of stimulation that a family provides is very important in connection with the development of maximum knowledge and intellectual potential. This may relate to the very earliest years of life as well as to issues during the school years (Skeels 1966). In homes where there are books, where the parents read, where there is an interest in cultural aspects of various sorts, the children learn that there is a reward through imitation and identification with the parents and ultimately may find some rewarding responses from the pursuits themselves.

6. EDUCATIONAL SYSTEM FACTORS

In recent decades, the educational system in this country has become two-tiered. The public schools have been equalled or outnumbered by private schools in some parts of the country. Though each is of variable quality in standards, teachers, and curriculum, the public schools are now looked down on by the private schools. Parental support is often unavailable in the public schools and may be less than optimal even in private schools as parents strain to meet private school fees.

Many youngsters are passed from grade to grade because of social consequences (the teacher fears "if that teenager were not promoted . . ." or believes the adolescent is "too big to remain in a lower grade"). Underachievement is almost the status quo and reflects a national apathy about keeping standards of achievement that are meaningful for students. For several decades, we have planted socially what we are now reaping academically. Lower academic standards, social promotions, and giveaway courses and grades have led to a mass educational state of underachievement by the young; one in five workers now is functionally illiterate and unable to undertake advanced training.

After eighteen months of study, the National Commission on Excellence in Education concluded that about twenty-three million American adults are functionally illiterate; about 13 to 40 percent of all seventeen-year-olds are functionally illiterate; more than half of gifted students do not achieve up to their tested ability; remedial math courses are now one-quarter of all maths taught in state colleges; and one-quarter of Navy recruits cannot read at the ninth-grade level, the minimum required to understand written safety instructions (see "A Nation at Risk: Education Report" in the *New Orleans Times— Picayune* 1983).

Poor grades in school are often seen as the equivalent of misbehavior. Youngsters who are distractible, impulsive, and disruptive have poor grades because they have difficulty concentrating in class. Their symptoms affect their classmates as well. If the teacher ridicules distractible or impulsive students or those who do not do as well as hoped, the youngsters may associate learning with pain and poor grades, which can lead to withdrawal, avoidance, and more poor grades.

An additional aspect of underachievement depends on the teacher's sensitivity and functioning. When teachers are unsympathetic, untrained to understand emotional needs, or have serious problems— such as being severely disturbed, psychotic, or incompetent—it affects students, so that the whole class may be underachieving for the year.

MINIMAL COMMUNICATION BETWEEN PARENTS AND SCHOOL

If communication is lacking between teachers and parents about students' attendance, conduct, attitude, and participation, even the report cards about grades may carry little weight for the student in need of help. The student may need testing for disabilities—physical, neurological, or emotional—but without a clear picture of the student in class, the teacher overlooks an opportunity to help the parent initiate further help. If absences are not brought to parental attention, the student may miss weeks or months without the working parents' knowledge and then be failed for lack of knowledge or for having less than the minimum required days in school.

Case Example 4

A fifteen-year-old boy of average intelligence had been truant without his parents being notified by the school. This youngster had had average grades in the preceding year without any conduct difficulties. He had been on drugs for more than two years. When the school term began, he increased his dealing and substance abuse. As he continued in this state, he hardly ate, lost weight, and slept fitfully and in fear. He fought verbally and physically with family and friends. After the parents discovered he had failed all subjects, they attempted a discussion, but he became enraged, fought with them, became more depressed, and then overdosed. Subsequently, he admitted his truancy and was referred for therapy.

Case Example 5

A youngster of sixteen years was failing in an excellent private school, after having passed the previous years satisfactorily. In the preceding grade, he had had a trip to the hospital emergency room after excessive use of alcohol and violence to the family. During exam week about a year later, he was severely inebriated. While out of contact and control, he was admitted to the psychiatric ward. From a discussion with the school personnel, the parents learned that their son had been seeing the school counselor for many months because of his poor grades. The counselor knew of the boy's history of heavy drinking and pot smoking but kept it from the parents because of the confidentiality involved.

Conclusions

Every average classroom can expect a high number of underachievers, given the broad range of potential causes. The burden is squarely on early detection, proper placement, and efforts to help these youngsters. Only one-fifth will need psychiatric treatment. The others need to be attended to by the family, society, teachers, improved education standards, detection of teachers' emotional and competence problems, proper nutrition, and good medical care.

If we can provide a healthy beginning for all children, starting in utero, and have this concept nurtured, broadened, and deepened so that they are ready to learn when they start the primary grades, then, perhaps—with a furthering of such aims to improve education along all societal tributaries—there will be fewer underachieving adolescents and youngsters will be able to achieve their maximum potential in learning.

438

REFERENCES

Baird, H. W.; John, E. R.; Ahn, H.; and Maisel, E. 1980. Neurometric evaluation of epileptic children who do well and poorly in school. *Electroencephalography and Neurophysiology* 48:683–693.

Blanchard, P. 1946. Psychoanalytic contributions to the problem of reading disability. *Psychoanalytic Study of the Child* 2:163–187.

Cartwright, J. D.; Rosin, M. F.; and Price, Y. 1980. A medical team approach to children who fail to progress in school. *South African Medical Journal* 57:248–251.

Cravioto, J. R. 1973. Nutritional deprivation and psychobiological development in children. In S. G. Sapir and A. C. Nitzburg, eds. *Children with Learning Problems*. New York: Brunner/Mazel.

Freud, S. 1905. Three essays on the theory of sexuality. *Standard Edition* 7:125–126. London: Hogarth, 1968.

Finucci, J. M., and Childs, B. 1983. Dyslexia: family studies. In C. Ludlow and G. Cooper, eds. *Genetic Aspects of Speech and Learning Disorder*. New York: Academic Press.

Galler, J. R.; Ramsey, F.; Solomano, G.; Lowell, W. E.; and Mason, E. 1983a. The influence of malnutrition on subsequent behavioral development. I. Degree of impairment in intellectual performance. *Journal of the American Academy of Child Psychiatry* 22:8–16.

Galler, J. R.; Ramsey, F.; Solomano, G.; Lowell, W. E.; and Mason, E. 1983b. The influence of malnutrition on subsequent behavioral development. II. Classroom behavior. *Journal of the American Academy of Child Psychiatry* 22:16–23.

Hier, D. B.; Atkins, L.; and Perlo, V. P. 1980. Learning disorders and sex chromosome aberrations. *Journal of Mental Deficiency Research* 24:17–26.

Holdsworth, L., and Whitmore, K. 1974. A study of children attending ordinary schools. I. Their seizure patterns, progress and behavior in school. *Developmental Medicine and Child Neurology* 16:746–758.

Levine, M. D.; Oberklaid, F.; and Meltzer, L. 1981. Developmental output failure: a study of low productivity in school-aged children. *Pediatrics* 67:18–25.

McKay, S., and Brumback, R. A. 1980. Relationship between learning disabilities and juvenile delinquency. *Perceptual and Motor Skills* 51:1223–1226.

439

A nation at risk: education report—a tide of mediocrity. 1983. *New Orleans Times—Picayune,* August 28, sec. 1, pp. 23–25.

Pavenstedt, E. 1967. *The Drifters: Children of Disorganized Lower-Class Families.* Boston: Little, Brown.

Piaget, J. 1952. *The Origins of Intelligence in Children.* New York: International Universities Press.

Silver, L. B. 1983. Introduction. In C. C. Brown, ed. *Childhood Learning Disabilities and Prenatal Risk.* Pediatric Roundtable no. 9. New York: Johnson & Co.

Skeels, H. M. 1966. Adult status of children with contrasting early life experiences. *Monograph of the Society for Research in Child Development* 31:1–65.

Sugar, M. 1968. Normal adolescent mourning. *American Journal of Psychotherapy* 22:258–269.

Sugar, M. 1970. Children of divorce. *Pediatrics* 46:588–595.

Sugar, M. 1982. *The Premature in Context.* New York: Spectrum.

Zinkus, P. M.; Gottlieb, L.; and Zinkus, C. B. 1979. The learning disabled juvenile delinquent: a case for early intervention of perceptually handicapped children. *American Journal of Occupational Therapy* 33:180–184.

29 UNDERACHIEVEMENT AND FAILURE IN COLLEGE: THE INTERACTION BETWEEN INTRAPSYCHIC AND INTERPERSONAL FACTORS FROM THE PERSPECTIVE OF SELF PSYCHOLOGY

HOWARD S. BAKER

The importance of childhood trauma is a subject of controversy within the psychoanalytic movement. Is the crucial etiology of adult psychopathology the actual traumas and failures of the childhood environment? Or is it the sexual and aggressive fantasies and drives directed toward parents and the conflicts that arise as a consequence of those drives and fantasies? Most psychiatrists probably would find both important and would add that biology, family interactions, and relations with the broader social network must also be considered. Despite widespread agreement that all of these factors interact, there is less consensus on how they interact. The purpose of this chapter is to offer an explanation of their interaction from the particular viewpoint of the psychology of the self.

The discussion begins with a brief summary of the psychology of the self that Kohut (1971, 1977, 1984) and others have formulated. Of necessity, this is a simplification of a complex subject and does not include the criticism that self psychology has provoked (see Curtis 1985; Levine 1985; Slapp and Levine 1978; and Wallerstein 1983). That summary is followed by case material of students with severe academic inhibition, which shows how the metapsychology of self psychology can explain some of the pathogenic interactions between psyche, family, and broader

441

social milieu. This material further demonstrates how a self psychological perspective adds a useful dimension to the treatment of some failing college students.

Summary of Self Psychological Theory

Kohut (1971, 1977) concluded that developmental and ongoing interpersonal interactions affect the formation and maintenance of one's basic identity. What actually happened developmentally and currently is happening between our patients and important others is the most salient factor in creating intrapsychic structures, in shaping and altering the drives, in developing the dynamics of conflict, and in producing symptomatology.

Repeated, significant failures on the part of parents and parental substitutes occupy a place of primary importance in the etiology of psychopathology. Kohut realized that the child's behavior, such as petulant withdrawal or aggressive behavior with siblings, might at times complicate matters. He believed, nevertheless, that it was most accurate and useful to see those responses as the child's best effort to preserve the integrity of his developing self.

He believed that problems in nurturing create intrapsychic difficulties that will almost always persist into the adolescent and adult lives of the people whom we end up seeing as patients. Initially (Kohut 1971), these opinions were limited to those with preoedipal psychopathology. Eventually Kohut (1984) came to believe that actual limitations on the part of parents in meeting the needs of their children were factors in the development of essentially all psychopathology. However, he did not believe that all or even most of these failures were incestuous in nature. Rather he considered them to be parental inabilities to respond empathically to certain crucial developmental needs of their children.

Kohut realized that parents must (and generally do) respond with developmentally appropriate, accurate empathy to the needs of their children. He divided these needs into three specific groups: (1) mirroring, (2) idealizing, and (3) twinship or alter ego. Parents will inevitably fail to some extent, but Kohut thought that adequately appropriate parental response would lead to the development of endopsychic structures that enable the person to (1) maintain self-esteem; (2) establish vigorous and appropriate self-assertive ambitions; (3) calm and soothe the self under circumstances of stress or upset; (4) channel and regulate the drives; (5) develop meaningful goals for living; and (6) maintain a sense of connectedness to other human beings. In the remainder of this essay, I shall refer to these six elements as the essential self-capabilities.

Mirroring is the term used to describe one aspect of parental response to the child's behavior. If the parent's response is appropriate delight and pride, this response will reflect back to the child (as a mirror reflects back our visual image) that the child is valuable and a source of pleasure. A consistent parental response of indifference, competitiveness, or hostility provides a reflection that is similar to a fun-house mirror— no matter where one stands or what one does, the reflection is unattractive. The parents' ability to respond to the child is distorted by their own limitations, but the child is unable to realize that the mirror provided by parents may be distorted. Instead, the child believes their reflection of him is true and that he is genuinely defective—that he is of little value, that he is intrusive and bothersome, and that his self-assertion is unlikely to be enjoyed or appreciated.

The child responds to parental empathic failures in mirroring by developing fantasies of himself as perfect and omnipotent. Kohut calls this the grandiose self. The child expects total perfection of himself and needs constant external approval of this perfection in order to tolerate himself. If the parents are genuinely "good enough parents" (Winnicott 1965), who provide a sufficient gratification balanced by appropriate frustration, the child tempers the grandiose self and replaces it with intrapsychic capabilities to maintain self-esteem, to have realistic ambitions, and to pursue those ambitions with vigor. He is then able to tolerate slights, criticism, and failure without serious disruption. If, however, the balance between good enough success and occasional failure to meet the mirroring needs of the child is tipped seriously in the direction of excessive deprivation or gratification, the child will continue to be plagued by the demands of the grandiose self and the resultant inability to tolerate the inevitable frustrations of life. Numerous symptomatic behaviors and feelings will probably eventuate.

The child needs, demands, and wants a positive or even extravagant mirroring response in a multitude of areas, one of which is libidinal drives. It is certainly not uncommon for a small boy to ask his mother to admire or perhaps even kiss his penis. Her response to this request, and her overall response to him, will be crucial in determining the fantasies and conflicts that he will develop regarding his penis. Shocked withdrawal, a seductive flirtation, or a calm "It's very nice" followed by going about her business—each response will each lead to quite different fantasies in the child. Other mirroring needs include age-appropriate admiration for developmentally salient tasks such as learning to skip or reciting the ABCs. Again, responses may be highly inappropriate. For example, one mother became hysterical over a first-grader's report card. "You'll never get into college!" she cried. Since this was typical of her behavior, deeply confusing and troubling fantasies resulted in her child. The overall appropriateness of the parental responses to the child's mirroring needs determines the extent to which the child is able to soften the demands of the grandiose self and to replace fantasies of perfection and omnipotence with internal abilities to regulate self-esteem and establish appropriate and vigorous ambitions.

The idealizing needs of the child require a person who is available, willing, and able to help in the face of difficulty. Because of the presence of the idealized parent, the child feels that the world is a reasonably safe place or, at least, that there is a solution to problems that arise. The obvious paradigm for this occurs when the toddler falls and bruises his knee. The parent responds by picking up and kissing the child. The calmness of the parent, the relaxed tone of the parent's muscles, and the affection rendered all combine to soothe the child. From thousands of these interactions the child develops internal mechanisms to calm and soothe the self.

Again, parental responses will not and cannot be perfect. The consequence of this imperfection is the development of the idealized parental imago. This term refers to the child's hope for and effort to find the fantasized parent who is always available and is always able to handle any difficulty with ease and perfection. Basch (1984) compares this to Aladdin, who had his ever-present, all-powerful genie.

When a child is unsettled by libidinal drives, the parents' calming responses will create an atmosphere in which the child will learn not to be frightened by his drives. He will be able to find ways to channel and regulate these feelings. However, an angry or anxious response to questions like "What do you and Mommy do in bed?" will have a disruptive effect.

Just as with the grandiose self, if the balance is sufficient between good enough success and phase-appropriate failures in meeting the idealizing need of the child, the search for the idealized parental imago will be tempered, and the individual generally will be able to calm the self under stress and feel the need for and seek only that external reassurance that is normally available in life.

Finally, Kohut (1984) considered twinship needs. This area has been thought of as a distinct aspect of the self only in his last work, *How Does Analysis Cure?* (which points out that self psychology is by no means a finished theory and remains in a state of flux). The twinship need is the need to feel a sense of similarity to or connectedness with other people. The little girl who "helps" her mother cook dinner establishes that sense of connectedness when the mother enjoys this so-called help. If, however, there is a consistent response of not wanting the child there because she interferes with a busy schedule, the child will feel isolated, lonely, and disconnected. If, on the other hand, the balance of parental response is favorable, the child develops a feeling of relatedness to others and, when an adult, enjoys the silent pleasure of collegial support and the sense that we are all a part of the human race—that we are at least trying to work together.

In terms of drive issues, Kohut thought it crucial that the parents' twinship responses communicate that the child is a "chip off the old block" rather than that the sensual feelings are peculiar or nasty. He came to believe that the child's sexual conflicts and fantasies were profoundly dependent on the patterns of parental mirroring, idealizing, and twinship responses. He did not consider the salient issue in pathogenesis to be primarily the intensity and the unavoidably conflicted nature of the child's aggressive and libidinal drives. Rather he considered the crucial factor to be the nature of the parental responses to those drives and fantasies. He believed that under the conditions of developmentally appropriate responses by parents, children would resolve their conflicts without serious difficulty.

The relationship in which the constituents of the self develop is described by Kohut as a selfobject relationship. Selfobjects assist the self in accomplishing certain functions that cannot be achieved entirely independently. They help the person maintain self-esteem, facilitate the restoration of calm in the face of upset, and aid in the other essential self-capabilities noted above. The selfobject serves a vital psychological function, just as the lungs serve a vital physiological function. Furthermore, while the extent of the self's dependence on its self-objects diminishes with maturity, Kohut believes that one can never be entirely without them any more than one can exist without oxygen. Furthermore, and in contradistinction to accepted object relations theory, who (or even what) meets the selfobject need is at least relatively independent of the particular individual who is meeting the need. That is to say, the self must meet its mirroring needs; but if the mother fails, the father, nurse, sibling, teacher, or others are sought as somewhat equivalent substitutes. For example, some patients—when frustrated by someone who is vital in helping maintain self-esteem—will be forced into a frantic search for other selfobject supplies, often resorting to promiscuity or other symptomatic behavior in the effort to obtain a selfobject relationship.

Selfobject needs follow a developmental course that is parallel to and different from object development. What the self requires of its selfobjects varies at different points in the life cycle (Wolf 1980). The toddler may need reassurance when he falls, while the adolescent may need tolerance and thoughtful limit setting in efforts to understand and regulate sexual feelings. The extent to which one needs selfobject assistance varies from absolute to modest. What determines the level of maturity is the responsiveness of the crucial selfobjects at each developmental level—and whether the person was able to use those selfobjects effectively in building endopsychic capabilities to do internally what the selfobject had done externally. Past selfobject failures leave deficits in internal structures that complicate all further developmental phases.

Since one is never without need of selfobject support, it is evident that parents have selfobject needs that can vary from modest to constant and desperate. Parents must turn to each other, to their friends, relatives, and jobs—and to their children—to meet these needs. Thus, when other sources fail, parents may make inappropriate demands on their children. Despite having genuine love for their children, parents may put their own requirements ahead of their children's developmental needs. Their doing so will yield problems for the growing child. For example, one father needed a son who was a fine athlete and pushed his son to be a hockey player despite the fact that the son had a deformed leg.

The success of the child-parent interaction in mirroring, idealizing, and twinship selfobject relationships enables the development of intrapsychic structures that provide the essential self-capabilities described, such as the independent maintenance of self-esteem. These structures facilitate the experience of a firm sense of self, one that is only minimally vulnerable to disappointments and failures.

Defining "self" is important, although very difficult. The dictionary states that the self is "the essential person distinct from all other persons in identity." Noshpitz (1984, p. 18) has noted, "Perhaps nothing is more real and immediate for each person than his subjective sense of self. At the same time, nothing is harder to describe." He clarifies the concept by describing the self as if it occupied space. Within that space are numerous characteristics. These include (1) the routine patterns by which self-esteem is maintained, tension is reduced, and drives are regulated and channeled; (2) the patterns of major ambitions and goals; and (3) the ways available skills are used to attempt to achieve these goals. These factors create a nuclear program that the self seeks to express or actualize through characteristic action.

Within this "territory," a vital essence exists—something that needs selfobject sustenance to thrive and is vulnerable to selfobject failure. With optimal selfobject responses, the child develops a healthy, vigorous self that is capable of withstanding even serious failure and selfobject loss without experiencing fragmentation or depression. In health, the nuclear program of the self is relatively internally based, or as Kohut and Wolf (1978, p. 414) put it, the self is an "independent center of initiative." However, a less fundamentally secure self is more reliant on selfobject supplies and may need to sacrifice its needs substantially in order to comply with demands made by the selfobjects. Then a conflict is created between maintaining selfobject supplies (which are needed to avoid fragmentation or depression) and unfolding the nuclear program of the self.

The experience of dissolution of the self is, according to Kohut (1984), the most profound anxiety known to mankind. While it is akin to the fear of death, he finds it more profound. It is the fear of psychological death. The abandonment so common as death approaches is often as troubling as the impending death itself, because it means that the dying person has lost vital, sustaining selfobjects at the very time they are most needed. The experience of self-dissolution was described by one patient in a recurrent fear known to him from childhood: "I am floating in space without oxygen, unable to touch anything solid, and no one is within millions of miles."

Because dissolution of the self is so impossible to tolerate, Kohut thought that maintenance of a coherent, vigorous self is the supraordinate motivation around which the structure of the personality is crystalized. People do what they do to maintain the cohesion of and enhance the development and expression of the self. Therefore, the individual must take action when disruptions occur in vital selfobject relationships. What are called symptoms are understood to be efforts to restore the sense of self. While symptoms may be unconstructive and shortsighted, they are perceived by the patient to be better than the experience of enfeeblement or fragmentation of the self.

Although not always successful, the self must and does take action to establish selfobject relationships that enable the full expression of its development. Buttressed by internal mechanisms to meet most mirroring, idealizing, and alterego needs, the mature person is generally able to obtain the remaining selfobject supplies from the average environment. Fragmentation and depleted depression are rare experiences; freedom exists for the development of the program of the self and for healthy object relationships, including object love.

The patient who has failed to develop effective intrapsychic mechanisms to calm the self and accomplish the other essential self-capabilities is, to some varying degree, excessively dependent on the environment to provide selfobject supplies. Exceptionally felicitous circumstances may occur, to enable further growth and substantial maturation of internal mechanisms. Far more likely, though, the environment will fail, and the self will experience frightening fragmentation and/or depression. Frantic efforts to reestablish selfobjects may result in self-destructive and/or indiscriminate object choices and a variety of symptoms.

Parents fail to meet the selfobject needs of their children for a variety of reasons. These failures are rarely caused by mean spiritedness, a wish to harm the child, or even lack of love for the child. They are most frequently a result of limitations in the parents' personalities that make it impossible for the parents to respond in the developmentally appropriate, empathic fashion. As noted, parents also have selfobject needs, and not infrequently their own selfobject needs take precedence over meeting the needs of their children. That is to say that narcissistically vulnerable parents are unable to respond as they might know they should when overwhelmed by their own needs. Kohut underscores this point by frequently stating that it is not so much what parents do—but rather who they are—that causes the failure in selfobject relatedness to their children.

Parents may also fail because certain inborn characteristics of the child interact with basic, normal character elements of the parents' personality in an unfortunate and unwholesome way (Thomas and Chess 1984). Some parents can enjoy an active child but are unable to respond to a passive one. Still other parents fail to respond sufficiently because unfortunate external events and/or the biology of the child make the child's needs difficult to meet. For example, some children have learning disabilities. With exceptional responsiveness, they can learn well and do not develop secondary narcissistic vulnerabilities. More often, the disability is not understood, and the child develops poor self-esteem and a tendency to avoid schoolwork. Thus, a parent might respond more than satisfactorily to a typical child but be unable to meet the needs of a special child.

In terms of treatment, self-psychologically based psychotherapy and psychoanalysis are engaged in an effort to understand (1) the nature of the disruptions in the ongoing selfobject milieu; (2) the consequences of these disruptions; (3) the vulnerabilities due to the lack of the internal structures needed to maintain the self; and (4) the genetic and dynamic origins of these structural deficits. The therapeutic alliance is understood to be a particular sort of selfobject relationship that satisfies the patient's need to be understood in depth. However, gratification of other selfobject needs is to be avoided. Disruptions in the selfobject relationships, particularly as they occur in the transference, are analyzed. If these disruptions are relatively small and manageable, the patient is provided with a manageable challenge and is offered a renewed opportunity to reinstitute development of the endopsychic structures. The patient may then accomplish the essential self-capabilities, such as the independent regulation of self-esteem.

Self psychology primarily conceptualizes psychopathology as resulting from deficits in internal structures not as the symbolic efforts to gratify or disavow drives complicated by unresolved conflicts. Although uncovering, clarifying, and resolving conflicts are important, these do not play a primary role. Instead, through the help of the therapeutic relationship, the patient creates new structures that protect and firm the self. These provide a solid foundation for object relations to develop and for the secondary resolution of conflict.

Self Psychology and Academic Underachievement

The internal life of adolescents is directly dependent on both the firmness of the intrapsychic mechanisms of the self and the responsiveness of their current milieu. While the intrapsychic and interpersonal worlds are different, they are interwoven into a fabric that can facilitate or interfere with personal growth and success. This interaction may be seen in many college students suffering from psychologically determined academic failure. They have satisfactory intellectual capability and sufficient developmental and academic cognitive preparation to enable them to function, but they do not.

As in all symptomatic behavior, four areas exist with varying degrees of importance—biological, sociological, familial (Baker 1975), and intrapsychic. The first three have an inevitable impact on the intrapsychic, leaving some individuals without a firm self. These weaknesses in the self make academic difficulties a certainty.

Academic success demands that students be able to maintain self-esteem in the face of the inevitable small failures that study insistently presents. They must be able to calm themselves sufficiently to sit quietly and read, take notes, and learn for long periods of time. They also need to have developed appropriate academic goals, possess self-assertive ambitions to pursue those goals, and have the technical skills required to accomplish them. While a certain amount of help from the selfobjects we call faculty, friends, and family is possible and necessary, students must be able to stand alone to a considerable extent, relying on already developed and sufficient intrapsychic capacities. If these internal capacities are deficient, symptomatic efforts to restore the sense of self will occur and the student will be unable to do the necessary academic work.

College demands mastery of a substantial body of knowledge. If a student is not able to tolerate the multitude of small frustrations that occur when reading a text and not understanding it immediately, problems are inevitable. If, because of the persistence of the unmodified grandiose self, a student demands absolute perfection of himself, he is certain to feel intolerably stupid and valueless almost every time he tries to study. The demands of this grandiosity, combined with the inability to regulate self-esteem internally, can then cause sufficient loss of self-esteem and precipitate frightening fragmentation or enfeeblement of the self. The student must then avoid the source of the threat and undertake steps to repair and restore the self.

In behavioral terms, this means one may spend hours in front of books without really studying. He may be so distracted by his internal needs that his ability to absorb material unrelated to those needs is diminished to almost nothing. He may be lost in grandiose daydreams, which may restore the sense of self temporarily. Another student might act out and seek something comfortable, such as watching TV, talking to friends, smoking marijuana, or indulging in sexual exploits. In any case, what does not get done is effective study. The obvious result is poor test results and inadequate grades.

As described, self psychology understands that the capability to regulate self-esteem develops in the context of mirroring relationships with selfobjects. The reason some students are unable to sit alone quietly for the prolonged periods of time that studying demands may not be primarily due to difficulties regulating self-esteem. Rather, when alone, tension or overstimulation builds. Without the internal capability to calm oneself, escalating affect (whatever its source) interferes with the ability to concentrate. According to self psychological theory, the internal ability to calm the self is developed in the nurturant ground of idealizing selfobject relationships. Again, without the ability to calm down, the danger to self-cohesiveness may grow to such an intolerable extent that some sort of emergency measures must be taken. Above all, one must avoid the source of the danger—studying. Solace may be sought in the comfort of a sexual relationship or in endless bull sessions in the dormitory. Obviously, the work does not get done, and the result is predictable.

For still other students with problems in the idealizing pole of the self, the issues are slightly different. In high school, under the strict supervision of teachers and parents, these students were told exactly what to do and when to do it, and they complied. In college, however, studying must be done on a self-motivated basis, without parental restrictions. In high school, phase-appropriate independence was never granted to them, so internal discipline did not develop. Furthermore, many became excellent at figuring out what the salient authority figures wanted and producing it and only it—not a prescription for independent thinking. When they encounter university-level teachers who demand independent analysis and evaluation, these students flounder. It is perhaps noteworthy that there are some disciplines that require much less independent thinking, and many students may do well in such areas. For example, certain aspects of accounting and engineering fall into the structured category, whereas theoretical physics and the humanities generally do not.

This last problem is closely related to still another problem that may occur because of disruptions in selfobject relationships. Most often, we see it toward the end of college or graduate school. The university

451

setting and/or the faculty advisor provides a substantial opportunity to meet both mirroring and idealizing needs. Without the related internal mechanisms to regulate self-esteem, pursue ambitions, calm the self, and set relevant personal goals, the student is unable to give up the advisor or the university, because he needs continued external self-object supplies to make up for internal deficits. Consequently, he may end up failing a course in the last semester or become unable to complete a dissertation.

In many of the mentioned circumstances, therapists understand the data in terms of conflicts related to oedipal competition or separation from the needed maternal object. Indeed, for some students, this explanation is entirely satisfactory. For others, the self psychological perspective may simply add an enriching dimension. However, for a number of students, I believe that what initially masquerades as conflict-related pathology is later revealed to be based on self pathology (Tolpin 1978). These students form both selfobject and object transferences (Wolf 1984/85), but the selfobject transference requires particular attention. They are exquisitely sensitive to insult and/or are unable to tolerate working alone. With these people, one must be ever alert to the selfobject failures that led to the intensification of the conflicts surrounding competition and/or separation and individuation. We may find, for example, a graduate student with an advisor well known to be an exceptionally competitive person, who in fact has tremendous difficulties dealing with the successes of students and colleagues. Such advisors may actively or passively interfere with their advisees' work in ways that are subtle or blatant. It comes as no surprise that individuals who have had highly competitive parents "mysteriously" seem to end up with such advisors.

As a consequence of early selfobject failures, many students have problems both in maintaining self-esteem and in calming themselves when under stress. Therefore, they have intensified needs to seek mirroring and idealized selfobjects in their current environment. If, to return to the same example, an advisor is not exceptionally sensitive and does not provide a great deal of affirmation and encouragement, selfobject needs will fail to be met. This failure enfeebles the self and precipitates danger of self-disintegration. As Kohut (1972) pointed out, the danger of self-disintegration precipitates narcissistic rage toward the failing selfobject. This rage can genuinely look like out-of-control competitiveness.

452

Unfortunately, interpreting a problem rooted in self pathology as competitiveness based on drive-related residuals from the Oedipus conflict may miss a deeper problem. The patient may then feel that oedipal or competitive interpretations simply miss the mark. However, a more serious problem may occur—one that can interfere with the therapeutic process. Since such interpretations do not describe what the patient is experiencing, they may leave him feeling misunderstood, demeaned, or even assaulted. The mirror that the therapist then provides is inaccurate and countertherapeutic. Such a well-intended interpretation may further reduce the patient's vulnerable self-esteem and might drive a wedge through the therapeutic alliance (Terman 1984/85). The patient may drop out of therapy feeling abandoned or betrayed, or—and this is far worse—he may feel compelled by his need for a selfobject relationship to continue therapy. But he goes underground. He avoids talking about issues and may even fake a cure to please the idealized person whom he needs. Of course, he needs the therapist to provide the understanding selfobject without which growth is impossible. In the absence of this understanding, he complies with what appears to be the therapeutic process. However, he has unwittingly colluded with and further confused the therapist. The misguided course of treatment gives the appearance of progress but leaves the underlying problems untouched.

Clinical Examples

Three cases illustrate the two major theses of this chapter—that self psychology offers one explanation for the relationship between intrapsychic and interpersonal aspects of human psychology and that it can also provide a useful framework for treating some students suffering from academic underachievement.

Tom became my patient many years ago, before publication of Kohut's first book. He was an undergraduate student at a prestigious and competitive eastern university. Despite genuine intellectual gifts, well demonstrated on standardized tests, he was in danger of flunking out. He complained that he was unable to study, became easily bored, and was dissatisfied with his performance.

Tom was the oldest of three brothers born into a troubled family. His parents' marriage was marred by constant conflict, and they had separated when Tom was five. His father returned when Tom was seven, but it was never possible for the two men to establish a positive relationship. The father would tell his wife about any affection Tom expressed to him, provoking jealousy in her and betraying Tom's confidence. The mother was a difficult woman, both intrusive and occasionally seductive. When Tom was fourteen, his parents again separated and divorced, completely rupturing the relationship between father and son. The father was unable to meet even his financial responsibilities due to his long-term, serious gambling problem. His meeting his emotional responsibilities to Tom was out of the question.

From this abbreviated history, one can easily discern serious conflicts for Tom surrounding both oedipal competition with his father and separation from his mother. Repeated interpretations based on that understanding were made in a thoughtful, kind manner. Whenever possible, transference data were used to clarify these conflicts. I thought I was offering correct, well-timed interpretations; my supervisors agreed; and the patient generally seemed to understand. The only problem was that neither his grades nor his object relations showed much improvement.

After familiarizing myself with Kohut's first book, "new" data emerged (which had undoubtedly been present all along but which I failed to appreciate). My attention turned to the unbridled demands of Tom's untamed grandiose self. His grades improved, and he took the Graduate Record Exams. He got all but one question correct, which placed him in the top of the ninety-ninth percentile. But our work was by no means done, since all he could experience was disappointment that he had failed to achieve a perfect score.

My interpretations shifted to deal with the disappointment he felt with both of his parents. His father was not effectively loving and helpful and would use Tom as a tool in arguments with his wife. He could not by example help Tom set adequate goals for a career or for life. Crippled by his own tensions, which led to his compulsive gambling, he could not comfort and calm Tom when he needed help in that area. Thus, Tom was unable to calm himself to study and was unable to set relevant goals.

Although Tom experienced no shortage of insults from his father, Tom's mother was even more problematic in her rapid shifts from excessive praise to inappropriate attack. Particularly during the repeated disruptions in her relationship with her husband, Tom's mother would turn to her son for sustenance. She idealized the boy and needed his presence to comfort her. As noted earlier, parents always gain some selfobject benefits from their children. Unable to gain support from her husband or her own parents, Tom's mother found it necessary to turn to Tom in ways that were primarily designed to meet her, but not his, needs.

Interpretations were directed primarily at examination of disruptions in selfobject relationships between Tom and his parents, girlfriends, peers, and others. We continued to work through the consequences in his daily life of the multitude of unreasonable, perfectionistic demands he made on himself. Most important, we tried to understand the ways he felt I failed him and how he reacted to disruptions in the selfobject relationship between us. He began to tolerate minor failures and felt that they taught him how to work more effectively.

Gradual progress occurred in all areas. Several years after our last therapeutic contact, a chance meeting revealed that Tom had completed graduate school, was apparently happily married, and was the father of two children.

Had Tom found a supportive selfobject relationship with a teacher, that relationship might have enabled him to repair some of the intrapsychic deficits on his own. Were the school less demanding, he might not have experienced the repeated assaults to his perfectionism. Opportunities for healing experiences were not sufficiently available to enable Tom to develop the essential intrapsychic capabilities to love and work. The demands of Tom's grandiose self and his needs for an idealizable parental imago were simply beyond the capabilities of his available environment, and therapeutic intervention was required.

Paul was another young man with abundant intellectual gifts, but his grades careened between F's and A's, and he always found himself on probation or very near it. If a problem arose when studying, he would immediately abandon the work. Unprepared, he would cut classes, fearing he would be called on and appear stupid. He would then be afraid he had annoyed the instructor and find it necessary to miss still more classes. If a particular professor did, in fact, tend to be critical or unsupportive, the problem was worse. If the subject matter seemed easily mastered, however, or if the teacher seemed kind, Paul would generally get an A.

Paul was obsessed with his physical appearance. He was panicked by the belief that he was going bald, although the casual observer would never have noticed that he was losing his hair. If he were upset, he would look into every available mirror to check his hair. If he was at a shopping center—filled as they are with mirrors—his despair might deepen to such an extent that he had to return home to a darkened room. If he were in a good mood, he would not even look in mirrors.

His relationships with women were also deeply tortured. He felt that the lot of women was infinitely superior to that of men. He was jealous that women could have multiple orgasms, and he believed that men had no choice but to satisfy women in any way they demanded. He claimed he would perform cunnilingus on his willing girlfriend for hours, maintaining an erection but never ejaculating.

Again, the interaction between intrapsychic deficits and the availability of selfobject sustenance in the patient's environment is evident. Most college women probably would not wish the sexual interaction described, but Paul found one who did. His obsession with his appearance and with mirrors varied as a direct, and eventually obvious, consequence of interactions between important others and himself. Consequently, kindly teachers got very different academic work from him than did aloof or critical ones.

Paul's mother was a severely, narcissistically self-involved woman. She spent untold hours on her appearance and was devoted to a part-time career as lead singer in a rock band (at age fifty-two). These preoccupations led to frequent neglect of the needs of the remainder of the family. The parents appeared to have a civil but unaffectionate and disengaged marriage. The father was rarely emotionally available to either his wife or Paul.

The therapy was conducted primarily along self psychological guidelines. Interpretations were directed at disruptions in and repair of critical selfobject relationships. I chose to address competitive difficulties from the vantage point of the demands of his grandiosity rather than to consider conflicts over aggression.

Paul also presented an exceptionally clear example of narcissism interfering with competition in an arena other than academics. He was a potential professional athlete in an individual sport that has accurately measured scores. He could easily beat many opponents and could perform well even against known professionals. In situations where he was pitted against an equal and beating his rival depended more on determination than on talent, however, he would freeze and lose. These failures might be explained reasonably as a derivative of unresolved castration anxiety. Close questioning revealed, however, that in these situations he would make a minor error and berate himself furiously.

He would then panic that the opponent or spectators would consider him a phoney and humiliate him. Interpretations focused on his grandiosity, which demanded positive mirroring from his athletic performance, spectators, and opponents—all of whom functioned as needed selfobjects. These interventions helped, and the improvement showed in his academic scores as well as his athletic performance.

Paul has a severe narcissistic personality disorder and remains in treatment. He has, however, graduated from college. When he began psychotherapy, his average was just under 2.0 (on a 4-point scale). For his last several semesters he got near a 3.0, and he finished with a 2.4 average. He has broken up with the first girlfriend and established a relationship with a more understanding and giving woman. While symptomatic improvement has occurred, fundamental weakness persists in his self-structure, which requires continued examination of the vicissitudes of his selfobject relationships, particularly within the transference. A phase may well occur toward the end of therapy in which the emphasis will shift to more drive- or conflict-related issues. Kohut (1977) noted that this occurs, but he found that it is relatively brief and that the patient does not find it to be a difficult phase of treatment.

A final case concerns another young man for whom issues of family, social class, and neighborhood peers provided serious complications. John is the son of immigrants from eastern Europe and the family structure was typical of the "old country." The father was a laborer—to be obeyed without question—and the mother was not permitted to work, although money was needed. They lived in a neighborhood surrounded by families of similar background and values. Until college, John attended parochial schools. As a college student, he continued to live at home.

The parents had no knowledge of what college life was like but insisted that John study essentially without a break for five or six hours each evening. Although John was not particularly interested in engineering, his parents demanded he pursue that major, believing it would assure him a lucrative job. It was necessary for him to work part-time to help finance his education. He was the only person at his job who attended college, and his co-workers constantly derided him for his "snobbish" pretensions.

John began his college education at a school that catered to the children of affluent parents. His daily commute lasted an hour and a half and passed through some of the most affluent neighborhoods in the city. The view from the commuter-train window was like looking into a mirror and seeing all he wished he was, but all he thought he was not. He felt out of touch with and envious of the other students. He was also alienated from his peers at work. His grades were poor, but not failing, and he transferred to another college that had more students from his socioeconomic background but was also more academically competitive. Unfortunately, at the first school, he had acquired a number of upper-class tastes and attitudes, and he looked down on the other working-class students as plodders who were ignorant of or cared nothing for important intellectual values. When his grades deteriorated, he sought counseling.

Again, an underlying perfectionism was present and was mainly dealt with using cognitive techniques. Repeated examination of his relationship with his parents enabled him to accept them and yet to change his major to one more suited to his interests. Support was offered concerning his anguish about loyalties to his peers in the neighborhood and at work. These therapeutic interventions, based on a self psychological perspective, produced felicitous results. His average grades before treatment were about 2.0 and after treatment were above 3.0. Recent contact revealed that he was about to graduate and was actively pursuing appropriate job opportunities.

Conclusions

Freud (1926, p. 195) noted that, "In psychology we can only describe things by the help of analogies. There is nothing peculiar in this; it is the case elsewhere as well. But we have constantly to keep changing these analogies, for none of them lasts us long enough." For some practitioners, self psychology offers a new set of analogies useful in explaining the interaction between intrapsychic and interpersonal variables relevant to a patient's psychopathology. It conceives of human interaction in terms of both object and selfobject relationships. When the internal structures necessary to maintain the cohesion of the self are poorly developed, a person must turn to important others. He may then act in such a way as to meet his own selfobject needs; but, at the same time, he may interfere with vital selfobject needs of the other. These behaviors, in turn, lead to an often endless chain of disappointments and create the sort of intrapsychic difficulties that often yield psychopathology.

The self psychological perspective has offered some clinical usefulness under a variety of conditions. Since relative outcome data comparing self psychological and neotraditional psychoanalytic approaches do not yet exist, sweeping claims about which approach is superior are inappropriate. My position, however, presented here and elsewhere (Baker 1979), is that a self psychological approach can be useful in the treatment of at least some students who are in serious academic difficulty. Self psychology can also provide a basis for interventions that range from psychoanalytically oriented psychotherapy to cognitive psychotherapy.

When psychoanalysis or psychoanalytically oriented psychotherapy is appropriate and available, self psychological interventions deal primarily with examination of disruptions and repairs in selfobject relationships. The therapist is concerned in this regard with both the transference and the ongoing relationships in the patient's environment. Examination of the origins and consequences of insufficient intrapsychic structures is also useful.

Although treatment of failing students often proves difficult, it is clear that individual cases show significant improvement when the principals of self psychology help to inform the treatment. The statement of Wolf (1983, p. 316) gives a helpful perspective: "As a physician, a scientist, and as a responsible human being I cannot ethically ignore the vistas opened up by self psychology. But this does not mean that classical psychoanalytic theory is wrong. Rather, classical theory is merely another way of looking at and organizing data, and for some patients it is the most useful and effective way of doing so."

REFERENCES

Baker, H. 1975. The treatment of academic underachievement. *Journal of the American College Health Association* 24:4–7.
Baker, H. 1979. The conquering hero quits: narcissistic factors in underachievement and failure. *American Journal of Psychotherapy* 33:418–427.
Basch, M. 1984. Selfobjects and the selfobject transference: theoretical implications. In P. Stapansky and A. Goldberg, eds. *Kohut's Legacy.* Hillsdale, N.J.: Analytic Press.
Curtis, H. 1985. Clinical perspectives on self psychology. *Psychoanalytic Quarterly* 56:339–378.

Freud, S. 1926. The question of lay analysis. *Standard Edition* 20:179–258. London: Hogarth, 1961.

Kohut, H. 1971. *The Analysis of the Self.* New York: International Universities Press.

Kohut, H. 1972. Thoughts on narcissism and narcissistic rage. *Psychoanalytic Study of the Child* 27:360–400.

Kohut, H. 1977. *The Restoration of the Self.* New York: International Universities Press.

Kohut, H. 1984. *How Does Analysis Cure?* Chicago: University of Chicago Press.

Kohut, H., and Wolf, E. 1978. The disorders of the self and their treatment: an outline. *International Journal of Psycho-Analysis* 59:413–424.

Levine, F. 1985. Self-psychology and the new narcissism in psychoanalysis. *Clinical Psychology Review* 5:215–229.

Noshpitz, J. 1984. Narcissism and aggression. *American Journal of Psychotherapy* 38:17–34.

Slapp, J. and Levine, F. 1978. On hybrid concepts in psychoanalysis. *Psychoanalytic Quarterly* 47:499–523.

Terman, D. 1984/85. The self and the Oedipus complex. *Annual of Psychoanalysis* 12/13:87–104.

Thomas, A., and Chess, S. 1984. Genesis and evolution of behavioral disorders: from infancy to early adult life. *American Journal of Psychiatry* 141:1–9.

Tolpin, M. 1978. Self-objects and oedipal objects. *Psychoanalytic Study of the Child* 33:167–184.

Wallerstein, R. 1983. Self psychology and "classical" psychoanalytic psychology: the nature of their relationship. In A. Goldberg, ed. *The Future of Psychoanalysis*. New York: International Universities Press.

Winnicott, D. 1965. *The Maturational Processes and the Facilitating Environment*. New York: International Universities Press.

Wolf, E. 1980. On the developmental line of selfobject relations. In A. Goldberg, ed. *Advances in Self Psychology*. New York: International Universities Press.

Wolf, E. 1983. Empathy and countertransference. In A. Goldberg, ed. *The Future of Psychoanalysis*. New York: International Universities Press.

Wolf, E. 1984/85. Self psychology and the neuroses. *Annual of Psychoanalysis* 12/13:57–68.

OBSERVATIONS FROM CLINICAL WORK
WITH HIGH SCHOOL AGED, DEAF
ADOLESCENTS ATTENDING
A RESIDENTIAL SCHOOL

CARL B. FEINSTEIN AND RICHARD LYTLE

It has long been recognized that psychiatric disorders are a major problem among hearing-impaired and deaf adolescents. Most previous writings in this area, however, have reported research on groups of children or have focused on general considerations regarding the personality traits of the deaf. This chapter will utilize a clinical, case-centered approach to focus on the common psychosocial problems of high school aged, deaf adolescents attending a residential school. Our objective is to describe the experiences and problems of a sector of our population about which many psychiatrists know very little. It is hoped that this approach will help familiarize clinicians who do not have regular contact with deaf individuals with issues they may encounter when called on to provide mental health services to those youngsters.

Review of the Literature

Many authors have reported a typical personality profile for the deaf that includes the characteristics of rigidity, egocentricity, absence of creativity, lack of empathy, deficits in inner controls, suggestibility, and impulsivity (Altshuler 1971; Freeman, Malkin, and Hastings 1975; Mindel and Vernon 1971; Schlesinger 1977; Vernon 1967). Several au-

461

thors, however, have disagreed with this notion. In a study of deaf children sent to a special school, Williams (1970) found that these children's maladjustments were similar in type to those of hearing children. Reivich and Rothrock (1972), using a behavior-problem checklist to survey students in a state school for the deaf, found that conduct, personality, and immaturity dimensions were similar to those in a normal hearing population. Only problems related to isolation and communication were more common.

Chess and Fernandez (1980) found that 75 percent of their cohort of teenagers with deafness secondary to rubella, but with no other handicapping condition, were free of the commonly reported characteristics of impulsivity, hyperactivity, rigidity, and suspiciousness. However, 69 percent of rubella-deaf adolescents with other handicaps had one or more of these traits. The deaf teenagers without other handicaps differed from normal children only with regard to the trait of impulsivity.

Lesser and Easser (1972) asserted that "one cannot adequately evaluate or classify congenitally deaf persons unless one includes the knowledge of the very different developmental and experiential tracks over which these children have advanced." They found that many social and academic situations were stressful for deaf children secondary to problems of communication. Moores (1978), in his text on the deaf adolescent, also stressed the need to study the naturalistic setting of the deaf teenager.

Recently, one of the authors (Feinstein 1983) reported his experiences as a psychiatric consultant and group therapist to a large, special day school for the deaf. The focus in that paper, however, was on the period of early adolescence. The youngsters described had many problems functioning socially, either in informal peer group settings or classroom situations, despite a clear interest and involvement with peers on a one-to-one basis. These difficulties derived from three factors: (1) experiential deprivation in the development of social skills, (2) low self-esteem, and (3) difficulties relating to communications by sign language in the group setting. Most of the students came from families in which no one knew sign language, although this was their only effective communication modality. The resulting extreme limitations in social communication in their home deprived these youngsters of most means of sharing thoughts and feelings with other members of their families. Many of them brought to school a devalued self-image, feelings of interpersonal futility, and a proneness to narcissistic rage outbursts.

For the first time in their lives they were grappling fully with the difficulties of finding their place in the larger hearing community. Choices they repeatedly faced involved such issues as whether to hide their deafness, pretend to understand spoken language, and conceal the use of sign language or to be open about their deafness and publicly communicate by signing. They experienced certain unique difficulties using sign language in informal social group situations. Principle among these was the need to gain the eye contact of the others in order to be "listened to" and the competition for attention within the group that ensued. The fact that only one person could be "heard" at the same time had a very disruptive effect on peer interactions. Those children who had less facility in signed communication were unable to compete effectively in the peer group milieu and were driven to maladaptive forms of behavior to attract attention, further impairing their self-esteem.

Because the school setting in which these observations took place draw from a predominantly underprivileged population, and because signing was the main form of communication while oral skills were very low, it is difficult to generalize these findings to the entire population of deaf early adolescents. However, problems in communication between deaf children and their families, the inevitable need to confront the issue of one's place in the hearing community, and the ongoing problems in communication resulting from deafness would likely be problems common to most deaf adolescents.

Data Collection

The findings related here are based on clinical data collected at a residential high school for the deaf. The school, a model program, is a highly endowed facility with a splendid physical plant and an excellent level of staffing. Its educational philosophy stresses the "total communication" approach. At the time this study was done, the total enrollment was 410. Of these 410 students, fifty-five were commuters who lived locally. The other 355 students lived in dormitories located on a large campus that included a special day elementary school and a university for the deaf. It should be noted that 40 percent of all school age children with severe bilateral hearing loss attended residential school.

These figures are substantially higher for the adolescent age range and for those with the most severe hearing loss (Karchmer and Trybus 1977). The experience of attending a residential school is not unusual or rare for deaf adolescents.

Admission to the school was competitive. The minimum reading skill to gain admission was third-grade level. This represents the mean reading level for deaf youngsters at the time they enter high school, reflecting the fact that reading is a greatly delayed process among deaf students (Moores 1978). Thus these deaf high school students represent a spectrum of academic attainment ranging from average to superior. While exact demographic data for the entire student body were not collected, Hollingshead-Redlich social class determinations for the entering class were as follows: class 1 (highest), 4 percent; class 2, 28 percent; class 3, 39 percent; class 4, 19 percent; and class 5, 8 percent. This social class distribution was representative of the student body and indicates that these adolescents came predominantly from middle-class backgrounds. Racial composition of the student body was approximately 75 percent white, 20 percent black, and 5 percent Hispanic or other.

The language and educational background of the youngsters varied widely. Some came from educational settings that emphasized oral communication and mainstreaming approaches. Others came from programs in which both methods had been used at one time or another, and some came from centers in which sign language was emphasized. While most of the youngsters came from hearing families, 9 percent came from families with one or more deaf parents.

The cause of deafness among these students varied widely. The largest group consisted of those with a history of maternal rubella. However, there were a substantial number for whom the etiology was either unknown, related to hereditary factors, or secondary to meningitis or encephalitis. The age of the high school population ranged from thirteen to twenty.

Not infrequently these students took longer than four years to complete the high school curriculum. Typically, 80–85 percent of the graduating class went on to some form of postsecondary, college, or vocational training. In the year in which the study was conducted, 59 percent of the graduating class went to four-year college programs, mostly to two highly regarded colleges for the deaf, Gallaudet College and National Technical Institute for the Deaf. Thirteen percent went to two-year colleges and 5 percent to vocational-training programs. Twelve percent had jobs. The status of 11 percent was not known.

Findings from the Counseling Service

Of the 410 students enrolled in the school during the academic year of the study, 326 (80 percent) were involved at one time or another with the counseling service. There are many features of this institution that should be reviewed to bring this astonishingly high figure into perspective, some of which will be addressed now and some later. It should be borne in mind, however, that the counseling service in this highly endowed school was not the front line of personnel available to the students. Beyond the classroom-teacher level, all the students were assigned an academic adviser. In the dormitory the students made frequent use of the resident advisers, many of whom were deaf, and all of whom had excellent mastery of sign language.

Referral sources for counseling are itemized in table 1. Data kept by the counseling service concerning the reasons for referral came from a checklist that accompanied each referral. This checklist was problem oriented rather than directed toward diagnosing psychopathology. Table 2 summarizes the findings from this survey. Since it was possible to check more than one of these categories when the referral was made, a total of 549 referral reasons were listed for the 326 students.

One factor related to the large number of referrals was the unusually high ratio of teachers and support staff to students. In this model program, a high degree of observation was directed toward the students, along with a corresponding readiness to refer to counseling. In a normal school setting, many of the more "minor" problems might not have come to the attention of a counseling service. Students with

TABLE 1
REFERRALS TO COUNSELING SERVICE

Referral Source	N
Academic adviser	87
Self	68
Teacher	16
Other	26
Continuation counseling	129
Total	326

NOTE.—Student body = 410.

465

TABLE 2
REASONS FOR REFERRALS TO
COUNSELING SERVICE

Reason	N
Self-concept	93
Classroom performance	48
Adjustment to the school	39
Peer interaction	81
Teacher/adviser interaction	27
Family/home situation	72
Postsecondary/career plans	95
Health needs	22
Financial needs	7
Other	65

more serious emotional disorders were referred by the counselors for psychiatric consultation. Although a wide variety of problems were presented, certain issues recurred with great frequency. These illustrate some of the important and sometimes unique psychosocial issues that impinge on this group of severely hearing-impaired students.

Entering the Residential School

Approximately 20 percent of the students had previously attended residential schools before arriving at this institution. Another 30 percent had attended special day schools for the deaf. Fifty percent came from a public school mainstream educational background. For the first time, many from this latter group were in a social setting in which their handicap did not isolate or distinguish them from their peers. They had entered the world of the deaf. Sign language replaced oral communication as the linqua franca, and, consequently, they were in twenty-four-hour contact with signing peers and adults. Since most acquired substantial signing skills within a few months, before long the communication barriers they had experienced their entire lives disappeared. Previously, many of them had been extremely isolated socially from peers. Now they were in an intense communications-rich twenty-four-hour peer environment. It should be noted that this opportunity to be part of a deaf community was often a major reason stated for the decision to attend this school.

Not surprisingly, the most common source of difficulty complicating the entry of these students into the new peer community was difficulty separating from parents, especially if the parent-child relationship prior to their departure had been problematic. The deaf child of hearing parents is almost invariably subject to some measure of isolation from family life. This problem had been greatest for the majority of students whose parents had never learned to sign.

The refusal of some parents to learn sign language often either reflected a failure to work through their deep-seated grief and disappointment at having a handicapped child or expressed underlying rejecting feelings. Some parents had responded punitively toward their child's effort to sign, generally forbidding it in public places. Often the nonsigning parents understood their child poorly and had great difficulty empathizing with his or her situation and handicap. Not infrequently, however, both parents and student would maintain that they understand each other well, although in family sessions counselors would observe massive communications problems and misunderstandings.

Case Example 1

Susan, a sixteen-year-old girl, was beginning her second year at the school. Her course of adjustment had been stormy from the outset. Much of the time she reported being preoccupied with her relationship with her parents, sending them long letters and becoming upset by their infrequent and irregular responses. Although initially she had been successful in forming friendships, her problematic behavior had eventually alienated many of the students. During her first year there had been two suicidal gestures consisting of marking her arms with superficial razor cuts. In addition, on a few occasions she had been in disciplinary trouble for marijuana use. The staff agreed that her use of drugs was not nearly so serious a problem as it was for some other students; however, she had behaved in a provocative way, calling attention to herself.

The suicidal gestures and disciplinary problems had led to a recurring scenario in which a counselor would call the parents to inform them of their daughter's last infraction. The question would then be raised as to whether Susan should be sent home for a period of "calming down." In response to these urgent phone calls the parents became critical of the school, blamed it for a lack of discipline, and declined to take her home. They would then give their daughter a "pep talk"

467

in which they promised to visit or telephone at some future time. As a rule they failed to keep these promises. Susan responded to having her hopes of support from her parents dashed by escalating her "emergency behavior" in order to reengage them. It became increasingly apparent that her parents were reluctant to have their daughter return home.

Susan was one of the three children from a well-to-do family who resided several hundred miles away. She was the only deaf person in her family. Her parents were ambitious and upwardly mobile. They placed great emphasis on conservative, proper, conforming behavior. Prior to her present placement they had sent Susan to strict oral schools for the deaf. They rigidly forbade her the use of sign language, which they considered disfiguring. When they found her signing with a deaf student from her school, they punished her. Although Susan had been unable to form meaningful relationships with nondeaf peers, they discouraged friendships with deaf classmates.

Susan presented clinically as an attractive girl with fairly good oral skills. Although her speech was intelligible, she tended to fake understanding of more complicated vocal communications. She seemed indifferent to the behavior that had gotten her into trouble, explaining only that she had been preoccupied with various family matters. Despite concerted therapeutic efforts by the counseling staff to engage her in new relationships at the school, Susan's behavior eventually resulted in a long psychiatric hospitalization. She was unable to abandon her futile efforts to reattach herself to her parents, who, in turn, never accepted her deafness and continued, indirectly, to expel her from the family.

Case Example 2

Jerry, a fifteen-year-old boy with a severe congenital bilateral hearing loss who had good academic strengths, was referred to counseling during his first year at school. The presenting problems involved some degree of distractibility and inattentiveness in the classroom, difficulty in understanding the concepts his teachers were explaining, a great deal of manifest anxiety, and a preoccupation with being a "bad" person and being "brain damaged." His parents had sent stimulant medication along with him to school, and he repeatedly expressed a concern that if he missed or was late taking his dose, his brain would become further damaged. This preoccupation had begun to extend itself into the dietary realm as well. He had understood his parents to say that some foods made his brain damage worse. After several months of work, the counselor had learned that Jerry felt even to look at a girl's body meant that he was bad. In the course of normal dormitory living and in physical education class he had had a few "explosions." These violent upsets occurred when he felt that girls had disrobed too much or that students were engaging in sexually provocative behavior.

Jerry came from a well-to-do home. His previous educational background was exclusively in the oral method. In his later school career he had been diagnosed as "hyperactive" and placed on stimulant medication. Despite these problems, he had achieved some measure of academic success, particularly in reading. In his mainstreaming program, however, he had never formed any friendships with a hearing youngster. Neither of his parents knew any sign language, and, prior to entering the school, Jerry had had remarkably little exposure to this modality. His parents insisted to the counselors that they experienced no difficulty communicating with Jerry. When the counseling staff explored this, it was found to be far from the truth. Jerry had fair speech intelligibility, but his lip-reading skills were poor. Generally, he faked understanding when in fact he grasped only a small fraction of what had been said to him. His parents informed the counselor that they had explained to Jerry that he took the medicine because he had "minimal brain damage." They had also told him that eating certain kinds of food tended to aggravate this problem. A review of his early childhood history confirmed hyperactive, restless behavior that might have justified a trial of stimulant medication. However, it was clear that, even though his behavior and academic work had never really been problematic, the parents tended to blame all Jerry's problems on the "minimal brain damage."

During the year prior to his arrival at the school, his mother had discovered girly magazines in his bedroom. His father had, at that point, given him a "sex education" talk, but it was evident to the staff that Jerry had merely pretended to understand and had, in fact, been unable to absorb most of what his father had said. His father, in addition, had told him that these magazines were a bad influence. As a result of trying to guess what his father had said, Jerry had developed the impression that this "badness" might be connected with his "brain damage." At the school Jerry came in contact with a number of students who were involved in fundamentalist religious sects. They spoke of how the devil got into people and made them do bad things. This became connected with the notion that the devil could damage his brain by making him behave badly.

Jerry presented as an anxious, awkward, but well-related boy in mid adolescence. It was evident that he had poor receptive language skills for vocal communication. While his speech was intelligible, he had considerable difficulty articulating complex thoughts. A greater problem, however, was his tendency to nod his head as though he had grasped the issue when this was clearly not the case. In addition, his sign language was relatively poor for the length of time he had attended the school. What gradually emerged was that, since his arrival at the school, he felt he had lost the support of his parents in combating his "badness" and "brain damage." He believed his medicine was protecting him from an advance of his brain damage and also helping fend off the devil. He viewed himself as defective and retarded. Many of his thoughts, especially about sexuality, appeared to be a mixture of superstition, taboos, and phobic concerns mixed in with misinformation, partially understood information, and fantasies.

Despite his degree of inner turmoil and confusion, there was very little evidence of formal thought disorder or poor reality testing. Although somewhat isolated socially, he very much wanted to develop friendships with peers and, in fact, got along well with his roommates. Unfortunately, these peers were continually confronting him with material he regarded as taboo. As a result of his great difficulty conceptualizing ambiguity or complex interactions, he clung desperately to the ideal of doing what he thought his absent parents wanted him to do. After overcoming the parents' reluctance to accept how poor the channel of communication with Jerry had been, they were relatively empathetic and certainly not the rigid moralists convinced of their son's brain damage that Jerry had made them out to be.

The nature of Jerry's language difficulties, even in signing, was difficult to elucidate. It seemed to result in a primary process quality of thinking much like that described by Lesser and Easser (1972) as characteristics of the deaf. We have encountered a number of students like this, and it is our clinical impression that in some rubella-deaf individuals there may exist a distinctive language-based communication disorder on which the deafness is superimposed. Jerry did well in long-term, supportive counseling, improving the quality of his peer relations and becoming more comfortable with sexuality.

Acting Out: Sex, Drugs, and Rebellion

As mentioned, many of the students had come from a background of social and communicative isolation to a milieu in which access to peers was continuous and in which everybody signed without self-consciousness. Many had great difficulty coping with the intense, peer group environment of the residential school. Some maintained their pattern of social isolation, a carryover of low esteem and feelings of interpersonal awkwardness from their prior experience. Others dealt with the separation from their parents by forming intense, dependent sexual attachments. These relationships were made easy by the twenty-four-hour contact the students had with each other. Both boys and girls had trouble dealing with sexuality, often rushing into intercourse prematurely. This problem was compounded by a common lack of information about sex and birth control.

Since the school was an island of deafness in the sea of a hearing world, students tended to pair off or to pass the time by "hanging around together" in small groups. Most avoided exploring the cultural and recreational resources of the large metropolitan area in which their program was located. Instead, they huddled together in the rich, intense, but limited milieu of the campus. Many of the dating relationships that ensued ended catastrophically. This was particularly the case when one member of the couple attempted to withdraw from a premature and overly intense relationship; the person being rejected often responded with intense depression or rage. On several occasions, girls physically attacked either their former boyfriends or the girls who had replaced them.

Both boys and girls turned to the counseling department for help in detaching themselves from such overly close relationships. Suicidal gestures after "breaking up" on the part of some of the girls were common. These not only created a crisis situation for the girl but often sent the boy into counseling as a result of intense guilt feelings. For some girls who were awkward, socially isolated, or unattractive, promiscuity or episodic interpersonal sex became a means for trying to achieve closeness or a feeling of belonging. This led to a few situations in which the question came up as to whether a younger girl had been raped or sexually exploited by a boy or a group of boys.

Despite vigorous administrative efforts to prohibit substance abuse, drug and alcohol use on campus was a widespread form of rebellion against authority, as were the various contemporary countercultural identifications. One of the most intriguing manifestations of adolescent rebellion, paralleling similar issues in the hearing world, involved a small group of students who became converts to a fundamentalist religious organization and whose proselytizing efforts often precipitated uproar and controversy within the school community. These controversies often pitted students against administration on issues of freedom of self-expression.

Case Example 3

Beverly, a seventeen-year-old white girl, maintained an academic level in the superior range and was also a student leader. She was referred to psychiatric consultation after she was implicated as a leading figure in repeated incidents of drug use, drug "busts," and drug dealing. Beverly herself had become frightened by her overuse of drugs and alcohol. She portrayed herself to the counselor as a victim of intense peer pressure in this regard.

Beverly's deafness was on an hereditary basis. By virtue of her good native intelligence, her early and continuous use of sign language, the absence of language communication barriers with her parents, and her parents' aspirations for her, Beverly was considered a likely prospect for success in both social and academic functioning at the school. However, she really had no close friends among the girls. Instead, she attached herself as the only girl to a small group of male students who were involved in drugs.

She revealed absolutely nothing about her heterosexual adjustment. No one seemed to know whether she had ever dated, and no one knew whether her relationships with any of the boys in her group were sexual. Although attractive and possessing good general social skills, she dressed in a boyish fashion and gave other subtle indications of difficulties with feminine identification. In counseling, it gradually emerged that she was often preoccupied with family strife (or with fantasies of the same) and, in particular, was tied into authority conflicts with her father. Her rebellious behavior and frequent disciplinary problems regarding drug use were vehicles for continuing her ambivalent struggle with her father. Since the deaf community nationwide is small and closely linked, news of her vituperative complaints about him to peers and staff, as well as her delinquent behavior, easily spread beyond the boundaries of the school and threatened to become a source of gossip about and embarrassment to the family.

Beverly's course at the school remained unstable until the very end. She continued periodically to be rounded up in drug busts, about which she would say nothing. From time to time, when questioned, she turned to her counselor in a bout of depression, stating that she hated herself for her drug use. At the same time she left the impression that she was in conflict about other activities, which she would not reveal. Despite all these problems, she eventually graduated. She had never wavered in her wish to be accepted at a four-year college program, and in this regard she was successful.

Case Example 4

Tod, a fifteen-year-old white student, had attended the school since age thirteen. At one time or another he had involved every level of the student body and administration in conflict and debate regarding his religious activities. Although he was a popular, academically successful young man, the school, nevertheless, considered suspending or expelling him for his intense religious proselytizing on campus. Off campus, the school in no way interfered with the students' participation in religious activities; however, after years of difficult experience, they had arrived at a policy of forbidding members of a particular religious organization to carry out proselytizing activities on campus.

Despite this, students who became members of the church in question felt themselves bound to spread the faith. Other students reported being told by them that God had made these proselytizers deaf specifically so as to bear his message to deaf people. Tod was particularly effective in this regard. He persuaded a number of other students into believing that they were damned until converted. The devil was described as lurking in the corridors, waiting to possess those who failed to see the light. On more than one occasion, students had panicked in the face of illusions (hallucinations?) of seeing the devil. When adversity would strike one of these students, Tod would be there, placing the blame on the student's lack of religious faith. As a consequence of Tod's success, the school was continually being called by irate parents, who threatened to withdraw their frightened or recently converted children. The school administration felt itself in a quandry, unable to reconcile the right of free speech with the real threat to the ongoing education of substantial numbers of students. There were many conferences with Tod. At times he agreed to desist from his conversion activities at school, but then he would continue his efforts in secret until another controversy arose.

Tod was the son of two hearing parents. At first his mother had been convinced that it was best to use the oral approach. She had forbidden him the use of sign language and at the age of four had sent him to a strict oral residential school. He remained there for several years, during which time he failed to make substantial academic progress and never developed a useful level of speech or lip-reading skills. Behaviorally, he was a major management problem, and his mother was told he was hyperactive and possibly brain damaged.

Eventually, his mother decided to abandon the oral approach and learned sign language herself. She enrolled him in a school that used the total communication approach. Eventually, Tod's father also became fluent in sign language. Tod himself described his current relationship with his parents as close. Recently, however, conflict had erupted when his mother attempted to dissuade him from his religious activities. She became convinced that he should be removed from the influence of this religious group, leave the school, and attend a setting near their home. Tod was obviously ambivalent toward this, torn between his intense devotion to his religious leader and unspoken but apparent wishes for closeness with his mother. In counseling it became clear that his crusading tendencies derived from profound feelings of unfairness and injustice at having been born deaf.

Conflicts about Graduation

As graduation approaches, each student in this school faces life choices that extend far beyond the question of vocation or education. Almost invariably the major conflict centers around whether or when the student will leave the cocoon of the residential school. Should he do so, he must face once again the hearing world, where his handicap will be manifest and where the barriers of communication and information will challenge his sense of self-esteem and confidence anew. For those students who are most successful and who go on to one of the colleges for the deaf, this problem is postponed. However, a substantial number of students meet the requirements for graduation but do not have the ability or inclination for postsecondary education. For these students, leaving the school is extremely stressful and anxiety provoking.

Case Example 5

Diane, a nineteen-year-old senior, was referred to psychiatric consultation for a number of problems. Though she possessed enough credits to graduate, she seemed to ignore that possibility altogether. In the past semester her grades had fallen precipitously. She had frequent temper outbursts and, on several occasions, had refused to cooperate with teachers. It was also noted that she was eating poorly, was borderline anorexic, and required daily monitoring by the student health service. Although always a loner, recently she had become irritable and hostile when others approached her. She was enrolled in dormitory and educational programs that provided her with training in "life skills" (such as budgeting money). Nonetheless, she repeatedly demonstrated a lack of competence inconsistent with her average intellectual abilities. As a decision about graduation approached, she began attacking her counselor for being overly critical and demanding.

Diane was the only deaf child of a working-class family from a predominantly rural area. Her parents had never really accepted her deafness. She especially felt rejected by her father, who, when she was at home, continually berated her for not doing enough work. Neither parent had shown any interest or motivation in learning sign language. Diane's early schooling was with an oral approach. This was moderately successful, and she developed some capacity for intelligible speech. However, she was painfully aware that her speech sounds were noticeably abnormal. In the hearing world, she tended to avoid speaking.

The community in which her family lived had very poor vocational training services and no program for the deaf. Her reading and writing skills, while adequate for graduation from the school, did not really bring her to a level at which she could compete for a clerical job. On the other hand, although she was eligible for a number of local technical vocational training programs, none of these were residential, and all would involve her living in the community on her own. The staff strove to prepare her with the various self-support skills; however, it was precisely in this area that Diane refused to cooperate. Clearly, she felt pressured to leave the residential school and return to a world where she saw for herself only the possibility of social isolation and handicapped status.

Conclusion

We have presented a range of descriptive and clinical material regarding the interactions between phase-appropriate adolescent issues and the unique psychosocial situation of deaf teenagers attending a residential school. Our experience at this model school attended by deaf teenagers of at least average intelligence and predominantly middle-class backgrounds suggests that these youngsters are, in fact, more vulnerable to problems of adjustment than are hearing teenagers. This increased vulnerability is due not to a characteristic "deaf personality" but rather to the greater stress on communication, family interaction, adjustment to the outer world, and other features of the special minority experience of being deaf. In addition, the life experience of attending a residential school, during which so many of the ongoing stresses of being deaf are removed, creates short-term challenges to adaptation and heightens some of these teenager's awareness of the potentially isolated and minority status they face in adulthood.

REFERENCES

Altshuler, K. Z. 1971. Studies of the deaf: relevance to psychiatric theory. *American Journal of Psychiatry* 127:1521–1526.

Chess, S., and Fernandez, P. 1980. Do deaf children have a typical personality? *Journal of the American Academy of Child Psychiatry* 19:654–664.

Feinstein, C. 1983. Early adolescent deaf boys: a biopsychosocial approach. *Adolescent Psychiatry* 11:147–162.

Freeman, R.; Malkin, S.; and Hastings, J. 1975. Psychosocial problems of deaf children and their families: a comparative study. *American Annals of the Deaf* 120:391–405.

Karchmer, M. A., and Trybus, R. J. 1977. *Who Are the Deaf Children in "Mainstream" Programs?* Office of Demographic Studies, Publication no. 4, Series R. Washington, D.C.: Gallaudet College.

Lesser, S., and Easser, R. 1972. Personality differences in the perceptually handicapped. *Journal of the American Academy of Child Psychiatry* 11:458–466.

Mindel, E. D., and Vernon, M. 1971. *They Grow in Silence: The Deaf Child and His Family.* Silver Spring, Md.: National Association of the Deaf.

Moores, D. F. 1978. *Educating the Deaf: Psychology, Principles, and Practices.* Boston: Houghton Mifflin.

Reivich, R. S., and Rothrock, I. A. 1972. Behavior problems of deaf children and adolescents: a factor-analytic study. *Speech and Hearing Research* 15:84–92.

Schlesinger, H. 1977. Treatment of the deaf child in the school setting. *Mental Health in Deafness* 1:77–84.

Vernon, M. 1967. Characteristics associated with post-rubella deaf children. *Volta Review* 69:176–185.

Williams, C. C. 1970. Some psychiatric observations on a group of maladjusted deaf children. *Journal of Child Psychology and Psychiatry* 11:1–18.

EDUCATIONAL ISSUES IN ADOLESCENTS: THERAPEUTIC POTENTIALS IN SCHOOL PROGRAMS: INTRODUCTION TO SPECIAL SECTION

IRVING H. BERKOVITZ

In the past forty years, there have been widespread efforts to improve mental health benefits in schools preventively, interventively, and postventively. Even earlier, Witmer (in 1896) and the Freuds—Sigmund (in 1910) and Anna (in 1936)—were active in trying to bring mental health knowledge and techniques to educators. Since the 1950s, Caplan, Berlin, Hollister, and others have elucidated and fostered more explicit consultative activities with school personnel.

The school experience is essential for adolescents to learn basic cognitive skills as well as the maintenance and repair of self-esteem, coping techniques, development of satisfying peer relations, and how to build self-sufficient and independent identities. Each individual enters school with strengths, vulnerabilities, and often psychopathology. These can operate to facilitate or impede receiving benefit from the school milieu. Some troubled adolescents will be fortunate enough to find necessary support. All could better weather developmental crises if there were available the assistance of empathic teachers, counselors, and other school specialists. Too many young people may not be able to receive any kind of support. Sometimes, there may be other community, religious, or family resources that can provide the necessary help. The public schools, however, are often the only resource available.

Society's financial support of and confidence in schools have not always been consistent. During the 1980s, there has been greater attention to the importance of schooling in the lives of children and youths, and, as a result, there has been some increase in funding for academic improvement but not necessarily for psychological support services. On the other hand, improvement of academic resources may indirectly raise performance, self-esteem, and the mental health of many young people. For example, an enriched counseling program for tenth graders was intended to improve high school performance and therefore the number of students that would graduate. The program included group counseling to look at academic programs. In the process, many emotional, behavioral, and familial factors were examined and remedied. The knowledgeable mental health professional often can optimize benefits from available programs, and the chapters in this section give some examples of what some schools do provide or could provide, especially with the assistance of mental health personnel.

The chapters presented here illustrate only a small segment of the myriad programs introduced into schools to influence the minds and emotions of students. Underlying and intermixed with the academic, cognitive program in schools is an informal curriculum shaping and modeling the emotional life of the young. An important aspect of this is the way the educational system deals with aggression—in staff as well as students. Equally relevant is the interplay with other emotions. In his chapter, Berkovitz describes the ways that aggression in students and school staff complicates the emotional-educational process.

The sources of adolescent depression are ubiquitous. The interplay between adolescent anger, self-esteem impairment, depression, substance abuse, and suicide is well known. Two chapters focus on some of these features; Berkovitz details some of the elements of the school setting that can potentially be of benefit to depressed and suicidal students, and Peck and Berkovitz present examples of the usefulness of mental health consultation for suicide prevention, intervention, and postvention.

Two chapters describe group counseling, which represents one of the more directly therapeutic features of school mental health services. Berkovitz provides a review of the current literature and points out the differences between group therapy in the clinical setting and group counseling in the schools. Fleisher, Berkovitz, Briones, Lovetro, and Morhar present examples of the value of group counseling to students who have experienced various losses but who would not have availed themselves of clinical services. Very often, the mental health consultant can be of great service in providing this form of assistance. The last contribution deals with the important role of peer influence in schools and in adolescence generally. To illustrate, Hansen, Malotte, and Fielding describe a project to mobilize peer influence to reduce the use of tobacco and alcohol. This reinforcement of peer influence has been a feature of other programs to help control of drug abuse and inappropriate sexual behavior.

This special section is offered with the hope that psychiatrists and others working with young people will regard the school milieu as less puzzling, alien, or repelling. It is imperative that educators and mental health professionals learn to understand and work with each other's frame of reference to bring earlier and more effective assistance to children and adolescents.

31 AGGRESSION, ADOLESCENCE, AND SCHOOLS

IRVING H. BERKOVITZ

The maturation of each individual and the strength of the impulses will determine whether aggression becomes effectively assertive, constructive, and task oriented (ego aggression) or inappropriate, destructive, and self-defeating (primary drive aggression). Ego strength, sense of self, and choice of defense mechanisms are intimately related to the quality and form of impulse regulation. While significant directions are determined in early childhood, during adolescence there is the recapitulation of separation-individuation dynamics (Blos 1967) and the reshaping of the superego. These events do affect the reworking of earlier psychic patterns, including the intensity, stimulus, and mode of expression of aggression. Kalogerakis (1974) identified several familial origins of violence and aggression. He established the importance of arbitrariness, injustice, cruelty, and sadism on the part of parents. "The bind of the child, who both needs his parents and is powerless against them is particularly apparent when he is being exploited and abused." He called for parents to "perform more adequately and to permit more give and take of angry feelings with their children" as a way to enhance "mutual love and respect."

Next to the family, those experiences most involved in the growth of adolescents are the peer group and school. The school includes important interactions with the peer group as well as with adults, educators, and other personnel. While the teachers' prime task is to expand cognitive skills, unavoidably they also become the transference recipients of conflicts with parents. This process can lead to further insight and reworking of earlier struggles, but acting out may aggravate previous problems. This collision of adolescent energy and the particular school structure can repeat conflicts already experienced in the youngster's family and result in new crises. While many expressions of aggression will have been internalized prior to the onset of adolescence, the emphasis in this chapter is on the interplay between the external structural influences of school and the adolescent intrapsychic forces.

Aggression and School

It would be unrealistic to expect the schools to manage and redirect all expressions of adolescent aggression. Yet the approaches that educators use to deal with that aggression are especially crucial as powerful models. In one way or another, however, educators do have to create a peaceful climate in which learning and cooperative interrelations can occur. The Safe School Study (1978) observed that school violence and vandalism increased during the 1960s but leveled off in the early 1970s. There are indications of a decline that has continued into the 1980s, but the level is still higher than society can tolerate. Violence, crime, and vandalism are evidences of aggression that has not found constructive channels. There are, in addition, other harmful internalized effects of aggression that have more of an individual than a group consequence, for example, depression, suicide, underachievement, absenteeism, apathy, and physical illness.

POSITIVE USES OF AGGRESSION

Derivatives of aggression are useful for the adolescent and the school when expressed in the form of assertiveness and determination, whether on an interpersonal level or when applied to a task such as learning. Aggression can be a stimulus for social and political change. It can be a response to agencies and institutions of society that are not meeting the needs of their members or are restricting some desirable freedoms. Distinguishing and fostering constructive expressions of aggression depend on the creativity of the participants, recipient, or onlooker. In the school setting, instantaneous defensive or offensive reactions often occur before anyone can take the time to differentiate. This is not to deny that at times aggression, especially from adolescents, can be spontaneous, dangerous, and require control. Quiet, thoughtful discussion may have to await more peaceful times.

With adolescents, especially, aggression often serves a developmental role reinforcing feelings of mastery and ego skills. It can be a necessary and potent form of communication. The verbally less-skilled young person may use aggression to try to establish an identity in the group. It can serve exhibitionistic purposes to win approval, publicity, or membership. It can serve to define submissive and domination positions. However, aggression can also become addictive and habitual for the individual who needs to maintain an angry level of bodily tension and avoid more frightening tender emotions such as love, depression, or sorrow. At times, of course, aggression may also be a form of appropriate self-defense against verbal or physical attack from peers or adults. Any, and all, of these varying motives and uses can operate in the school setting as well as in the family or elsewhere.

CASE EXAMPLE 1

The following example shows the dynamics of interplay between adolescent aggression, a family, and the school milieu in one particular young adolescent.

Mike, a bright, handsome, thirteen-year-old eighth grader, in a small private secondary school (250 students), repeatedly baited and insulted his teachers, especially his science teacher. The science teacher, who liked Mike, did not appreciate the hostility, did not punish inappropriately, and tried to talk with Mike. Mike also enjoyed fights with peers and was proud of his fighting ability as well as his skill in team sports. At home, Mike similarly insulted his mother and defied her demands. She would explode, almost out of control, and punish him. Father, usually at work, was occasionally called in by mother. A negative recriminatory climate prevailed at home, compounded by Mike's domination of a younger brother. This continuous, unresolved anger in the family and school contexts was building a negative path for Mike. Parenthetically, the private school had no effective psychological staff.

Mike entered therapy at this point. He slowly built trust with the therapist, after only a brief expression of mild hostility. He spoke proudly of his anger at teachers, peers, and mother. Focus turned to his ambitions to become a lawyer or doctor and earn high salaries. The need for education and the wish to excel, also a part of his ego ideal, came to the fore and were reinforced. By May, Mike had attenuated his expressions of anger at teachers and peers and had improved academically. The faculty recognized his improvement and was willing for him to stay in the school, but the headmaster did not concur. Mike was made aware of this. His parents came to his aid as well, but this only partially salved his hurt feelings. In the next school year he enrolled at the larger public junior high school's eighth grade. The work was easier for him, but he proceeded to do less. He avoided hostility with teachers or peers, but his grades began to decline. He looked depressed and seemed to be internalizing the anger from his rejection. Complicating the situation was that the junior high school would not enroll him in more advanced academic classes until he had been in the school one year. The therapist's intervention was to no avail. The therapist reiterated to him his need for challenge to maintain and develop his good intellectual powers and advised the parents to seek another private school. This was considered, especially because Mike voiced wishes to leave home for a school on the East Coast, where his father had attended school. After a year of successful schooling in the East, he did return to the local high school and was able to live at home and attend school with greater harmony.

This example shows how a negative interaction at home had been reproduced in school, resulting in a potentially damaging school expulsion. A contributing factor was the inflexibility of the school's administration, the absence of a helpful school psychological staff, and an inflexible emphasis on academic standards. Mike's postpubertal emancipatory strivings had been stalled due to his own ambivalence, mother's difficulty loosening attachments to her firstborn son, and a school milieu that could not respond to the developmental significance of his anger. It is a moot question if some other type of school resources could have responded better, thus avoiding the need for therapy. It is my opinion that it was more likely that Mike's problems, especially the family component, did require the time and expertise of professional therapy. Very often the therapy of a teenager does require intervention or advice about more effective and appropriate schooling. In Mike's case, psychotherapy did help him progress through the separation-individuation process of early adolescence with less anger invested in futile chronic combat with the school milieu and his family. In many cases such combat does ultimately result in emancipation, but not without scars and residual impediments to future development.

SCHOOL MILIEU SOURCES OF AGGRESSION

The previous example showed the importance of the school milieu's interplay with a teenager's aggression. On any secondary school campus there is a delicate balance beween the energies of the adults and adolescents. At times, the anger of the adults can fuel anger in younger people and vice versa. Adult fears of aggression from young people can promote a readiness to overreact and inhibit the adult's ability to be able to see options for defusing or redirecting the reaction.

CASE EXAMPLE 2

The following incident occurred in one secondary school (DeCecco and Richards 1974):

Gail came storming down the hall yelling that someone has stolen her pen. The language is unbearable. A teacher stops her and starts to yell at her about her language. They both yell at each other for a short period of time. Students gather. The teacher grabs the student by the arm to take her to the office. She resists, calling the teacher names. In fact she attempts to hit the teacher and finally does. Other teachers join in and take the girl to the office. The principal, on hearing the story, suspends Gail because of her language and because she struck the teacher. Parents, teachers union, civil rights leaders, etc. enter the situation until finally Gail is reinstated.

SOURCES OF AGGRESSION

One may consider the level of aggression and its various sources in at least three categories: (1) from outside the school, that is, individual pathology derived from family problems, child abuse, poverty, crime in the neighborhood, and gangs; (2) from inside the school, that is, inappropriate rules, unsympathetic authority, unrealistic academic expectations, inadequate facilities, and staff stress or pathology; and (3) from the wider society, that is, conditions of war, unemployment, and media violence among others.

The world outside the school does demand major attention at times, but the school's ability to intervene effectively is limited. An example of the special role of the school in a situation of war or community chaos and violence has been described in the schools of Northern Ireland, Israel, and New York (Schwartz 1982). In Northern Ireland, many children came to school showing effects of constant exposure to danger, violence, and death. They were also seen to be suffering internally—insecure and frightened to the point of requiring high dosages of tranquilizing medication.

The school was generally regarded as "a place set apart in which to learn lessons." The teachers were divided about whether to provide a sanctuary from life or to explore the difficult emotions of the children (and themselves). Most chose to attempt to provide a sanctuary. Under some conditions, exploration of feelings might be more helpful. In some Israeli schools, teachers did participate in group discussion of the life and death experience they were witnessing during the Six-Day War, with consequent reduction in feelings of helplessness (Abraham 1978).

Another dimension of aggression is aggression among the involved individuals and/or groups in the school setting: (1) aggression between students and teachers or other staff; (2) aggression among students; (3) aggression among school personnel; (4) anger between staff and parents; and (5) anger between community members and the school community.

AGGRESSION OF STUDENTS TOWARD TEACHERS AND TEACHERS TOWARD STUDENTS

There has been an unprecedented increase in the incidence of murder, rape, and other violence against teachers. The classroom in some schools has been compared to a battlefield (Bloch 1972). Complicated security devices have been installed to help teachers summon help. Security police have become a feature of most campuses, especially in secondary schools. The genesis of this change involves society as a whole. However, the school milieu is a social microcosm and includes its share (or more) of disruptive social events and conditions. Fortunately, just as in families, there is the possibility of more positive responses.

Too often teachers and other school staff, without intention or awareness, may make depreciating remarks to students either to encourage better performance, as a form of humor, or because they are irritated and need a target. Most students will absorb this and later complain about it to peers or family members outside class. However, a small number will react physically immediately or brood and react later against the teacher or against school property. Occasionally, teachers will use physical actions with students, ranging from an affectionate embrace to a restraining grip, or at times even an angry blow. DeCecco and Richards (1974) analyzed 1,284 incidents that involved the use of violence by students against school authorities and by school authorities against students. The findings were disturbing; school authorities used force in 716 incidents (about 56 percent). Students used force against school authorities in 192 incidents (about 15 percent). Many school personnel are not always aware of their touching a student, especially in a heated moment. This action may be misinterpreted by the student as more hostile than may have been intended.

If corporal punishment is practiced as part of the school's disciplinary program, some precariously balanced students may be provoked into violence. This is especially risky if the youngster has already experienced bodily punishment at home. Use of this form of discipline could well contradict and make more difficult the attempt to teach that words can be used to express anger and lead to better resolution of conflict situations.

VANDALISM

Rutter, Maughan, Mortimore, and Ouston (1979) found that in high schools when the "ethos" was positive (teachers used a respectful attitude toward students, teachers expected students to perform well, and teachers were conscientious), student achievement and behavior improved.

Goldstein, Apter, and Harootunian (1984) brought together some relevant features about students responsible for vandalism: the school vandal is just as likely to be white as nonwhite (Goldmeir 1974), middle class as lower class (Howard 1978), and (at least for graffiti and similar acts) female as male (Richards 1976). Most vandals are eleven to sixteen years old (Ellison 1973), are no more disturbed on formal psychological

489

evaluations than youngsters who do not vandalize (Richards 1976), are frequently students who have been held back (Nowakowski 1966), are often truant (Greenberg 1974), and have frequently been suspended from school altogether (Yankelovich 1975).

DEALING WITH AGGRESSION IN THE CLASSROOM

Classroom interactions are a prime place for positive or negative transactions to occur between student and teacher. A well-managed classroom where the teacher has command of teaching methods and presentation of material and knowledge of classroom group dynamics will often result in a happier experience for all concerned. In the absence of these, many students get restless and disinterested and often create or contribute to situations of classroom conflict.

Some students act as if they do not care. They may never have done well in school and may have become dedicated to failure patterns. They may be inflicting these on the rest of the class as well as on the teacher. The teacher may then have the dilemma of direct confrontation or exclusion and referral. There may not be sufficient support staff available to accept referral, and administrative staff may not be supportive of referrals. Direct confrontation and/or persuasion by the teacher may be the only approach available.

There are several possible ingredients and safeguards involved in such a classroom confrontation. First to consider is the mood of the teacher that day and moment. Many teachers often are not aware of being in a bad mood until a confrontation occurs. Some students are sensitive to their teacher's negative state of emotions and may become insecure or helpful. On the other hand, some students may be waiting for an opportunity to increase the teacher's distress. Introspection by the teacher to determine mood or possible bias about the provoking student is desirable but not always possible. Mental health consultation when available can at times improve this ability. A second factor to be considered is the student. Is this a student always in difficulty and showing defiance, or is this a rare occurrence? Is this possibly an off day for the student, and is the confrontation a way for the student to blow off steam, avoid depression, or regain self-esteem? Would it be helpful or destructive to discipline this student? A third factor is the presence of other members of the class. If the teacher is aware, he or she may ask, Is it wise to have the confrontation in the class before the students' peers or to have it in private where neither has to be concerned about losing prestige in the eyes of the other students? The student may be trying to gain a certain advantage with peers rather than make a valid point. At times, some adolescent students are just beginning to learn ways to feel equal to adults and to feel less intimidated by parents (or other adults). The classroom confrontation may be chosen by the student as the arena for practicing these new skills. This behavior, if accepted and kept within reasonable bounds, may often be short-lived. Humor is often useful at such moments, especially if the aggression is in the service of mastery.

INTIMIDATION OF TEACHERS BY STUDENTS

Some students have learned to intimidate teachers, whether to bolster a poor sense of self, defeat the adult, indulge sadistic urges, or other motives. Pickhardt (1978) believes that fear and lack of its recognition are one of the most destructive occurrences in many schools. He feels that fear enters "through the student's need to assert power and the teacher's need not to lose power in their relationship with each other." He states that teachers have three interpersonal adequacy needs with students—to be liked, to be effective, and to be in control. When these adequacy needs become frustrated, they transform into adequacy fears. For their part, students are irresistibly drawn to asserting interpersonal power as part of their social development. Pickhardt interviewed several of the more defiant students and learned from them some of the "fear games" they employed to frighten teachers.

CLASSROOM INTERVENTION

At times, consultants may be available to intervene and change the climate in a classroom. In one high school math class, the counselor was called in to assist the teacher with a class that did not seem to want to learn. The counselor conducted three meetings with each half of the class, eliciting open, frank discussion, especially attitudes about the subject and the teacher. Students returned to class with a more positive attitude (Thomsen and Jones 1975).

In a sixth-grade class, the teacher felt there was an atmosphere of excessive anger. The teacher and the counselor were able to have a consulting psychiatrist conduct weekly thirty-minute class discussions over a four-month period about negative feelings, relationships, and other matters (Berkovitz and Estabrook 1987). This procedure seemed to reestablish a climate of cooperativeness and better relations among the class. Often a teacher may be able to have this kind of discussion with a class and establish a new, more productive classroom atmosphere.

GROUP COUNSELING

In group counseling, one of the most frequent topics is the way to moderate, to understand, and to express aggressive feelings more effectively generally but especially to teachers (Bates 1975). A successful counseling experience has often led to a reduction of anger in students and better learning in class. A very impressive example of this occurred in a junior high school where angry feelings had been aroused during a year of mandatory desegregation. The group consisted of those students who were considered leaders by the counselors but also the ones who had been referred most often for disciplinary problems on campus. For two months, this group met weekly. The discussions were frequently heated, to show the learning of verbal expression and understanding as an alternative to physical violence. As one might predict, some of the students had been subjected to physical abuse in their families. This seemed to encourage the use of physical violence as a solution to tension and threat on campus. In the group discussions, however, they did explain to each other the risk of these physical responses. For example, one black boy said, "If that teacher bothers me one more time, I'm going to pop off and hit him." A formerly overly aggressive Caucasian boy then said, "Don't do that, man. You'll be the one who gets hurt." They recommended that there be more groups next year: "If there's a chance to talk, then you don't have to fight" (Berkovitz, Carr, and Anderson 1983).

INFLUENCES FROM OUTSIDE THE CLASSROOM

While the teacher most often will be the first to interact with angry students, the attitudes and interactions of other staff personnel are of import as well. One school superintendent (Green 1969) detailed some ways in which staff unknowingly can contribute to student unrest— tendency to talk more than listen; tendency to impose, unconsciously, the prevailing value system on youngsters who neither understand it

492

nor accept it; tendency to overemphasize rules, regulations, and other rigid school controls; tendency to see pupils not as individuals but as a group; tendency to "turn off" students who display deviant behavior in terms of class performance, grooming, and dress; tendency to "lock" students into a category of ability or aptitude (self-fulfilling prophecy); tendency to convey through a look, tone of voice, or gesture "silent contempt" for some deviant characteristic of the student.

The other important areas of aggression in the school setting are relations between students and the teacher-administrator relationship. The teacher-administrator relationship will often feature controlled, concealed, and/or disguised expressions of anger, which occasionally may reverberate into the clasroom and provoke more open expressions there.

AGGRESSION AMONG STUDENTS

Aggression between peers may arise from many of the same sources as aggression toward adults—poor sense of self, frustration, fear of fusion in the closeness, chronic use of anger as a defense, and family models of violence. The particular quality of the school's features and psychological climate can affect peer interaction and level of hostility. Also, the postpubertal years involve greater competitive urges, concern about popularity, appearance, conformity, and other differences.

Young persons are frequently in motion whether on the playground on in class. Collisions will occur, which can cause arguments and fights. With the prevalence of weapons in society and on campuses, there will even be shootings or stabbings, especially in secondary schools. At times, these differences can be settled peacefully by negotiation sponsored by the adults, teachers, administrators, support staff, and even peers. All manner of differences can contribute to and aggravate aggression between young people, whether cultural, ethnic, language, or economic. The adults in the school can help young people to learn that differences can coexist with mutual benefit and respect rather than with antagonism and hostility.

Large urban secondary (or elementary) schools may engender conflict and violence by the more prevalent sense of isolation and alienation, lower proportions of adults, and difficult learning conditions. In the larger schools, it is more difficult for the educator to intervene productively in disputes among students. Many educators and mental health experts feel that smaller units allow for better learning of harmonious group relations (Miller 1970). In organized school sports, there can be some attention given to individuals having difficulty handling aggression in competitive situations. Providing the athletic coaches with an opportunity for mental health consultation can be useful (Beisser 1987).

During the desegregation efforts of many school systems in the 1970s, there was friction among peers of different races as well as faculty members and parents. Several schools initiated dialogue groups to include students and parents of minority groups and school staff to help convert physical anger to verbal anger so that negotiation and resolution could take place. Consultant mental health personnel were of assistance (Zegans, Schwartz, and Dumas 1969). On occasion, groups of parents with professional expertise were able to work with administrators and faculty to set up discussion forums. In one senior high school, an antagonistic, boiling group of students, who were ready to attack the authority represented by the new principal, was able to displace these feelings to the forum leader. Progressively, the militancy abated with improved communication between generations and races (Sugar 1975).

AGGRESSION AMONG SCHOOL PERSONNEL

While this chapter has focused mainly on the adolescent, one must realize that the adults in the school have their own aggressive processes that give rise to anger, which may then effect students individually and collectively. Any group of adults working together can experience antagonisms, enmities, misunderstandings, and feuds. When adults work with children or adolescents, this is all the more likely because the intensities and immaturities of provocative young people can arouse unresolved childhood behavior patterns and conflicts in the adults. The new found strength of teacher unions and the increase of adversarial relationships between administrators and teachers have also aggravated tensions among school personnel.

Adults, unlike children, tend to moderate their aggressive feelings and express them in disguised or covert ways that often complicate and interfere with task performance, job satisfaction, optimum communication, or even bodily health. Many communication exercises have been devised to help faculties or other groupings of school personnel

494

to bring these buried antagonisms safely to the surface. Not all of these antagonisms can be resolved easily, and often anger does continue to exist in concealed ways, interfering with amicable staff relationships. At times, the anger can be reasonable and amenable to easy clarification. Other times, it may require the transfer or resignation of some personnel. The relationship between the principal of a school and the teachers in the school is a crucial one. This is especially so as far as the satisfaction of the teachers and the relation between the teachers and the students is concerned. Several studies have correlated principal leadership style, teacher style, and student learning outcome (Lieberman 1973).

A program designed to improve communication between the principals and superintendent in a district of twelve schools found that some principals improved their communication skills with teachers such that the following statements were made after two years: "I can take criticism more easily. As a result, I developed rap sessions with my staff and I found that my staff perceived me differently from how I perceived myself." "I was a new principal at a school. When I first arrived there were some days when as many as eighteen or nineteen students were lined up outside my door awaiting disciplinary action. Now there are none." "I have taught my teachers to become better listeners. As a result of my leveling with teachers and comparing philosophies of child management, we've become better able to work together."

CONFLICT BETWEEN PARENTS AND TEACHERS

Often teachers are not prepared to deal with angry or distraught parents. The teacher, who may be younger, unmarried, or without children, may be made to feel less adequate than the parent in question. The parent may have felt angry at and ashamed of the poorly performing child for years and is not willing to hear a poor report one more time. Such a parent may be ready to place the guilt on the teacher, especially if the teacher is feeling uncertain about his own competency or performance with this particular child. Parents who performed poorly or had bad experiences in school may come to visit the teacher of their child with trepidation or anger. Parents with college-level education or teaching experience may come prepared to do battle for their own ideas of the proper education of their child. Some parents have done physical harm to teachers or other personnel. Workshops to help teachers better understand and work with parents have been well received in many schools. Advisory councils and PTA groups often facilitate a more peaceful dialogue with parents.

AGGRESSION BETWEEN COMMUNITY MEMBERS AND SCHOOL PERSONNEL

That part of the community that does not include parents of students in the schools is often a potential source of aggression against schools. Some of these may resent the children's more uncontrolled energy circulating in the neighborhood—teenagers smoking marijuana in alleys, children shoplifting or simply noisily filling the aisles in the stores or buses. Community members who serve on school advisory councils provide input on community reactions and happenings. Schools would do well to invite community members to school events.

In recent years, disturbed or criminal individuals have entered schools to register protests, commit crimes, or even to seek closeness to children in an environment that once might have meant comfort and love to them. A troublesome event is the occasional violence committed against school property or persons. Disturbed individuals have vented their anger against children and personnel in schools, killing and wounding innocent persons. This type of event can disrupt a school program for months, endangering future learning and mental health. Crisis teams have been developed to help survivors, children, and adults to surface their feelings to help reduce posttraumatic emotional symptomatology (Eth, Arroyo, and Silverstein 1985).

AGGRESSION IN WORK SETTINGS

It is difficult for aggression to surface in a close working or living setting unless there is a format for its acceptance and resolution. Most people's feelings are sensitive and easily subject to hurt. Role play simulations can be very helpful as can "confrontation" groups under proper conditions. These procedures involve temporary suspension of the usual rules of social decorum and openness. Such exercises can come to grief when the statements made are so close to primary aggression that the participants cannot comfortably integrate what they perceive as an attack.

How to allow anger to surface with fairness and less feeling of hurt is a skill not easily acquired, either in families or in schools. Debate societies in secondary schools come close to this but in a highly intellectualized format. The "roast" is an example of the stage presentation of very destructive statements said with laughter and, therefore, "not really true." However, in the minds of the roastees, there must be some memory of how one's "flaws" were seen and tolerated in the eyes of others. Humor can be a valuable ingredient for communication of anger—again, if done with skill and sensitivity. The disclaimer, "it was only a joke," often may not erase the hurt of a humorous barb. The ability to see oneself truly as others see one is most difficult, whether due to normal or exaggerated narcissism. The presence of a facilitative, empathic, and nonjudgmental third party often does allow the surfacing of these difficult self-awarenesses and a return to a smoother working (or other) relationship.

Disappointment is inevitable as long as this world is populated with imperfect beings and situations of unequal distribution of material things and personal attributes. Some skill, format, aids, or other facilitation of the resolution of interpersonal tensions is essential. The need for such skills exists at all levels of society, interpersonal and organizational. The learning may well proceed in the schools as well as in families, churches, courts, and playgrounds.

Conclusions

Aggression and its modes of expression are crucial issues in adolescence because of the developmental significance and psychosocial consequences. This emphasis is not meant to overlook the equal importance of love and affection. Schools are places where, while intellectual skills are being strengthened, adolescent relations to adults, other adolescents, and the self are being determined, usually through experiences with the less intellectual sets of affects—anger, love, and sorrow. The school as an organization has certain demands during which aggression is more likely and does receive attention, deliberate or inadvertent. These points are (1) tension between student and staff, especially in the classroom where student-teacher confrontations are likely; (2) anger between students; (3) anger between school personnel; (4) anger between staff and parents; and (5) anger between community members and the school community. In some cases, learning may occur, but more often control and defensiveness take priority.

497

REFERENCES

Abraham, A. 1978. Group intervention for teachers in time of war. *Group* 2(1): 40–53.

Bates, M. 1975. Themes in group counseling with adolescents. In I. H. Berkovitz, ed. *When Schools Care.* New York: Brunner/Mazel.

Beisser, A. R. 1987. Broadening goals of physical education teachers and coaches. In I. H. Berkovitz and J. S. Seliger, eds. *Expanding Mental Health Interventions in Schools,* vol. 2. Dubuque, Iowa: Kendall/Hunt.

Berkovitz, I. H.; Carr, E.; and Anderson, G. 1983. Attending to the emotional needs of junior high school students and staff during desegregation. In G. J. Powell, ed. *The Psychosocial Development of Minority Group Children.* New York: Brunner/Mazel.

Berkovitz, I. H., and Estabrook, W. 1987. Multiple functions of a consulting psychiatrist in the elementary school. In S. Leung, ed. *Mental Health and Schools.* Chicago: Eterna International.

Bloch, A. 1972. The battered teacher. *Today's Education* 66:58–62.

Blos, P. 1967. The second individuation process of adolescence. *Psychoanalytic Study of the Child* 22:162–186.

DeCecco, J. P., and Richards, A. K. 1974. *Growing Pains: Uses of School Conflict.* New York: Aberdeen.

Ellison, W. S. 1973. School vandalism: 100 million dollar challenge. *Community Education Journal* 3:27–33.

Eth, S.; Arroyo, W.; and Silverstein, S. 1985. A psychiatric crisis team response to violence in elementary schools. In I. H. Berkovitz and J. S. Seliger, eds. *Expanding Mental Health Interventions in Schools,* vol. I. Dubuque, Iowa: Kendall/Hunt.

Goldmeir, H. 1974. Vandalism: the effects of unmanageable confrontations. *Adolescence* 9:49–56.

Goldstein, A. P.; Apter, S. J.; and Harootunian, B. 1984. *School Violence.* Englewood Cliffs, N.J.: Prentice-Hall.

Green, N. 1969. High school student unrest. *Education U.S.A.: Special Report.* Washington, D.C.: National School Public Relations Association.

Greenberg, B. 1974. School vandalism: its effects and paradoxical solutions. *Crime Prevention Review* 1:11–18.

Howard, J. L. 1978. Factors in school vandalism. *Journal of Research and Development in Education* 11:13–18.

Kalogerakis, M. S. 1974. The sources of individual violence. *Adolescent Psychiatry* 3:323–339.

Lieberman, A. 1973. The power of the principal: research findings. In C. M. Culver and G. Hoban, eds. *The Power to Change*. New York: McGraw-Hill.

Miller, D. 1970. Adolescents and the high school system. *Community Mental Health Journal* 6:483–491.

Nowakowski, R. 1966. Vandals and vandalism in the schools: an analysis of vandalism in large school systems and a description of 93 vandals in Dade County schools. Ph.D. dissertation, University of Miami.

Pickhardt, C. E. 1978. Fear in the schools: how students make teachers afraid. *Educational Leadership* 35:107–112.

Richards, P. 1976. Patterns of middle class vandalism: a case study of suburban adolescence. Ph.D. dissertation, Northwestern University.

Rutter, M.; Maughan, B.; Mortimore, P.; and Ouston, J. 1979. *Fifteen Thousand Hours*. Cambridge, Mass.: Harvard University Press.

Schwartz, R. E. 1982. Children under fire: the role of the schools. *American Journal of Orthopsychiatry* 52(3): 409–419.

Sugar, M. 1975. Modified group process in the management of a high school crisis. In I. H. Berkovitz, ed. *When Schools Care*. New York: Brunner/Mazel.

Thomsen, M., and Jones, G. F. 1975. An experiment in the use of group guidance to improve classroom control. In I. H. Berkovitz, ed. *When Schools Care*. New York: Brunner/Mazel.

Violent Schools—Safe Schools. 1978. Washington, D.C.: U.S. Department of Health, Education and Welfare, National Institute of Education.

Yankelovich, D. 1975. How students control their drug crisis. *Psychology Today* 9:39–42.

Zegans, L. S.; Schwartz, M. S.; and Dumas, R. 1969. Mental health centers' response to racial crisis in an urban high school. *Psychiatry* 32:252–264.

32   BUILDING A SUICIDE PREVENTION
CLIMATE IN SCHOOLS

IRVING H. BERKOVITZ

Although many causes of suicide in adolescents precede school entry or are not significantly influenced by events in school, some young persons are emotionally vulnerable and events in school, especially relationships with peers or adults, can play a life-influencing role.

In a survey of 101 school children aged six to twelve using interviews and questionnaires, Pfeffer, Zuckerman, Plutchik, and Mizruchi (1984) found that twelve (11.9 percent) had suicidal ideas or had made threats and attempts. There were significant differences in nine variables between the twelve children and the rest of the group. They had a higher level of recent depressive symptoms, recent aggression, preoccupation with death, parental suicidal tendencies, parental separation, and parental depression. In another study, 385 junior and senior high school students were surveyed using only the Beck Depression Inventory questionnaire (Kaplan, Hong, and Weinhold 1984). Depression in this group was described as mild in fifty-two (13.5 percent), moderate in twenty-eight (7.3 percent), and severe in five (1.3 percent). Lower-social-class adolescents were more depressed than higher; younger adolescents were less depressed than older. Unlike other studies, no difference in statistics was found between boys and girls of the group. Of the group, seventy-eight (20.2 percent) had had suicidal ideas, four (1 percent) more severely, and twenty-two (5.0 percent) very severely. An evaluation of these data raises the question of whether an interview

Parts of this article were published in an earlier version, *Expanding Mental Health Interventions in Schools,* edited by Irving H. Berkovitz and Jerome S. Seliger, published by Kendall/Hunt Publishing Co. in 1985.

survey is more likely to reach concealed feelings than use of a questionnaire alone.

School problems have been implicated in adolescent suicide and attempts. Adolescents who attempt suicide often have relatively poor academic records despite average or above-average capacities. A large percentage drop out of school for other than academic reasons (Husain and Vandiver 1984). Many students are one to four years behind, and most have had long-standing school problems that have antedated the suicidal attempt by at least two years (Finch and Poznanski 1971). Both Finch and Poznanski (1971) and Otto (1972) believe that it is unusual for school to be the direct cause of a suicide attempt. In late high school and college, however, adolescents may find themselves unable to maintain the standards of academic work they have set for themselves and may think they are failing themselves and their parents. Adolescents who indicate "school" as the reason for their suicide attempt most commonly specify "unsatisfactory school result" as the reason (Otto 1972).

During a two-year study, a total of sixty-five youngsters who attempted suicide were identified in the emergency room at the University of Maryland Hospital. Seventy-five percent were girls, ranging in age from seven to nineteen years. Social isolation was a major characteristic, with 50 percent being described as loners. Seventy-five percent had exceptionally poor school grades; 19 percent had failed one or more grades; and 35 percent were dropouts or truants. The other 35 percent were also recorded as having more than a large number of behavior or discipline problems such as class disruption and fighting. Twenty percent had results in testing consistent with minimal brain dysfunction (using the criteria of the Bender-Gestalt Test) (Rohn, Sarles, Kenny, Reynolds, and Heald 1977).

Components for a Suicide Prevention Climate

General and specific components that school personnel can use to help adolescents who are at risk for suicide are, generally, a positive mental health atmosphere along with an optimum psychological services staff and organization and, specifically, a suicide prevention program, adequate health services for effective suicide intervention, and a suicide postvention program.

The first two general components, which should be a part of all school

501

districts for all students, are unfortunately not always available for a variety of reasons, financial and philosophic. Without them, the three more specific elements may not always be as effective. In addition, in providing these programs, one must consider the different needs for the various age levels (elementary, junior, and senior high schools) and pay attention to special attitudes about death and life after death of various ethnic, religious, or racial belief systems of the students and their families.

A POSITIVE MENTAL HEALTH ATMOSPHERE

Ideally, a school should have a humane, understanding, supportive, and challenging environment that can provide validation, growth, support, training, and enhancement for children. Some may think that this is more than one can or should expect, especially from public schools. Yet, with the family instabilities and deficiencies currently prevalent for so many teenagers, schools may be the last public agency that can provide some rescue or repair before other social or legal agencies need to be called in.

Schools can provide a bolstering element to give the child a positive learning experience, a sense of mastery and self-esteem, and a positive view of self and the world. This element unfortunately is not possible for all children in all schools nor for all children in all families. Although preventive assistance is certainly necessary in families as much as in schools, schools can repair some of the disability or at least sound an alarm so that somewhere in the community or in the family the child at risk can receive the needed special attention and help before disability and/or more serious illness develop. The mandated reporting of suspected or actual child abuse in most states is an example of such help.

Through in-service training and emphasis, the staff can be made to appreciate levels of depression, loneliness, and apathy in adolescent students as well as aggressive outbursts and student concerns over grade-point averages, college admissions, and job prospects. It can be of crucial importance, at times, to know which students have experienced divorce or the death of a parent, suicide of a friend or relative, or other tragedy, without this information being misused to stigmatize, coddle, or unduly mark a student. Even more sensitively, it may be of importance to know which students have parents who are depressed, alcoholic, abusive, or suicidal. Perhaps teachers should have more extensive mental health training and understanding to be able to use this information appropriately without distracting from their academic duties. Often these data are known to many of the faculty but may be items of gossip rather than optimally helpful. Consultative assistance may help educators to use the data more appropriately.

Pedersen, Faucher, and Eaton (1978) showed that a significant correlation existed between the care and support of learning provided by a warm, conscientious but also challenging first-grade teacher and her students' better achievement as adults twenty-five years later. Certainly, such a teacher's positive influence would be beneficial for all children, but especially for those at risk for suicide. This degree of concern and involvement is more possible in early grades than in later because in the high school years it is too often assumed that students have or should have achieved successful autonomy and independence and do not need, nor will they accept, special assistance and caring. Occasionally, ingenious efforts may be needed to support or nurture proud, sensitive teenagers.

The climate in a particular school is often determined by the attitude of the principal and the other administrators. A principal who is comfortable with adults and likes young people—even if they are defiant at times—can often help, while moving through a school, without being considered intrusive or judgmental. This administrative style usually promotes a more positive, cooperative staff and school atmosphere. A secondary school of 800 to 2,500 students usually has a large administrative staff and requires that the principal have leadership as well as psychological skills.

The withdrawn, apathetic, depressed, or drug-dependent adolescent is frequently conspicuous in the classroom. Some teachers may respond to the nonverbal cry for help, whereas others try to proceed with the academic task and ignore or remove the needy student. Some flexible and sensitive teachers may allow and promote free discussions about emotions and significant current events alongside the day's educational tasks, conveying an interest and appreciation for the student's welfare and concerns without sacrificing a proper concern for the curriculum. In secondary schools, teachers are divided into those who focus on the cognitive and the smaller number who recognize the important emotional issues being faced during puberty and adolescence. Smaller school units can facilitate better interaction (Berkovitz 1980a).

503

When the teacher is comfortable and skilled with free discussions, the opportunity is greater than in the more controlled classroom for input on attitudes and values. This technique can be a way to influence student attitudes more positively, to improve student-teacher relations, and often to become aware of students who are having emotional as well as academic difficulties. Occasionally, such less structured and more effective types of discussion have been facilitated in the classroom by school psychological personnel or a consultant from an agency outside the school. In such a situation, the arrangements are made with the teacher's full agreement, otherwise the class's loyalty and later attentiveness to the teacher might be compromised.

At one time, teachers paid more attention to the aggressive, disruptive student and less to the uninvolved, withdrawn loner (Wickman 1928). Now, however, teachers are still concerned about the angry, disruptive student but have developed a greater awareness of the needs of the quiet and withdrawn. Although in-class efforts can be of assistance, referral to the school's psychological services is probably necessary for most of the needy adolescents.

SCHOOL PSYCHOLOGICAL SERVICES

Most school districts need more and better psychological services, including the assistance of mental health consultants from outside agencies (Berkovitz 1980b). In secondary schools, the psychological or support staff usually includes school psychologists, counselors, a nurse, and, in some schools, resource specialists. In addition, the dean of boys or girls may be psychologically trained and skilled. Certain teachers may be known as more interested in and sensitive to students, especially in their willingness to listen. At times, custodians, cafeteria workers, and secretarial staff can provide important nurturance and assistance to students. If peer counseling is a part of the school's program, this group of students may be utilized as a resource. Occasionally, there is a resource room where personnel may serve urgent needs. Most secondary school campuses have security personnel who at times are empathetic and available. Ideally, every adult on a school campus, elementary or secondary, should be available for helping purposes even if not skilled for more extensive psychological assistance. In many schools, volunteer parents assist school personnel and, at times, students.

School psychological staff, if properly attuned and not overloaded with other responsibilities, can be attentive to the emotional needs in students. Unfortunately, each counselor often has a responsibility for 300 to 500 students per year as well as other tasks. A load of this size precludes effective individual attention. Ross (1980) showed the value of a highly involved group-counseling program for dealing with suicidal ideation and attempts. Often it takes a suicide to mobilize faculty, support staff, community, and students to provide more effective in-school attention to the needs of depressed, alienated, or otherwise needy students.

Certain procedures still available in many school districts can be called into play when depression, undue withdrawal, unusual drop in performance, or other pathological behavior are recognized in a particular student. In schools where parents are able to afford the expense, students may be referred to clinical facilities. Unfortunately, as is too common, there may be concern that the district may have to pay the expense of each treatment under the provisions of Public Law 94-142. This fear, often unjustified, has prevented many appropriate referrals. More usually, when resources permit, the young person will be seen for evaluation by the school counselor, briefly. If interference with school performance is minimal, little more may be done unless the counselor feels the compunction to inform the parents or refer the student to school therapeutic facilities. Some counselors do occasionally get involved with certain students and may even carry on a weekly individual counseling program. The psychologist, nurse, or resource specialist may be less able to give such individual attention, beyond brief contacts.

In some schools, group and/or peer counseling may be available (Hamburg and Varenhorst 1972). These modalities may allow for a more prolonged and possibly more effective intervention. Usually, the psychologist, counselor, or other counseling-oriented personnel leads such a group. Occasionally, a motivated teacher—optimally with support and consultation—will lead a group.

TEACHERS AND THE EMOTIONAL COMPONENT

In secondary schools, the teacher who has many classes, with numerous students in each class, usually must be interested primarily in academic progress, achievement difficulties, and college or vocational prospects as well as in maintaining order in the class. Often, little time is left for consideration of mental health issues. With proper training and backup from consultants in the school system or from agencies outside the school, the teacher may be helped to assess which students seem depressed, which students are isolates, and which students show other kinds of unique emotional behavior. These students can then be offered assistance if they so desire it. Often they do.

An especially helpful form of group counseling intervention has been developed in some secondary schools, especially by some dedicated teachers who have had available expert psychological support. It operates somewhat as follows. After appropriate assessment, the teacher invites a certain number of the isolates or those with other disturbing behavior to enter a group called a "discussion" or "growth" group. Attending such a group might not necessarily be considered a stigma, especially if a certain amount of fun is connected with it along with providing a useful place to discuss growth problems of adolescence. Most teenagers—even perhaps some with ongoing suicidal ideation—desire this contact. Needless to say, such a group would have to be led with skill and sensitivity in a noncoercive atmosphere.

In one successful high school program, teachers and psychology trainees based at a nearby community mental health center were co-leaders of the groups. Teachers were able to keep separate the didactic and counseling roles, so that material from each role did not intrude inappropriately into the other (Sperber and Aguado 1975). Usually, the classroom teacher is the one who knows best the mental health makeup of a class, especially if there is an awareness and interest in this component of student behavior.

An especially effective step in increasing group counseling services in a high school was provided by a school social worker (Natterson, personal communication, 1983). This worker, with the sanction of the principal, was able to recruit social work students who, as a part of their placement while in training, led counseling groups in the high school. The school social worker instructed and supervised as well as helped to form the groups. This way of increasing the number of trained personnel available to provide for the serious mental health needs of high school students is probably possible wherever there are nearby schools of graduate training in social work, psychology, nursing, or child psychiatry. It does require the presence of an insider with the respect, skill, and assertiveness to innovate and defend a new organizational change. Occasionally, a respected consultant from an outside agency may be able to do this as well (Kandler 1979).

Another place in schools where young persons may communicate depressive or suicidal concerns is in creative writing classes. Especially in secondary schools, many students write and think in a depressive, pessimistic vein about the future, at times focusing on death, without being at risk for suicide. Undue concern by the adult may at times be harmful. Most English teachers are more often concerned with sentence structure and language than with mental health diagnostics. Very often, expressing these feelings in writing and neutral discussion is therapeutic. How to distinguish which depressive or death-focused writing should receive special attention may need to be discussed with the counselor or psychologist at the school. This person may then make a sensitive intervention, if deemed necessary.

Equal in importance to the teacher—especially in elementary schools but also in secondary schools—is the school nurse. She often can be the stimulus for beneficial mental health activities on campus, for example, group counseling programs (Elkin 1975) or suicide prevention programs. Some nurses can provide early recognition of psychosomatic issues such as anorexia, bulimia, premenstrual syndrome, pregnancy, etc. In addition, the nurse can function as a consultant to the administration and teachers in integrating mental health concepts into the curriculum (Blomquist 1974).

A most obvious role of the nurse is to give medical assistance to the suicidal victim. Hart and Keidel (1979) discuss as well the function of the nurse after the return of the suicide attemptor to the school setting.

SPECIAL SCHOOL UNITS

The continuation high school is yet another level of secondary school structure in which depressed young persons can often be helped. Here the students work individually or in small groups. They attend school for a shorter day and meet in a building usually separated from the larger high school. These students may not have adjusted well to the large high school classes. They often do better in the smaller continuation high school setting where there may be only one or two teachers and only a small number of students per class.

Some continuation high schools include group and family counseling. The goal is to reconnect these isolated, failure-oriented, disruptive, or apathetic students and develop better verbal communication with teachers, peers, and parents. These schools represent for many students the last contact with any kind of organized assistance or, for that matter, any real hope about their futures. The better schools do convey an attitude of hopefulness and the positive view that a previously negative pattern of behavior or thinking can be reversed.

Already mentioned are the special classes for severely emotionally disturbed students under Public Law 94-142. Providing assistance to the staff of these units is crucial to improving efforts with this group of students. Unfortunately, even the minimal psychological resources available in most school systems are frequently less available to these special units, although the need is greater.

PREVENTION PROGRAMS

The previously described programs to improve school mental health attention to depression, alienation, and suicide as well as other student behavior do not exclude the use of more focused suicide prevention programs. Suicide awareness will not operate well without a sensitive psychological services network in place. For example, students made aware of depressive, suicidal ruminations through suicide prevention programs would have no ready support system available once the prevention program has left the school unless regular staff is ready to assist.

Referral to community resources often may not be possible or may not take place for various reasons. Unfortunately, some parents do not wish to seek therapy for a suicidal child. They resent the child's demands and fear public exposure of family problems. In such cases, child protection agencies may need to be called for the protection of the child, but in the meantime, the support and empathy of the school staff may be the child's prime resource.

Conclusions

Many suicidal adolescents may be helped in the school setting. To provide this help the school needs a positive mental health atmosphere and adequate psychological services. The effectiveness of more specific suicide preventive, interventive, and postventive programs may depend on the availability of these two more general features in a school. The ingredients and personnel involved in providing these features have been described, including the usefulness of consultant assistance from outside agencies. Many specific school personnel are essential to providing these elements to help depressed and presuicidal young persons. Most important are teachers, psychologists, counselors, nurses, and administrators. Some of the special school units have been described where assistance could be provided to poorly achieving suicidal students, such as the continuation high school and classes for severely emotionally disturbed students.

REFERENCES

Berkovitz, I. H. 1980a. Improving the relevance of secondary schools for adolescent developmental tasks. In M. Sugar, ed. *Responding to Adolescent Needs*. New York: Brunner/Mazel.

Berkovitz, I. H. 1980b. School interventions: case management and school mental health consultation. In G. P. Sholevar, R. M. Benson, and B. J. Blinder, eds. *Treatment of Emotional Disorders in Children and Adolescents*. New York: S. P. Medical and Scientific Books.

Blomquist, K. R. 1974. Nurse, I need help. *Journal of Psychiatric Nursing and Mental Health Services*. 12(1): 22–26.

Elkin, M. 1975. The school nurse organizes a group counseling program in a high school. In I. H. Berkovitz, ed. *When Schools Care*. New York: Brunner/Mazel.

Finch, S. M., and Poznanski, E. R. 1971. *Adolescent Suicide*. Springfield, Ill.: Charles C. Thomas.

Hamburg, B. A., and Varenhorst, B. B. 1972. Peer counseling in the secondary schools. *American Journal of Orthopsychiatry* 42:566–581.

Hart, N. A., and Keidel, G. C. 1979. The suicidal adolescent. *American Journal of Nursing* 79:80–84.

Husain, S. A., and Vandiver, T. 1984. *Suicide in Children and Adolescents*. New York: S. P. Medical and Scientific Books.

Kandler, H. O. 1979. Comprehensive mental health consultation in high schools. *Adolescent Psychiatry* 7:85–111.

Kaplan, S. L.; Hong, G. K.; and Weinhold, C. 1984. Epidemiology of depressive symptomatology in adolescents. *Journal of the American Academy of Child Psychiatry* 23:91–98.

Otto, U. 1972. Suicidal acts by children and adolescents: a follow-up study. *Acta Psychiatrica Scandinavica* (Supplement) 233:5–123.

Pedersen, E.; Faucher, T. A.; and Eaton, W. N. 1978. A new perspective on the effects of first grade teachers on children's subsequent adult status. *Harvard Educational Review* 48:1–30.

Pfeffer, C. R.; Zuckerman, S.; Plutchik, R.; and Mizruchi, M. S. 1984. Suicidal behavior of normal school children: a comparison with child psychiatric inpatients. *Journal of the American Academy of Child Psychiatry* 23:416–423.

Rohn, R. D.; Sarles, R. M.; Kenny, T. J.; Reynolds, B. J.; and Heald, F. P. 1977. Adolescents who attempt suicide. *Journal of Pediatrics* 90:636–638.

Ross, C. P. 1980. Mobilizing schools for suicide prevention. *Suicide and Life-Threatening Behavior* 6:239–243.

Ross, C. P. 1984. Teaching children the facts of life and death: suicide prevention in the schools. In H. Sudak, ed. *Suicide in Children and Adolescents*. London: Wright.

Sperber, Z., and Aguado, D. 1975. Teachers and mental health professionals as co-leaders in high school groups. In I. H. Berkovitz, ed. *When Schools Care*. New York: Brunner/Mazel.

Wickman, E. K. 1928. *Children's Behavior and Teachers' Attitudes*. New York: The Commonwealth Fund.

MICHAEL L. PECK AND IRVING H. BERKOVITZ

At a conference called to consider an alarming number of suicides in Vienna's secondary schools, Sigmund Freud made the following statement: "A secondary school should achieve more than not driving its pupils to suicide. It should give them a desire to live and should offer them support and backing at a time in life at which the conditions of their development compel them to relax their ties with their parental home and their family. The school must never forget it has to deal with immature individuals who cannot be denied a right to linger at certain stages of their development and even at certain disagreeable ones" (Freud 1910).

This statement may seem to place too large a responsibility on secondary schools. Yet despite the lapse of seventy years and the cultural differences from turn-of-the-century Vienna, the concerns are still present. Youth suicide is with us today in higher numbers than ever. One difference is that several states have developed new programs in schools to meet this crisis. However, other changes in the schools' psychological support system may be desirable as well (Berkovitz 1987).

The following data may serve to show the scope of the problem. More than 5,000 young people, age twenty-four and under, commit suicide each year. These numbers are the official figures. The actual numbers are likely to be much higher. Suicide represents the third leading cause of death for this age group and the second leading cause of death for white males.

From the years 1961 to 1975, the suicide rate among fifteen- to twenty-four-year-olds increased 131 percent, while the suicide rate of the population as a whole increased only 22 percent (Holinger 1979). Even the very young, age fourteen and under, showed a dramatic rise of 150 percent during this period. Suicide rates generally increase in the teen years, reaching a peak sometime in the twenties, taper off and drop slightly in the thirties and forties, and then go up again in the sixties and seventies (Peck and Litman 1974). Studies of ethnic and sex differences of youthful suicides reveal that in 1975 the suicide rates for males in the United States age fifteen to twenty-four was four times higher than females and the suicide rate of whites was consistently higher than that of blacks and other nonwhites. A recent finding by Peck (1982) suggests that the suicide rate of young Latinos is even lower than that of the black youth population.

An equally dramatic finding is that suicide attempt rates of young persons are considerably higher than those of people in the older age groups. It has been estimated that among adolescents, there are as many as fifty to one hundred suicide attempts for every completed suicide (Jacobziner 1965). There are many more suicide attempts by females than by males. Some have estimated the ratio to be as high as nine to one. On the other hand, the numbers of the very young (fourteen or less) who commit suicide are relatively small (approximately 190 in the U.S. as a whole). Recent data by Peck (1982) suggest that there is a relationship between learning disabilities and suicide in this age group.

Data from Holinger (1979) suggests that from 1961 to 1976 the suicide rate among this very young age group increased 150 percent. We have also seen a slow increase in completed suicides and attempted suicides in this age group. The Los Angeles Suicide Prevention Center, after reviewing fourteen suicide cases ages fourteen and under, found that 50 percent of the children involved had been previously diagnosed as having some kind of learning disability (Diller 1979). The principal diagnoses in these cases were hyperkinetic disorder, dyslexia, and perceptual disorder. This suggests that learning-disabled youngsters may be at enormous risk for suicide and other self-destructive behaviors.

The remarkable fact was that the seven youngsters who committed suicide had been diagnosed as learning disabled by the schools and were in some form of remedial treatment through the schools. They were also under the care of pediatricians and, in some cases, were receiving stimulants (methylphenidate) for their hyperactivity. These youngsters' unacceptable behavior and slow learning were treated. Their self-esteem, however, which decreased over the years as they fell farther behind their peers in terms of academic work, coordination, and social skills, received less remediation. The schools are in the best position to deal with the painful loss of self-esteem that many learning-disabled youngsters experience.

School personnel for the most part have been less familiar with the dynamics of suicide than clinicians, especially those active in suicide prevention and therapy. Therefore, these professionals based outside the schools have often been called on to supply their expertise. These consultants have provided assistance primarily in three areas: prevention, intervention, and postvention.

Prevention activities center on providing information and support, either to persons who are in high-risk groups for suicide or to so-called gatekeepers who work with high-risk groups. These activities are designed to provide people with the self-knowledge, skills, and sensitivity to prevent suicidal behavior before it occurs. Intervention refers to the classical treatment and therapeutic processes. Telephone hot lines and telephone crisis services are familiar intervention tools. Crisis intervention centers, emergency walk-in centers, psychiatric emergency rooms, and emergency treatment rooms in hospitals are additional intervention methods. Postvention activities usually center on counseling persons who are suffering grief over the loss of a loved one. This may take the form of a crisis bereavement session, group sessions for families or significant others, or group meetings with persons at institutions, such as schools, who may have suffered a loss through suicide.

Suicide Prevention

The major thrust of prevention in the schools usually centers on a lecture and group discussion format. This will vary depending on the categories of persons in the audience and especially on their particular roles. For example, there have been presentations of prevention material to students, classroom teachers, school nurses, counselors, school administrators, and parent-teacher groups. The level of presentation of the particular material given and the particular skills imparted to the audience may differ as a function of the age, training, sophistication, and goals of the particular audience. In response to this crucial opportunity to assist troubled children, several mental health professionals have designed and implemented educational approaches. These include curricular, lecture, and student-oriented features. However,

513

there are staff-oriented features as well and certainly case-oriented consultation for staff.

Victoroff (1977) designed a lecture and slide show on suicide for high school students. His idea was to present to the students actual cases of young people who had committed suicide and impress on the students the increase in incidence of youth suicide. This lecture approach was followed by a question-and-answer period during which the students were encouraged to talk about their own feelings. Victoroff's assumption was that this program would encourage students to become sensitized to their own needs and then request help if needed.

Hart (1976) presented a model for a "death education course" that stressed teaching young people to cope with loss, particularly loss of those things to which one has a high degree of emotional attachment. Hart pointed out that effective suicide prevention in the schools could not be implemented without an understanding of the meaning of life and death. This attention to suicidal thought, behavior, and ideation in the schools appears to be important.

Howze (1979) observed that 18 percent of youngsters in Detroit classrooms reported some kind of suicidal feelings, while Peck (1979) observed that up to 10 percent of youngsters in any public school classroom may be considered at some risk for suicide.

Suicide Intervention

There have been a number of systematic attempts to combine intervention techniques with prevention efforts among young people in schools. Ross (1980) reported on efforts in the San Mateo (California) schools. Discussion groups were set up to talk about issues related to life, death, loss, depression, and suicide. A trained discussion leader helped the youngsters better understand their own feelings about these matters, attempting at the same time to help them increase coping skills. If, during the discussions, serious suicide concerns emerged from one of the youngsters, he or she could be worked with intensively and referred for immediate help. In this way, both prevention and intervention could occur in the school setting.

Yet another approach for prevention and education in the classroom was presented by Colish (1979). She presented a series of options whereby the concepts of death and suicide could be discussed in the classroom within the framework of health education, social problems, mental health, and community health. Colish listed a number of concepts that needed to be communicated to the youngsters. Under each concept were a series of objectives and how to go about reaching them. The concepts were as follows: while death is a natural part of human existence, suicide is an act of self-destruction and involves an individual's intolerable unhappiness; although there is no such thing as a suicide type, the suicidal person gives clues and warnings of his intention to end his life; and most people who attempt suicide are ambivalent about ending their lives—if their cry for help is heard, many suicides could be prevented.

Concerned by the youth suicide epidemic of the past twenty years, some state legislatures have begun to fund prevention programs. In California, a youth suicide prevention bill gave funding to the State Department of Education, in collaboration with two suicide prevention centers, to develop a curriculum for high schools. This curriculum embodies many of the concepts and teaching of the previously described prevention programs but includes also the emphasis that a good friend will not keep secret another friend's suicide intentions. The friend is urged to confide this to a trusted adult to prevent the suicide. An additional important message is that depression is time-limited and not forever as many adolescents fear.

To be effective, suicide prevention education should begin at even earlier ages. Recently, several junior high schools (grades 7-9) have noted increased incidents of suicide threats and attempts. Fortunately, few completed suicides have yet been reported (Berkovitz 1986).

Many suicide prevention programs, however, are still developed on an ad hoc basis in response to a crisis. The following examples illustrate some specific consultations undertaken by the senior author to help develop such programs.

EXAMPLE 1

A small school district had been concerned about suicidal behavior among high school students. The school psychologist and one of the senior administrators organized a conference for administrators and counseling personnel in the school district. It was held away from the school in a community meeting hall. The author presented a lecture on recognizing the early stages of suicidal behavior in young people. A film on the subject was shown followed by a question period. Later there was a panel discussion that included the author and other mental health specialists from the community.

EXAMPLE 2

A meeting was held at a large metropolitan high school that had seen some suicides in the past. The administrators of the school were expressing concern about current behaviors of the students. The meetings were attended by school counselors, the school nurse, and key administrators. Since it was a small group, the format was informal. The author presented facts and information on youth suicide as well as on a number of case examples and early warning signs. Several examples were presented of youngsters' school behavior that had aroused concern. After lengthy discussion, recommendations by the group members as well as by the author were used to develop steps to be taken.

EXAMPLE 3

Two tenth-grade health classes in a large metropolitan high school were discussing the topic of depression and suicide. The classes met with the author to receive information about youth suicide and depression and to see a film on the subject. The focus of the formal input was to acquaint the young audience with the fact (1) that depressive feelings are universal, (2) that everyone experiences them at one time or another, and (3) that the daily depressive experiences that most of us have are different from the clinical depression that often precedes suicide. Examples were given. The questions from students helped to clarify even further the variables involved in differentiating people who are at risk for suicide from those who are going through a temporary upset. A sheet was passed around for students to make written comments, both about the presentation and the film. A wide variety of comments were made—some perceptive, some silly, and some obscene. Six students of the seventy in the group volunteered the information that they themselves were feeling suicidal or at least had suicide thoughts and were concerned about themselves. All of them voluntarily signed their names and, in one way or another, asked for help. A follow-up was done in all of these cases.

In these consultation illustrations, there was an effort to discuss suicide among people in an at-risk category. Also, a more active effort was made, which to some degree succeeded, to identify and respond to suicidal ruminations among students.

THE EMERGENCY CASE CONSULTATION

Most typically, suicide interventions in schools occurred in the following way. A call would come from a school psychologist, a school nurse, or a principal concerning a youngster who had moved into a suicide risk category. The concern centered on the youngster's symptoms and the request was to evaluate the danger and make recommendations. Occasionally, an appointment was made with the youngster. After evaluation, ongoing therapy might be recommended. More often, consultation was given to school personnel, frequently the school psychologist or counselor, who may already have developed a relationship with the suicidal youngster. Under these circumstances, supportive measures were used as part of the consultative procedures, to enable the school personnel to deal more effectively with the problem. Some case examples follow.

CASE EXAMPLE 1

A school psychologist contacted the senior author with information about a fifteen-year-old girl who cut herself in the shower during physical education. She was bandaged by the nurse and was sitting in the nurse's office. An appointment was made immediately for the girl and her mother to come and see the consultant. The girl was found to have psychiatric symptoms and was at the moment not in touch with reality. She was a definite suicide risk, and her mother was encouraged to seek hospitalization for the girl. She was hospitalized for one week, treated, released, and returned to school.

During this time, the author met the teacher, principal, and nurse to discuss the most effective course of action. We also discussed the various symptoms this girl had demonstrated that had not been recognized by the school personnel. They were sensitized as a result of this experience and became more able to recognize suicidal and psychotic symptoms. Intensive therapy, combined with supportive treatment in the school, assisted the girl to return to relatively normal functioning. In this case, ongoing case consultation by the consultant was an important part of a supportive function that the school was able to play.

517

A frantic phone call was received regarding a crisis situation in an elementary school. A twelve-year-old boy, in a state of high distress, was threatening to jump from an upper-floor window. Over the telephone, the principal was given specific instructions on how the situation could be handled in an effective way. The consultant came to the school shortly thereafter, at which time the boy was under control. A conference was held immediately with the boy's mother and the staff. It was decided that that particular school was an inappropriate setting for this boy, because he was unable to handle the high level of work required, and he was placed in another school. At the same time, his mother and he were referred for family therapy to a community agency. The school personnel were quite shaken by this event and additional meetings helped them to deal with much of the residual emotional upset.

Suicide Postvention

Postvention in schools centers primarily on helping school personnel deal with the death of a student or staff member through suicide. This usually occurs in a high school or junior high school. If a violent death occurs with a gunshot or drug ingestion, the school often becomes a mass of rumors. Sometimes other students become overtly suicidal. The staff may become anxious and depressed as intense feelings develop and frightened confusion sets in. The role of the consultant is to bring key people together, have discussions, present facts, and clarify information. When it is clear the death was a suicide, it is important to talk specifically about factors involved in suicide, such as how it occurred and why it occurred. The basic goal of the consultation is to reduce confusion, rumor, anxiety, and suicidal behavior. A major thrust is to reduce secrecy, externalize as many facts as possible about the death, and facilitate the mourning process. Sometimes a large assembly helps to initiate the bereavement.

CASE EXAMPLE 1

In 1984, in an affluent, suburban, southern California high school, three student suicides occurred during one three-month period. One was a female junior who died by gunshot. Another was a male junior who had just dropped out of school. He died in a motor vehicle crash. The third was a male senior whose death was also motor vehicle related. These three deaths traumatized the school community.

The senior author, as a consultant to the school, in conjunction with a local community mental health center and a school psychologist, formulated the following plan of action. Parent groups and faculty members were talked with to reassure them that this was "not their fault" and to provide them with crisis intervention skills. Students were addressed in a variety of ways. General information about youth suicide was provided, and rap groups were set up where friends of the three deceased students could gather to discuss their feelings. As a result of this, many students who might have otherwise been overlooked were identified as potential suicides and referred for help. The student body and the school community were given facts, disabused of rumors, and, eventually, grew closer. A school-based classroom suicide prevention program was instituted the following year.

CASE EXAMPLE 2

An eighteen-year-old college student committed suicide by jumping off the upper floor of his college dormitory. The other students in the dorm were upset. Many rumors began to spread about the deceased and the reasons for his action. The family was understandably shaken and tended to blame the school. The school authorities, in searching for a way to calm the turmoil and satisfy the family, asked the author to come to the dormitory. He was asked to consult with the resident counselors, some students who were closest to the decedent, and some of the staff who were experiencing considerable guilt.

The meeting began with the dean of students reading a prepared statement exonerating the school of all responsibility for the death. The dean left and the vice-chancellor announced that the author would discuss some suicide cases from the Suicide Prevention Center. It was clear that this approach would merely add to the secrecy and stigma already attached to the event. The author therefore proceeded to point out that the real reason for the meeting was to discuss the suicidal death of the young student, and that only by understanding that death could further tragedies be avoided. Refocusing the meeting toward the goal of understanding and future-oriented prevention enabled some of the stigma and blame to be reduced. People began to speak—cautiously at first and then more candidly. Significant catharsis occurred. At the conclusion, there was an attempt to summarize the group's understanding of what happened, review the clues that might have been present, and provide structure for reorganizing and preventing such behavior in the future.

Similar postvention consultations have been of value in several high schools.

Conclusions

Suicidal behavior among young people results in much stigma, chaos, and confusion. When it occurs in the context of the school community, an emotional decompensation process often occurs. It is in this highly charged atmosphere that the consultant who specializes in adolescent suicidal behavior can provide a most important service. Not only does the consultant help the staff of a school deal with a specific suicidal problem, he or she helps to provide structure and support for the school personnel. The consultant can reduce the tension and rumor in the school community that often may result in additional suicidal behaviors. Facilitating the mourning process can be a powerful outcome of the various approaches described, and it is our contention that proper mourning can result in significant growth and development.

REFERENCES

Berkovitz, I. H. 1986. Multiple suicide attempts in a junior high school. Unpublished manuscript.

Berkovitz, I. H. 1987. Improving the suicide prevention climate in schools. *Adolescent Psychiatry* (in this volume).

Colish, H. 1979. *Suicide Prevention in the Classroom: A Teacher's Guide to Curriculum.* West Point, Pa.: Merck, Sharpe & Dohme.

Diller, J. 1979. The psychological autopsy in equivocal deaths. *Perspectives in Psychiatric Care* 17:156–161.

Freud, S. 1910. Symposium on suicide. In P. Friedman, ed. *On Suicide: Discussion of the Vienna Psychoanalytic Society, 1910.* New York: International Universities Press, 1967.

Hart, J. 1976. Death, education and mental health. *Journal of School Health* 46(7): 407–412.

Holinger, P. C. 1979. Violent death among the young: recent trends in suicide, homicide and accidents. *American Journal of Psychiatry* 136:1144–1147.

Howze, B. 1979. A cross-cultural approach to the study of predisposing characteristics to suicide in a group of urban Detroit youth. Unpublished manuscript.

Jacobziner, H. 1965. Attempted suicide in adolescents. *Journal of the American Medical Association* 19(1): 7–11.

Peck, M. L. 1982. Youth suicide. *Death Education* 6:29–47.

Peck, M. L., and Litman, R. E. 1974. Current trends in youthful suicide. In J. Bush, ed. *Suicide and Blacks*. Los Angeles: Charles R. Drew Post-graduate Medical Center. (Issued by the Fanon Research and Development Center.)

Ross, C. P. 1980. Mobilizing schools for suicide prevention. *Suicide and Life Threatening Behavior* 6:239–243.

Victoroff, V. 1977. A means of preventing teenage suicide. *Family Health* 9(4): 22–24.

34   VALUE OF GROUP COUNSELING IN SECONDARY SCHOOLS

IRVING H. BERKOVITZ

When treating an adolescent, it is often useful to know the details of any group counseling available in the individual's school. Occasionally, one's patient may already have been referred by school personnel to the available group, or there could be benefit if the therapist knew enough to recommend such referral. On another level, the clinician interested in the general welfare of children in schools may wish to help to establish more and better group treatment facilities in schools. School personnel often appreciate and make good use of consultation with knowledgeable mental health professionals. This chapter should help the clinician know the limitations and potentials of such groups. Often, suitable groups are not available elsewhere in the community, and a well-run group in the schools can be a valuable therapeutic component.

Most early authors and practitioners derived many of the procedures and concepts used in school group counseling from clinical group therapy (Driver 1958; Gazda 1975; Glass 1969; Mahler 1969; Ohlsen 1970). While many concepts and practices are similar, several important modifications are necessary in the school setting. General counseling groups as well as task-oriented groups are useful in schools. Task-oriented groups can be set up to focus on sex education, problems of transition from junior to senior high school to high school graduation, issues of entering college, and leadership classes (Berkovitz 1987). In addition, some educators of necessity use group process in the classroom. There are differences in size of group, length of meeting, allowed spontaneity,

Parts of this article were published in an earlier version, *The Adolescent Group Therapies*, published by International Universities Press in 1987.

severity of problems, responsibilities of leader, range of topics, and other features of counseling and task-oriented groups.

Advantages of Group Counseling in the School Setting

Groups in the school setting have several advantages. (1) Young persons (and their families) who would not accept or follow through on referral to a community agency will often be able and willing to accept a school counseling group. There is not the usual implication of illness with school groups, and there is no financial obstacle. As a result, this may be the only setting where some severely disturbed adolescents will receive original assistance without having to deal with the resistance or transference issues of psychotherapy. (2) As in the traditional clinic or office setting, ego dystonic insights and confrontations in the group sessions may occasionally result in a member's abrupt departure or nonattendance. In school groups, continued contact in the course of the school day with other group members and leaders may provide reassurance and clarification, so that the young person can continue with the group without anger or fear. School absence to avoid such contact is rare; rather, school groups have usually improved school attendance (Awerbuch and Fraser 1975). (3) Facts and attitudes about each group member are often generally known by the other adolescents or the school personnel in the group. This information may be useful in the sessions if this can be provided without undue hurt and antagonism. Often the additional information will shorten and deepen the process. (4) Other school personnel, outside the group, will often have information or observations about group members that could be useful in that young person's counseling. In a clinic setting, proper confidentiality safeguards have to be followed, with all the attendant communication difficulties. In the school setting, the school group leader has more immediate availability to this data. (5) Teacher comments about positive change in the group members who are in their classes—when communicated to the members directly or to the group leaders—can be an important reinforcing influence to maintain group attendance as well as to bolster self- esteem.

Disadvantages of Group Counseling

The disadvantages of groups in schools, although less common than the advantages, stem from lack of control of the transference-countertransference that is standard in psychotherapy. (1) On occasion, a group session can lessen emotional control such that inappropriate disruptive behavior can occur. (2) Sensitive material may be leaked from the group to persons outside the group. This breaking of the rules for confidentiality can damage an individual's reputation, disturb the sense of privacy, and depreciate the group in the school context. (3) Faculty can be scapegoated in a session, especially if insufficient control is maintained. (4) School staff may resent the group, feeling that disturbed children should not be rewarded with all this attention, or some may reject counseling in general. (5) Interruptions may occur during sessions that may prevent the development of a useful group process attitude for considering behavior. (6) Noisy interaction during sessions can disturb nearby classrooms or offices and result in criticism or require undue moderation of spontaneous energy. (7) Parents, who may come to resent the groups, can complain to the school board or other authorities, cast the entire group program into disrepute, and, in some cases, have it canceled. (8) Summer and other school vacation periods may interrupt the life of the group, cutting off therapeutic momentum for some students. For others, it may be a useful respite.

Case Illustrations

Several case illustrations of the benefits to young persons are offered. An example of improved self-awareness occurred in a high school group conducted by the dean of girls.

CASE EXAMPLE 1

Cynthia would probably have been classified as a school phobic. Her problem was at home more than at school. She talked about the leniency of her mother and her fearfulness of her father. One day she came in furious at a teacher. As she was ranting on and on about this teacher, one of the group members noted a similarity between the way she described the teacher and the way she described her father. I suggested role playing. Cynthia was to play her father or the teacher, and Lucy played Cynthia. Cynthia was delighted at the opportunity to show how really awful her father was. Lucy portrayed Cynthia accurately, and Cynthia got the message. She said, "Do I really push him like that?" [Evans 1975, p. 100]

CASE EXAMPLE 2

An example of likely characterological change emerged from a confrontation that occurred in a high school group conducted by a social worker on the school staff.

Bernice, ready to run away from home because of constant battling with her mother, had a history of intense fighting with parents, teachers, and peers.

Bernice's participation in the group for the first few months was minimal. When others spoke, she giggled, acted silly, whispered, or discourteously interrupted. When members criticized her disruptive behavior, she became defensive and threatened to leave. Her pattern was to arrive late—sometimes by a whole period— barge in, and self-righteously justify her lateness by claiming she had needed to attend the previous class.

I learned from her teachers that Bernice's grades were, indeed, caused by her absences from classes. The teachers also reported the same provocative behavior and immaturity in the classroom, such as giggling when others made a serious effort. School behavior paralleled group behavior; peers and teachers were provoked.

One day, when Bernice arrived a full hour late, an important encounter was occurring between two members of the group. She found it interesting and wished to be included. She loudly and intrusively asked what was going on.

My answer was that if she'd come on time she'd know. A reaction followed. Bernice cried and had hysterics. She had rightly observed my annoyance, but saw my confrontation as rejection. She defensively insisted that this time she had a good reason for being late; she'd been at home talking with her mother. She accused us of picking on her, singling her out for attack, and protested that she could not understand the reason.

I interpreted to her how she had invited the attack by repeatedly coming in late and disrupting the others, a characteristic action on her part, resulting in the negative reaction of others to her. Bernice wanted to leave the group after this encounter, but she requested two individual sessions. In these, I encouraged her to return and work out her negative feelings before discontinuing. When she came back to the group, the members supported her staying—and she stayed. She began to participate more realistically, and she

525

faced the part she had played in provoking others. Serendipitously, Bernice's outbursts provided the stimulus for another member of the group to get in touch with his own angry feelings. [Natterson 1975, pp. 53–54]

CASE EXAMPLE 3

Two group leaders with special sensitivity and clinical skills combined to lead a school group. A clinical agency provided a staff social worker to colead this school group with a school counselor.

A bright, capable, and attractive black girl had come from an almost wholly black elementary school to a junior high school comprising many ethnic groups. When she entered the group, she was underachieving and in difficulty because of open hostility to her teachers, who she felt were prejudiced. She expressed hatred for her new school and a desire to go to an all-black junior high school. The group, which was ethnically mixed and coled by a black counselor and a white social worker, repeatedly discussed the whole problem, separating out its various aspects and focusing on what Althea herself could do about it.

The school counselor was aware of prejudiced attitudes on the part of some teachers, yet she did not permit this to be used as an excuse for self-destructive defiance or withdrawal. She both supported and confronted Althea in group and out. Eventually, Althea became much more self-assured and comfortable in dealing with students and teachers of other ethnic backgrounds. Her academic work improved, and she eventually emerged as one of the natural leaders of the school. In all of this, the ongoing understanding and intervention of the school counselor was of crucial importance. [Kaplan 1975a, p. 179]

Some students with severe psychosocial difficulties may need more than school group counseling alone, as evidenced by a member of an inner city high school group.

CASE EXAMPLE 4

Nothing could be done about Carol's problems: an alcoholic mother, runaway father, brothers and sisters who were drug addicts, gang members, thieves, and constantly in and out of trouble with the police. All she could do was tell us about it. All we could do was listen and offer whatever we could. She must have gleaned something from the sessions, because she came every week for two years, except for illness. She often came to school just to attend group and left immediately afterward. [Leong 1975, p. 82]

Group Management Procedures

There are many technical details to be considered in discussing the inception and maintenance of effective groups in schools. While many procedures will be similar to those which should be followed in office or clinic groups, many details may need attention that do not pertain in the clinical context (Berkovitz 1972, 1987).

Process in Groups

Very often, groups—whether short or long lasting—will go through definable stages. Clark (1975) described a sequence in groups of fourteen- to fifteen-year-old, undisturbed students in a large, mixed, comprehensive school in London. The groups were balanced and met for ten to twelve sessions. His description possibly provides a baseline for how a group might be expected to operate with minimally disturbed young people. A group of more disturbed young persons might have shown more motoric expression of anxiety and less cooperation.

CASE EXAMPLE 5

First stage. Members remained highly dependent on the teacher or fragmented into a collection of unrelated subgroups or conflicting individuals. Silences often occurred, or solidarity developed through an attack on the leader or a group member. They were "unable or unwilling to treat each other as persons especially if they belonged to the opposite sex, while at the same time feeling the extensive frustration of themselves being ignored or rejected by the group."
Second (developing) stage. Pupils sought solidarity in subgroups but reached out to establish contact with the group as a whole. The search for significance and autonomy was pursued with great

527

confidence and more respect for what others have to contribute. Sex groupings occur with teasing, pranks, games, refreshments, and joke telling. A heightening of individuality occurred with emergence of leaders who at times were "autocratic" but other times could lead constructively.

Third (mature) stage. Pupils discover a sense of solidarity that permeated the whole group while at the same time each member felt that his presence and his contribution were genuinely valued by the others. This stage was characterized by spontaneous enjoyment and fun and especially playing games, verbal and physical. The relationship between boys and girls was much freer and unself-conscious. Participation was on an equal footing and pairing was open and enjoyed by all. Sexual questions were asked freely. Imaginative ideas for group activities emerged. No one member dominated.

The leader's task was to give "freedom for self-discovery and self-determination in the company of others," to "intervene only when this assists self-determination," but to avoid too much detachment or allowing pupils to "wallow in passivity and dependence." When there was complaint of boredom, the leader pointed out very forcibly that "the group was what we all made it."

Termination Techniques

Orderly termination of a group is a phase of importance to emotional learning. Here, young persons will learn to experience loss and grief—crucial emotions in the lives of children. Each group's style of termination will differ. For example, the following occurred in a junior high school, once-per-week group of boys meeting voluntarily.

CASE EXAMPLE 6

During the tenth meeting, the psychiatrist announced that the group would terminate after a few more meetings. The boys dealt with this in a rather elaborate way. They became convinced that the reason the adult leader had the interest to start such a group was to see "how stupid" they were. Another time, one boy started hitting the psychiatrist "in fun."

In the next-to-the-last meeting they decided to have a round robin of dirty jokes. This made it more apparent that they once

528

again wanted to reassure themselves that they could be with an adult and indulge in expressing sexual fantasies without being severely punished. Many of the jokes were rather typical, concrete sexual jokes.

Elaborate plans were made for a party for the last meeting. Food was brought in by the mothers. The food and drink were gorged. Then everyone sat around deliberating what was going to happen to close the last group meeting. They again decided to tell dirty jokes, and an exact repetition of all the jokes of the previous session ensued. Handling of loss and separation was done by different boys in their own different ways. One boy eulogized the psychiatrist as if he had died. Some of the more kinetic boys started acting up. One boy, who was going to move out of the community shortly, acted this out by isolating himself in a tent-like structure in the room. [Vanderpol and Suescum 1975, pp. 280–281]

Older teenagers will usually be more verbal and less "kinetic" and occasionally discuss other loss experiences.

In clinical groups, and occasionally school groups, termination is usually an individual matter, occurring as each individual reaches his or her own point of optimum benefit or tolerance. The last session(s) of any departing member, especially with older teenagers, can often be very poignant for the entire group, with tears and declarations of love. Occasionally there may be anger or withdrawal.

In school groups, the group often ends together at the end of a semester or the end of the school year. This does miss the possibility of an individual having a more focused grief reaction. Also, the grief reaction often is cushioned by the group's having a party or other orally gratifying culmination. This may be regarded by some as a lost therapeutic opportunity, but there is often sufficient opportunity to examine feelings about losses during the previous period of the group experience (Fleisher, Berkovitz, Briones, Lovetro, and Morhar 1987). School adolescent groups usually cannot sustain the prolongation of painful feelings, as might some clinical groups.

Leadership in a Group

While the group style will evolve from the personalities of the members in the group, the leader still sets the rules and the tone, and the young people look to the leader for expected boundaries. The type of leadership for groups is different from that needed in a classroom. This can be a difficulty for some school personnel whose training has been only for the classroom. Group counseling usually needs to allow for more spontaneous, less structured kinds of discussion than the classroom.

The following is an example of a social worker from a clinical setting using clarification of feelings to engage the attention of anxious students.

CASE EXAMPLE 7

Our first group meeting of seventh grade girls was in a laboratory; no other space was available. I had never met the girls who had been interviewed and selected by the grade counselor who was coleader—a warm, strong woman whom the girls obviously liked. As we seated ourselves in a circle, some of the girls began fooling around with the lab equipment, and Mrs. H told them firmly that they could not handle it. Several of them then began to flick their fingers and hands on each other's arms and legs, while a general air of restlessness pervaded the circle. Mrs. H looked at me, and I read her question clearly. Should she intervene again? I asked if the girls knew why they were here. Some said Mrs. H had asked them. More flicking, changing into hitting. I asked what they were saying with their hands and feet. This appeared to startle them. One girl said "Nothing! We do it all the time." I pressed further, and a discussion developed about how they express friendliness this way. They also agreed maybe it was a way of handling embarrassment at being here. This moved into a further discussion of how sometimes it ends in fights (which was one of the reasons some of the girls had been referred for group). Meanwhile, as the group talked about it, the actual behavior ceased. I breathed a sigh of relief that what I thought I knew about group process and feelings had worked at this crucial moment. [Kaplan 1975a]

Ideally, the counselor should not dominate group sessions except for a specific reason (e.g., to decrease the anxiety of the group). If the group is functioning well, it may be concluded that members are providing each other some significant new awareness. Such awareness is often better accepted from peers than from the counselor. If a problem is presented that may be contrary to the principles of the counselor, the counselor should be tolerant. However, if an antisocial point of view is being espoused by a majority of the group members, it may be important for the counselor to present an alternative view, though not necessarily in a strongly judgmental way. For example, one junior high school group was defending the justification of stealing. It was as if these students had never before heard the pros and cons of stealing as a way of acquiring material things in life. It was unlikely that strong criticism or contradiction by the middle-class counselor would have received a receptive hearing. It was more likely that a parable or some attempt to develop an orientation toward the future might have influenced some of them. In most school groups there will be one or more members of the group who will present the alternative point of view, but in the absence of these the counselor may be required to do so.

Usually, it is important for the counselor not to ally with the child against the parent. If the parent is glaringly at fault, the counselor may need to comment. Often other members of the group may criticize that parent or empathize with the youngster in a way that may help. If child abuse examples are disclosed by members, the leader may have no choice, since it is legally required in many states that such instances be reported.

Occasionally, some youngsters may have to be given individual counseling instead of or in addition to the group. While some familiarity with teenage vocabulary, interests, and current fads may be important for the counselor to establish empathy and understanding, generally students do not want the counselor to be one of the group. They may want friendliness, kindness, and respect, but not another teenager.

Some readers may wish to identify a consistent stance desirable for leaders of school groups. For better or worse, most leaders of school groups in reality have a wide range of styles and philosophies depending on their training, personalities, and attitude about children or adolescents. Fortunately, all approaches—analytic, behavioral, or cognitive—can be helpful if applied in a humanistic, nonrigid, less authoritarian, but somewhat consistent manner.

Usually, more empathic, less detached involvement is desirable than in office or clinic groups, especially since the leader is seen on campus often at informal moments. Most young people are so desirous and needing of a small group setting in which to relate that a wide range of positive styles can be facilitating.

In working with adolescents, a continuous monitoring of countertransference is essential. Most school personnel do not receive as intensive training in this regard as do clinically trained professionals.

531

The leader, at times, may have to moderate the amount and intensity of feelings surfaced about more difficult home problems, unless there is also concomitant family intervention or possibly referral to clinical facilities. The degree and type of activity necessary to involve more isolated students is another matter of judgment and skill. A description of desirable parameters would require at least an additional chapter.

Training of Group Leaders

While I have talked thus far as if the school counselor will be the leader of most group counseling, staff other than counselors have often served as group leaders as well. These may be the school psychologist, vice-principals or deans of students (Evans 1975), the nurse (Elkin 1975), and occasionally teachers (Sperber and Aguado 1975).

There are many examples of nonschool personnel being invited onto campus to conduct groups, usually in collaboration with school personnel but occasionally without such collaboration (Berkovitz 1975a, 1975b). Most school personnel, including those in the psychological services, are usually more familiar with one-to-one counseling than with group counseling. There are needs for in-service training to help school personnel reorient themselves and develop the expertise to lead groups. In addition to introductory in-service training, it is desirable to have ongoing supervision and support, where there is a chance to discuss the various crises and vicissitudes that may arise during the life of the group. This can be provided by experienced in-school personnel, if such are available, or by outside consultants (Jacobs and Deigh 1975; Vogel 1975). At times, there may have to be basic discussion of adolescent psychological processes for school personnel who have not had wide clinical experience (Berkovitz 1980a).

Of equal importance in group counseling programs is the ability of the leader to relate well to personnel, especially administrators and teachers. Without this capacity, there may be resistance to instituting effective group programs, at least under school psychology auspices. Psychological services personnel are often as much targets of fear and suspicion from other school personnel as mental health professionals from outside the school.

The school counselor is usually the overworked, frontline mental health person in schools. Though less clinically trained than the psychologist, a counselor frequently has a case load of hundreds of students. Therefore, it is often difficult for counselors to make time in their schedules to do group counseling. In schools where a counselor has been given the time to be in full- or part-time charge of group counseling, there has been greater success for the program (Leong 1975).

The school nurse is often very cognizant of mental health needs in a school. When sufficiently motivated and given time in her schedule, she also can become a valuable leader of a group-counseling program (Elkin 1975).

Teachers, administrators, and teacher aides have been enlisted to lead group counseling during free periods, with proper supervision. In one project, teachers and psychologist-trainees from a nearby clinic were coleaders of counseling groups, especially those composed of students selected by classroom teachers. Some deans of students (Evans 1975; Evans, Johnson, and Thompson 1975) and occasionally principals (Robinson 1975) have conducted groups very effectively.

Role of Consultants

When professionals from agencies outside of schools enter a campus to conduct groups, there is a need for a close liaison with at least one school person to arrange for referrals, administrative sanction, room assignment, and other relationships. These outside professionals can be from all of the mental health disciplines: psychiatrists, psychologists, social workers, psychiatric nurses, rehabilitation counselors, and so on, as well as probation workers, welfare department workers, police officers, or even volunteers without formal training.

The matter of financing these outside resources is frequently of concern. Some school districts are prepared to pay a small part of the cost of these group leaders on campus, when such funds are available (Kaplan 1975a). At other times, public agencies or corporations have been willing to help fund the services of some nonschool professionals conducting groups on school campuses.

Types of Referrals

The types of students referred to or seeking groups may vary from (1) those who have nonpathological problems of adolescence, such as shyness, parental conflict, or desire for discussion of growth issues;

533

(2) those who have identified problems, that is, are emotionally disturbed, are underachieving, or have behavior or adjustment disorders; and (3) special education groups involving those students with mental retardation, deafness, blindness, cerebral palsy, physical handicaps, and more severe emotional problems.

The most pathological groups may involve a leader's time outside the group in relating with parents, other agencies, and personnel within the school. Parent groups may be more necessary for certain groups of students than for others. These groups may be conducted by knowledgeable personnel within the school or in cooperation with community agencies.

Types of Groups

The junior high school years (grades 7–9, ages twelve to fourteen) are frequently difficult for the pubescent teenager. Awkwardness, embarrassment, and confusion occur in at least 50 percent of these children (Offer and Offer 1975). Teachers are often not sure if they are babysitters or academicians. Group counseling at this age is most difficult but very crucial and exciting when successful. Senior high school groups (grades 9–12, ages fourteen to seventeen) may be more attentive and productive compared to junior high school groups, but there will be some immature students in these as well. High school groups often can become more task oriented. These may be leadership groups, groups for pregnant adolescents, groups for weight reduction, career planning, and so on. After-school clubs, while directed toward specific interests, can certainly involve some elements of new emotional learning and interpersonal assistance, especially from knowledgeable faculty advisers or students.

Various styles and techniques may prevail with different group leaders, involving psychodrama or role playing, behavioral contingencies, use of recordings, films, trips, and guest speakers. Some groups may be a mixture of informational and psychological orientation. For example, some groups have been offered to teach coping and study skills, assertiveness and social skills, reality therapy, and transactional analysis.

At times, it is helpful for leaders to have different activities available with which to engage the interest and the attention of the otherwise disruptive, anxious young people. These can be art materials, a game, or a structured exercise. Bates (1975) has divided certain techniques into mild and moderate. Among the mild techniques she has described are discussions of birth order, territoriality, interaction diagrams, first memories, free association, stereotyping, and human potential. Among the moderate techniques she has classified the magic shop, role playing, identifying emotions, authority syndrome, autobiographies, the group sociogram, rejection, significant experiences, new ways of behaving, and psychodrama. Other authors have introduced discussion topics, such as boy-girl relationships, speaking to one's parents, making friends, and spending time alone, but stress it should not be a closely structured, "keep to the subject" type of discussion. Otherwise it could become too close to a classroom atmosphere and sacrifice the values of an interactive, participatory experience.

Especially with very active younger adolescents, behaviorally reinforced kinds of groups have been reported. These would usually require an observer to measure each member's interaction in order to give rewards for positive kinds of behavior (Bardill 1977). Some groups in clinical settings have used the lyrics of currently popular teenage music as a stimulus to discuss feelings such as sadness, jealousy, and anger (Vanderkolk 1976).

Groups for Special Problems

Groups have been designed to attempt to raise the grade-point average (GPA) of underachieving students. Low GPA can often be an accompaniment of transient or chronic emotional disorder but can be related as well to poor study habits, poor home facilities for studying, test anxiety, or problems between teacher and student. As a result, many types of groups will achieve a rise in GPA. Other changes in aspects of feeling and behavior are harder to quantify.

Desirable gains other than a rise in GPA may occur after some group interventions. For example, sixty-nine gifted, underachieving high school sophomores were given four semesters of weekly group counseling. Compared with a control group of eighty-five, no difference was found in the GPA, but the counseled students were rated by teachers as being less resistive and more cooperative in the classroom and less frequently absent from class (Finney and Van Dalsem 1969). Goodstein (1967), in his group, found that initial gain in GPA was completely negated five

535

years later. In fact, higher proportions of control subjects graduated than did counseled subjects. This is the only study reporting such an outcome.

Gurman (1967) stated that leader-structured groups appeared to be the most effective group method for the counseling of underachievers. If this is so—and the evidence in this regard is not yet clear—it implies that insight, as it is defined by psychoanalytically oriented counselors and therapists, is not essential to the successful treatment of underachievers.

Roth, Mauksch, and Peiser (1967) reported that 174 selected failing students were provided group counseling as a condition of their remaining in school. The results indicated that the counseled group increased their GPA significantly and that these changes held over time. The GPA of the comparison group did not increase significantly.

Empey (1977) reported that test anxiety desensitization at the junior high school level—using eight sessions of relaxations, visualization, and discussion—significantly improved GPA. Both a self-management approach—teaching the principles of behavior modification and self-control—and a group discussion technique—involving discussion of study habits and problems—led to improvements in GPA compared with a no-treatment control group for low-achieving junior high school students (Harris and Trujillo 1975). In a controlled study, Hamelberg (1981) demonstrated that coping skills training as a cognitive-behavioral intervention significantly reduced manifestations of inappropriate classroom behavior and improved social skills of youngsters with serious learning problems.

There have been several studies of groups to help ethnic minorities. A short-term school group for six Hispanic, eighth-grade girls reported that a major accomplishment was the participants' increased ability to tolerate anxiety, to verbalize cross-cultural conflicts, and to be able to turn to each other for support (Hardy-Fanta and Montana 1982). A group of thirty black students was compared to a control group using precounseling and postcounseling. After one year of group counseling, the experimental groups showed significant gains in vocabulary, reading, English usage, occupational aspiration, and vocational maturity (Gilliland 1968).

A group of twenty ninth-grade Mexican-American students of college potential in a minority high school in a low socioeconomic area met for a lunchtime conference daily during their freshman year, twice per week in the sophomore year, and occasionally during the junior and senior years. Topics of discussion ranged far and wide, although the primary focus was on why education was important, how to get into college, and special problems of Mexican-American students. The group was very informal and developed excellent rapport. Of the thirty-five, thirty entered college and did well; seven received scholarships (Klitgaard 1969).

In a junior high school subject to student friction during desegregation, a group was formed that provided important aid in the processing of angry feelings. The group consisted of twelve students who were considered "natural leaders" by the counselors. These were the ones who had most often been referred to the counseling office for disciplinary problems on campus. The composition was equally black, Hispanic, and Caucasian. For two months this group met weekly. These were the informal leaders among the students who had known of each other but had never sat down to talk to each other. The discussions were frequently heated. Especially notable was the learning of verbal expression and understanding, as an alternative to physical violence. Several of the students had been subjected to physical abuse in their families. This seemed to encourage their use of physical violence as a solution to tension and threats on campus. In the group discussions, however, they were able to explain to each other the risk of these physical responses. For example, one black boy said, "If that teacher bothers me one more time, I'm going to pop off and hit him." A formerly overly aggressive Caucasian boy then said, "Don't do that man! You'll be the one who gets hurt." The members of the groups began to be helpful to each other on campus. When they saw one of them about to get into trouble, they would help each other to avoid fighting. One even began to break up interracial fights on campus. They recommended that there be more groups next year: "If there's a chance to talk, then you don't have to fight." It was interesting to note that for almost all of the sessions, the members of each ethnic group sat separately in three segregated groupings. In the last meeting, however, there was some spontaneous mixed seating, which seemed to attest to the success of the communication achieved (Berkovitz, Carr, and Anderson 1983).

Many groups have been established on campuses to deal with drug abuse (Flacy, Goda, and Schwartz 1975). Some school systems have set up counseling groups for pregnant adolescents to try to improve

537

understanding and decrease the number of repeat pregnancies. In peer counseling programs, the training groups—in which older high school students are taught to counsel younger students—often provide a form of group counseling for the older students (Hamburg and Varenhorst 1972). Multiple-family group therapy has been useful in some school settings (Durrell 1969), as well as simultaneous group counseling with adolescents and their parents (Shaw and Mahler 1975).

Special education units for handicapped students use group counseling with varying effectiveness and special adaptations. Groups have been effective with adolescents who are educable mentally retarded (i.e., IQ 53–77) (Humes 1971; Humes, Adamczyk, and Myco 1969; Lee 1977; Lodato, Sokoloff, and Schwartz 1964; Mann, Beaber, and Jacobson 1964; Ringelheim and Polatsek 1935; Stacey and De Martino 1957), with those who are diagnosed as having autism or schizophrenia (Epstein 1977), and with those with multihandicaps (Empey 1977), epilepsy (Appolone and Gibson 1980), muscular dystrophy (Bayrakal 1975), stammering (Laeder and Francis 1968; Rustin 1972), or deafness (Bonham, Armstrong, and Bonham 1981; Sarlin and Altshuler 1968).

Evaluation

As mentioned in previous studies, criteria used for evaluation vary widely and include change in GPA, school attendance, disruptiveness, and empathy. Kaplan (1975b) evaluated twenty junior high school and seven senior high school groups conducted in eleven schools, with 310 students involved. Groups met weekly during the school year. The group discussions were fairly unstructured but focused on problems of achievement and difficulties with adult authority. Groups were coled by an agency social worker and, usually, a school counselor. Junior high students were referred for poor school performance, poor school attendance, problems with school authority, and immature behavior in school. Ten percent had difficulties in family relations. Changes in these referral criteria were then evaluated at the end of that school year.

Change was determined by ratings from group leaders and collateral school personnel, usually a grade counselor, vice principal, school nurse, or the teacher. It was of interest that compared to similar groups in elementary and high schools, the junior high school groups had the lowest percentage of students considered improved. There was a 57.6 percent improvement as seen by coleaders and collateral personnel, and a 60.6 percent improvement as seen by coleaders only. The percentage of group members showing improvement rose steadily in proportion to the number of group meetings attended at all three school levels. The highest was 84 percent improved for those attending twenty meetings. The most difficult problem area was acting-out, impulse-ridden, and/or antisocial behavior. A comparatively high percentage of students were judged improved in family problems; this totaled 71.8 percent and ran slightly higher for junior and senior high school group members. School-centered problems show a similar level of improvement—71.9 percent for all three school levels combined. Evaluation one year or more later would have been of value.

Use of Groups in Colleges

Group counseling is quite prevalent in college student mental health clinics. Swarr and Ewing (1977), in describing a long-term group therapy program in a four-year college, showed that significant positive change occurred in personality characteristics of self-esteem variables—anxiety, motivation and self-discipline, and activity, interest, and outgoing behavior levels in the first half ($M = 10.3$ sessions) of treatment. In contrast, poor interpersonal functioning and related feelings of distrustfulness, hostility, unassertiveness, and excessive status achievement needs resisted change, but they did change by the end of treatment ($M = 20.5$ sessions).

Many colleges offer classes that involve personal discussion with a learning and therapeutic goal. Evaluation of a community college laboratory course group ascertained that the course group developed a high sensitivity to their own needs and feelings. The participants became more assertive and less fearful of expressing feelings behaviorally (White 1974).

Several behaviorally oriented studies have been published describing efforts aimed at improving dating skills, especially in male college students. To what degree exploration of attitudes about women can be excluded from a program and still make a significant change in a man's conflict about dating seems questionable. One study found significant reduction in dating inhibition using either behavioral rehearsal in (1) an office group and (2) a natural environment group or (3) a discussion group without behavioral rehearsal (McGovern, Arkowitz, and Gilmore 1972).

The college-age adolescent faces problems and issues different than in the earlier years, especially issues of separation-individuation, leaving home, choosing a career, commitment to a belief system, general values, and relationships. Group experiences will have a special quality at this stage that is unlike those described in earlier years.

Conclusions

Group counseling in secondary schools—junior and senior high—is of special usefulness for (1) disturbed adolescents (other than the very psychotic), especially those who may not avail themselves of treatment in clinical settings; (2) adolescents experiencing moderate crises of growth or familial adjustment; and (3) adolescents with physical disabilities served in special education programs. Groups in schools need to differ from groups in clinical settings, but situations have been described where the school-setting group was the only therapeutic input or added to the impact of the clinical therapeutic program. Various examples have been given of individual benefit, group process, and activities of the group leader. All categories of school personnel—teacher, administrator, nurse, counselor, and psychologist—have conducted successful groups. Consultant mental health professionals, from outside the schools, have been effective as coleaders, in-service trainers, supervisors, and, occasionally, solo leaders. Some of the problems of the young persons who have received help in groups have included behavioral problems, underachievement, poor study habits, poor social skills, drug abuse, teenage pregnancy, and various physical handicaps.

REFERENCES

Appolone, C., and Gibson, P. 1980. Group work with young adult epilepsy patients. *Social Work in Health Care* 6(2): 23–32.
Awerbuch, W., and Fraser, K. 1975. Chronic absenteeism decreased by group counseling. In I. H. Berkovitz, ed. *When Schools Care: Creative Use of Groups in Secondary Schools*. New York: Brunner/Mazel.
Bardill, D. R. 1977. A behavior-contracting program of group treatment for early adolescents in a residential treatment setting. *International Journal of Group Psychotherapy* 27:389–400.

Bates, M. 1975. Themes in group counseling with adolescents. In I. H. Berkovitz, ed. *When Schools Care: Creative Use of Groups in Secondary Schools*. New York: Brunner/Mazel.

Bayrakal, S. 1975. A group experience with chronically disabled adolescents. *American Journal of Psychiatry* 132(12): 1291–1294.

Berkovitz, I. H. 1972. On growing a group: some thoughts on structure, process, and setting. In I. H. Berkovitz, ed. *Adolescents Grow in Groups: Experiences in Adolescent Group Psychotherapy*. New York: Brunner/Mazel.

Berkovitz, I. H. 1975a. Indications for use of groups in secondary schools and review of literature. In I. H. Berkovitz, ed. *When Schools Care: Creative Use of Groups in Secondary Schools*. New York: Brunner/Mazel.

Berkovitz, I. H., ed. 1975b. *When Schools Care: Creative Use of Groups in Secondary Schools*. New York: Brunner/Mazel.

Berkovitz, I. H. 1980a. Improving the relevance of secondary education for adolescent developmental tasks. In M. Sugar, ed. *Responding to Adolescent Needs*. New York: Spectrum.

Berkovitz, I. H. 1980b. School interventions: case management and school mental health consultation. In G. P. Sholevar, R. M. Benson, and B. J. Blinder, eds. *Treatment of Emotional Disorders in Children and Adolescents*. New York: SP Medical & Scientific Books.

Berkovitz, I. H. 1987. Application of group therapy in secondary schools. In F. J. Cramer-Azima and L. Richmond, eds. *The Group Therapies for Adolescents*. New York: International Universities Press.

Berkovitz, I. H.; Carr, E.; and Anderson, G. 1983. Attending to the emotional needs of junior high school students and staff during school desegregation: contributions of mental health consultants. In G. J. Powell, ed. *The Psychosocial Development of Minority Group Children*. New York: Brunner/Mazel.

Bonham, H. E. E.; Armstrong, T. D.; and Bonham, G. M. 1981. Group psychotherapy with deaf adolescents. *American Annals of the Deaf* 126:806–809.

Clark, D. B. 1975. Group work with early school leavers. *Journal of Current Studies* 7:42–54.

Driver, H. I. 1958. *Multiple Counseling: A Small Group Discussion Method for Personal Growth*. Madison, Wis.: Morona.

Durell, V. G. 1969. Adolescents in multiple-family group therapy in a school setting. *International Journal of Group Psychotherapy* 19:44–52.

Elkin, M. 1975. The school nurse organizes a group counseling program in a high school. In I. H. Berkovitz, ed. *When Schools Care: Creative Use of Groups in Secondary Schools*. New York: Brunner/Mazel.

Empey, L. J. 1977. Clinical work with multihandicapped adolescents. *Social Casework* 58:593–599.

Epstein, N. 1977. Group therapy with autistic schizophrenic adolescents. *Social Casework* 58:350–358.

Evans, A. 1975. The administrator as group counselor. In I. H. Berkovitz, ed. *When Schools Care: Creative Use of Groups in Secondary Schools*. New York: Brunner/Mazel.

Evans, A.; Johnson, A. V.; and Thomson, M. 1975. An administrator team as group counselors to an opportunity class. In I. H. Berkovitz, ed. *When Schools Care: Creative Use of Groups in Secondary Schools*. New York: Brunner/Mazel.

Finney, B. C., and Van Dalsem, E. 1969. Group counseling for gifted underachieving high school students. *Journal of Counseling Psychology* 16:87–94.

Flacy, D.; Goda, A.; and Schwartz, R. 1975. Assisting teachers in group counseling with drug-abusing students. In I. H. Berkovitz, ed. *When Schools Care: Creative Use of Groups in Secondary Schools*. New York: Brunner/Mazel.

Fleisher, S. J.; Berkovitz, I. H.; Briones, L.; Lovetro, K.; and Morhar, N. 1987. Antisocial behavior, school performance, and reactions to loss: the value of group counseling and communication skills training. *Adolescent Psychiatry* (in this volume).

Gazda, G. M. 1975. *Basic Approaches to Group Psychotherapy and Group Counseling*. 2d ed. Springfield, Mass.: Thomas.

Gilliland, B. D. 1968. Small group counseling with negro adolescents in a public high school. *Journal of Counseling Psychology* 15:147–152.

Glass, S. D. 1969. *Practical Handbook of Group Counseling*. Baltimore: B. C. S.

Goodstein, L. D. 1967. Group counseling with male underachieving college volunteers. *Personnel and Guidance Journal* 45(5): 469–476.

Gurman, A. S. 1967. Group counseling with underachievers: a review and evaluation of methodology. *International Journal of Psychotherapy* 14:463–473.

Hamburg, B. A., and Varenhorst, B. B. 1972. Peer counseling in the secondary schools: a community mental health project for youth. *American Journal of Orthopsychiatry* 42(4): 566–581.

Hamelberg, L. 1981. The effect of coping skills training on the classroom behaviors of students with serious learning problems. *Dissertation Abstract International* 41:4979-A.

Hardy-Fanta, C., and Montana, P. 1982. The Hispanic female adolescent: a group therapy model. *International Journal of Group Psychotherapy* 32(3): 351–366.

Harris, M. B., and Trujillo, A. E. 1975. Improving study habits of junior high school students through self-management versus group discussion. *Journal of Counseling Psychology* 22:513–517.

Humes, C. W., Jr. 1971. A novel group approach to school counseling of educable retardates. *Training School Bulletin* 67:164–171.

Humes, C. W., Jr.; Adamczyk, J. S.; and Myco, R. W. 1969. A school study of group counseling with educable retarded adolescents. *American Journal of Mental Deficiency* 74:191–195.

Jacobs, S. M., and Deigh, M. 1975. The use of demonstration student groups in teaching group counseling. In I. H. Berkovitz, ed. *When Schools Care: Creative Use of Groups in Secondary Schools.* New York: Brunner/Mazel.

Kaplan, C. 1975a. Advantages and problems of interdisciplinary collaboration in school group counseling. In I. H. Berkovitz, ed. *When Schools Care: Creative Use of Groups in Secondary Schools.* New York: Brunner/Mazel.

Kaplan, C. 1975b. Evaluation: twenty-seven agency-school counseling groups in junior and senior high schools. In I. H. Berkovitz, ed. *When Schools Care: Creative Use of Groups in Secondary Schools.* New York: Brunner/Mazel.

Klitgaard, G. C. 1969. A gap is bridged. *Journal of Secondary Education* 44:55–57.

Laeder, R., and Francis, W. C. 1968. Stuttering workshops: group therapy in a rural high school setting. *Journal of Speech and Hearing Disorders* 33(1): 38–41.

Lee, J. A. 1977. Group work with mentally retarded foster adolescents. *Social Casework* 58:164–173.

Leong, W. 1975. A total commitment group counseling program in an inner city high school. In I. H. Berkovitz, ed. *When Schools Care: Creative Use of Groups in Secondary Schools.* New York: Brunner/Mazel.

Lodato, F. J.; Sokoloff, M. A.; and Schwartz, L. J. 1964. Group counseling as a method of modifying attitudes in slow learners. *School Counselor* 12:27–29.

McGovern, K. B.; Arkowitz, H.; and Gilmore, S. K. 1972. Evaluation of social skill training programs for college dating inhibitions. *International Journal of Group Psychotherapy* 22:505–512.

Mahler, C. A. 1969. *Group Counseling in the Schools*. Boston: Houghton Mifflin.

Mann, R. H.; Beaber, J. D.; and Jacobson, M. D. 1964. The effect of group counseling on educable mentally retarded boys' self-concepts. *Exceptional Children* 35:359–366.

Natterson, I. 1975. Special advantages of group counseling in the school setting. In I. H. Berkovitz, ed. *When Schools Care: Creative Use of Groups in Secondary Schools*. New York: Brunner/Mazel.

Offer, D., and Offer, J. B. 1975. *From Teenage to Young Manhood*. New York: Basic.

Ohlsen, M. M. 1970. *Group Counseling*. New York: Holt, Rinehart & Winston.

Ringelheim, D., and Polatsek, I. 1935. Group therapy with a male defective group. *American Journal of Mental Deficiency* 60:157–162.

Robinson, F. W. 1975. A principal benefits from weekly meetings with a selected group of students. In I. H. Berkovitz, ed. *When Schools Care: Creative Use of Groups in Secondary Schools*. New York: Brunner/Mazel.

Roth, R. M.; Mauksch, H. O.; and Peiser, K. 1967. The non-achievement syndrome, group therapy, and achievement change. *Personnel and Guidance Journal* 46:393–398.

Rustin, L. 1972. An intensive group programme for adolescent stammerers. *British Journal of Disorders of Communication* 13(3):85–92.

Sarlin, M. B., and Altshuler, K. 1968. Group psychotherapy with deaf adolescents in a school setting. *International Journal of Psychotherapy* 18:337–344.

Shaw, M. C., and Mahler, C. A. 1975. Simultaneous group counseling with underachieving adolescents and their parents. In I. H. Berkovitz, ed. *When Schools Care: Creative Use of Groups in Secondary Schools*. New York: Brunner/Mazel.

Sperber, Z., and Aguado, D. K. 1975. Teachers and mental health professionals as co-leaders in high school groups. In I. H. Berkovitz, ed. *When Schools Care: Creative Use of Groups in Secondary Schools*. New York: Brunner/Mazel.

Stacey, C., and De Martino, M. 1957. *Counseling and Psychotherapy with the Mentally Retarded.* Glencoe, Ill.: Free Press.

Swarr, R. R., and Ewing, T. N. 1977. Outcome effects of eclectic interpersonal-learning-based group psychotherapy with college student neurotics. *Journal of Consultation in Clinical Psychology* 45:1029–1035.

Vanderkolk, C. 1976. Popular music in group counseling. *School Counselor* 23:206–210.

Vanderpol, M., and Suescum, A. T. 1975. Discussion groups: research into normal adolescent behavior in a junior high school. In I. H. Berkovitz, ed. *When Schools Care: Creative Use of Groups in Secondary Schools.* New York: Brunner/Mazel.

Vogel, L. B. 1975. Support of group counselors' feelings. In I. H. Berkovitz, ed. *When Schools Care: Creative Use of Groups in Secondary Schools.* New York: Brunner/Mazel.

White, J. 1974. The human potential laboratory in the community college. *Journal of College Student Personnel* 15:96–100.

35   ANTISOCIAL BEHAVIOR, SCHOOL
PERFORMANCE, AND REACTIONS TO LOSS:
THE VALUE OF GROUP COUNSELING AND
COMMUNICATION SKILLS TRAINING

STEPHAN J. FLEISHER, IRVING H. BERKOVITZ, LUIS BRIONES,
KIM LOVETRO, AND NORMA MORHAR

Experiences of loss are among the most prevalent and painful events in the history of most human beings. Losses may be from death or desertion of loved ones, natural or manmade disasters, forced migration, or due to movement from one state of security to a less secure stage in the course of individual growth and development. Coping with these losses can provide the ground for pathological (or occasionally creative) psychic reactions, using any of the defense mechanisms known to mental health. Early childhood losses exert the most crucial effect on later development and may be difficult to repair, even in individual or group therapies. One of the salutory benefits of therapy is the opportunity to bring loss experiences more into focus so that the person can better release anger and/or grief, which may have been blocking development.

Young persons in the process of coping with losses earlier in life may show internalized symptoms as well as disturbing behaviors. These behaviors can disrupt school environments and interfere with school performance. Certainly, in many cases, current difficult living conditions—familial or societal—may be reinforcing and compounding the effects of the earlier loss experiences. A variety of programs have been provided in schools, directed at alleviating the disturbing behavior or symptomatology. In one such program, not specifically directed at reaching loss experiences, an outstanding benefit seemed to have been the opportunity and enhanced ability for several of the students to verbalize feelings about past loss experiences. These feelings had been necessarily suppressed in the course of surviving in difficult home and community settings, where there were few empathic, interested adults. While some empathic adults are available in the schools, often their time or skill is not sufficient to allow them to make productive contact and dialogue with students, especially with the angrier, more delinquent youngsters.

We present here the details of a program that was available to children who would have been less likely to receive treatment at traditional outpatient clinics. The program allowed the entry of knowledgeable mental health personnel, from a community child guidance clinic, into two local schools to provide a range of services previously not available. Though this service was available for only thirteen weeks each school year, the opportunity was provided to begin therapeutic repair for some students. Unfortunately, only a brief glimpse of possible benefit occurred for others. Due to the nature of the funding agency, the focus of the program was on assisting delinquent youth.

No doubt many other school programs consisting of only group counseling do provide similar opportunities (Berkovitz 1987). The program reported on here included also social skills and communication training. It is possible that this feature helped provide a stronger impact, despite the briefness of the program, by facilitating a better use of the group-counseling component.

The Program

The program had three components. (1) The first involved training teachers to identify predelinquent youths who, despite average ability, were achieving substantially below grade level, were disruptive in class, aggressive toward peers, frequently truant, and at times came to school under the influence of alcohol and/or drugs. (2) The second involved training teachers to refer youths to the program, since many tended to experience anxiety in referring students and failed to inform them about the reasons for referral; thus, they arrived feeling defensive, anxious, and expecting to be punished, which made it difficult to involve them in the program. (3) The third component involved groups of elementary, junior high, and senior high youths meeting one hour per week for

547

thirteen weeks. The first six-week period dealt with teaching communication skills (Gordon 1970), and the second period dealt with improving assertion skills.

The communication classes dealt with common roadblocks to communication used by parents and teachers. Youths identified these roadblocks readily and, in many cases, were able to add others that they had experienced. They studied how they had incorporated these roadblocks into their own style and soon began to point out roadblocks in each other's communication styles. A classroom setting seemed to lower resistance and defenses and facilitated learning new modes of communication.

Components of listening skills were taught: (1) acknowledging feelings by maintaining eye contact—responding "uh huh," nodding the head, or saying "I understand"; (2) passive listening through taking in the communications of the speaker; and (3) active listening, empathizing with the speaker by acknowledging the speaker's feelings. The entire class, usually ten students, took part in role-playing listening skills. The role playing stopped frequently to reward or correct students' use of acknowledgment, passive listening, or active listening and to give immediate feedback on performance.

Role plays were based on situations that were occurring in each youth's life, at home or in school. Intake interviews prior to the group enabled the teacher or psychologist to diagnose each youth's problem area. Students frequently came from chaotic homes characterized by divorce, separation, alcoholism, child abuse, spousal abuse, parent abuse, parental criminalty (including drug dealing), and frequent abandonment. Role plays describing such situations were typed on index cards so students could practice communicating to parents more effectively regarding these troublesome issues.

Once communication skills were mastered, assertion training began. Students were taught to discriminate between nonassertive, assertive, and aggressive behaviors. They easily understood the nature of nonassertiveness but tended to confuse aggression with assertion.

Nonassertive behavior was described as behavior in which one violated one's own rights. Assertive behavior was described as behavior in which one stood up for one's own rights without violating the rights of others. Aggressive behavior was described as behavior in which one stood up for one's rights while violating the rights of others. Students tended not to perceive themselves as violating the rights of others. At home, their rights were frequently violated, so violating others' rights seemed egosyntonic. Gradually, peer pressure and feedback from the teacher enabled them to become aware of their persistent aggressiveness. Their mounting internal discomfort over their aggressiveness led to a moderation of their behavior at home and in school.

A structure was provided for assertive behavior. Lange and Jacobowski's (1979) approach was followed. The "When . . . I feel . . . I prefer . . ." model was used. Students used each of these to introduce their remarks. "When" introduced a description of a behavior that annoyed the youth. For example, "When you drink too much" could introduce a confrontation with an alcohol-abusing parent. Next, "I feel" introduced an "I" message about the youth's feelings regarding the offending behavior. Finally, "I prefer" introduced the youth's preference regarding an alternative behavior that the parent or other adult could manifest.

Students were taught that assertive skills did not guarantee results. However, they were becoming aware of how roadblocks and aggressiveness interfered with getting what they wanted. As with the communication modules, role plays based on the intake interview were typed on index cards to enable the youths to learn how to handle problematic situations at school and at home. Since nearly all of the youths were from similarly chaotic backgrounds, the role plays generated considerable mutual support, sharing of problems, and development of alternative coping behavior.

With high school students, a third module was added—namely, career planning. The high school students were all twelfth graders, on the verge of graduation, who had very little parental assistance in planning for careers. Questions to guide the discussions were drawn from Berne (1973) and McCormick (1971).

Sample questions were: What happens to people such as yourselves? If things keep on going for you the way they are now, what will you be doing in ten years? What did your mother or father do when things got tough? What do you do when things get tough? What do you want out of life? What is the best thing that could happen to you? What is the worst thing that could happen to you?

A difficulty that students encountered in planning for their future was "superoptimism," a phenomenon described by Yochelson and Samenow (1977), namely, the belief that "thinking makes it so." For example, students would daydream about high wages as if they were

549

actually earning them, although they had no job experience whatsoever. The youths were unaccustomed to putting out effort. Gradually, peer pressure in the classroom motivated them to work harder and to perceive their situations more realistically.

Many of the youths tended to identify with maladaptive aspects of parents' behavior, such as alcohol or drug abuse and criminality. By helping students to discriminate between adaptive and maladaptive aspects of their parents' behavior, it was hoped that students would identify more with parents' adaptive behavior, such as their employment.

Students were quite chagrined to hear from peers how they appeared to be repeating their parents' mistakes. This proved to be a powerful impetus toward change. Students realized that they were separating from their parents by becoming involved with peers who were involved with alcohol, drugs, or crime, but that they were not truly individuating from their parents in such a way as to be able to live independently. Several students felt helpless in this regard and saw themselves as fated to repeat their parents' lives. These students required more than the one-semester class that was offered.

Secondary School Groups: Feelings of Loss

Two major themes emerged in the junior high school groups—feelings of loss and the use of gang involvement. Many students had lost a parent (or parents) through separation, divorce, or abandonment. Devastated and bewildered, these youths often blamed themselves. Discussion uncovered the feelings that they had caused the disruption and were obligated to repair it. These efforts often led to symptom formation—acting out, school problems, and gang involvement.

The formal structures of the project classes provided a framework for surfacing the loss issues. Discussion broke through youths' defenses around their depression, releasing sadness, anger, and bitterness. Although this experience was too brief to be of certain long-range value, perhaps some decreased rigidity of characterological defenses occurred. It was emphasized that they could succeed and feel high levels of self-esteem no matter what their parents' traits. School offered numerous opportunities for the enhancement of self-esteem—academic, sports, arts, and responsible roles within the system.

Numerous youths had experienced multiple losses from gang murders, including relatives and close friends. While the improvement rate for these students was lower than for nongang groups, some members did improve their study habits and behavior. Gang violence increased the likelihood of gang membership. As these youths lost friends and family members, they repeated the violence they had experienced. Deprived of relationships, they joined gangs, which restored a sense of being wanted. Trust was a major issue. Not expecting care, the youths would reject the school group as they expected to be rejected by it. Some youths would spar verbally to dominate the group. It was stressed that true leadership was possible only through education.

Most of the youths had very limited career expectations. This was not surprising in view of the shortened life spans they had observed. The option to make choices was always emphasized, as was their ability to plan for the future, to be a different kind of parent than those they were experiencing, and how unresolved feelings of loss and anger can result in difficulties in school and with the police. The absence of constructive adult models was certainly of importance. The brief group experience may have supplied new models as well as a place to surface embarrassing, painful feelings in an accepting and empathic setting.

Senior High Groups: Identity Diffusion

These groups were very similar to those in the junior high schools except that the youths were more alienated, aggressive, and underachieving. Again, youths were attempting to cope with absent parents, often with fathers in prison. Youths identified with any meager available scraps of information regarding parents. Often the information concerned the most negative aspect of the parents' behavior. Youths perpetuated parents' aggressive behaviors in order not to let them down and to keep their memories alive.

Students were encouraged to broaden knowledge of their parents to enlarge the scope of their identifications. They were encouraged to learn verbal, problem-solving skills, which their parents had not acquired. They were also encouraged to accept their parents' limitations and to seek extraparental adults. As many youths had low self-esteem, this was difficult to achieve. They tended to defend their inept parents, since they felt they had little else to fall back on.

Group Members

The following vignettes give examples of the types of young persons who were able to get some benefit in the junior high school groups.

551

Each seventh-grade student was seen for an individual session prior to the thirteen-session group.

Jane was unconcerned about suspensions in sixth and seventh grades for disruption, fighting, talking, tardiness, and arguing with teachers. She was earning grades of F and D and had seven unsatisfactories. Twice per year she visited her father, whom her mother had divorced.

Richard's parents abandoned him at age one. Then his alcoholic, adoptive father left at age seven. Adoptive mother withheld information regarding his natural parents. Richard experienced school adjustment problems starting in the first grade.

John was expelled from his elementary school in sixth grade and was repeating seventh grade, which he was failing for the second time. He was suspended several times for truancy, fighting, and arguing with teachers. John was able to "laugh this off," especially since his parents' only response was a brief period of grounding. He had several police contacts for traffic offenses on a motorcycle, as well as arrests for stealing bicycle locks at school.

When Miguel was five, his father abandoned him following an argument with mother when she insisted on money for food. Soon mother placed him with aunt and left Nicaragua for the United States. Father wrote the patient annually. Since the patient never worked through his abandonments and anger, placement with his aunt was unsuccessful and he began a delinquent career in Nicaragua. He now had arrests for drugs, grand theft auto, assault, and possession of a deadly weapon. Drug arrests prompted three school expulsions.

Tim's parents divorced when he was five. His father lived 500 miles away and saw Tim three times a year. Mother remarried three times and had several live-in boyfriends. She had also changed jobs and moved several times. Tim was an excellent student until fourth grade when he began to fail and was placed in a military school.

Ernest was expelled from a private-school kindergarten class at five for hitting a teacher. He was bewildered by his mother's "vacations." She never explained to him that she was serving jail sentences for drug addiction and parole violation. Father had similar "trips" until he was killed by a friend in a drunken brawl. Mother had a nervous breakdown following this incident and was not able to assist her son through the grief process. Ernest experienced severe separation anxiety, likely related to his parents' unexplained absences.

Group Process

In group, Jane disclosed that she had not seen her father for two years. She revealed that he had been married five times and felt furious at him for his "hypocrisy," as she put it, since he was a preacher. With group support, she reached out to her father and established visitation twice per month. She wanted weekly visits and was negotiating for contact by mail, if visits could not be arranged. Her grades remained unsatisfactory since her mother was too exhausted by her chronic acting up to ground her anymore. However, her behavior did improve on campus. This may have reflected the gains she made in working through the feelings around her abandonment and her parents' divorce.

Richard disclosed that his natural mother was a "biker" who had been divorced "five or six times." She had had triplets, including Richard, at age seventeen and had put them up for adoption. He never knew his brother and sister, since they were adopted by another family. Feeling deprived of his siblings, he imagined seeing them speed by on a bus that he could not stop. He had seen his natural mother once when she was dying as a result of several motorcycle accidents. The patient identified with the few scraps of information about mother provided by his maternal grandmother and later crashed into barbed wire fences several times. In group, Richard was able to broaden his understanding of his natural mother. He understood that mother's giving him up for adoption was an expression of her concern that he have a better life. He realized that mother had had interests in school and sports. Richard played football and was involved in ballet and aerobics to improve his coordination. Unfortunately, he lost his eligibility due to failing grades. After the group experience, his self-destructive identification with mother was modified. He avoided fights. Prior to group, he would wander in alleys looking to be mugged and then get into a fight. He no longer acted out his angry feelings in this sadomasochistic ritual.

Ernest also suffered from unresolved losses. Mother never discussed father's being killed when the patient was two. He was angry and hurt regarding his loss and encouraged the aggression of others. Mother married another criminal who was in prison for assault. Throughout the sessions, he insisted that mother had taken him often to visit father's grave. During the final session, he was able to disclose that this was untrue; instead, mother would visit stepfather in prison. At the end of

553

the thirteen weeks of group, Ernest's teachers observed an improvement in his work habits in several subjects, although he still failed several classes. He began to formulate career plans related to his grandfather, who had retired as a police officer and had become chief of security at a local junior college. This could be seen as his attempt to sublimate anger at his mother, father, and stepfather and to find a more suitable object for identification.

John largely continued his delinquent career, although some improvement was noted. He developed feelings of depression regarding his constant acting up, improved his impulse control, and raised his grades. However, for the most part, he remained beyond parental control, although his family never sought help. He manifested criminal thinking errors (Yochelson and Samenow 1979). The district did not place him in a special classroom, although he was failing several classes. He was an award-winning bicycle and motorcycle racer and planned to continue in that field.

Although Miguel's aunt valued academic achievement, he experienced rage regarding his placement with her. This could be seen as anger displaced from when his parents abandoned him. Thus he did not identify with his aunt's values and instead joined a gang. She became enraged and responded punitively. When he did rejoin his mother in the United States, he became involved in several shootings and was wounded. He perceived mother as overwhelmed by her children's numerous difficulties but worked through his fatalism regarding his chances in life. When he joined the group, he was failing all six courses. At the end of the program, he was failing only one.

Tim had difficulty dealing with the loss of his father. He had seen him only three times a year. He was enraged at his mother's neglect as she attempted to pursue a Hollywood career. He rarely saw his stepfather, who worked overtime. Mother finally gave his guardianship to a neighbor. Like Ernest, Tim developed an interest in pursuing a career in law enforcement as a sharpshooter or helicopter pilot. He failed fewer courses following the group sessions. As he became more motivated, he experienced more internal discomfort regarding his underachievement.

It was impressive to see how even the minimal input of this group experience was able to achieve significant results for several young persons. There still may be tragedy ahead for most of them, but one hopes that the school system or other helping agencies can begin to see the long-range and cost-effective salvage values in even these minimal efforts.

Conclusions

Many young persons in the schools could benefit from even minimal opportunities to share their feelings about losses of significant persons—parents, siblings, and friends. The opportunity to have an empathic listener in a school group can often lessen anger and violent actions, improve school performance, and even reduce delinquent gang involvement. These results did occur in a thirteen-week school intervention program funded by the Office of Criminal Justice Planning. The program consisted of social skills training and group counseling in junior and senior high schools. Several vignettes of the life crises in some adolescent members have been described along with the impact of this brief intervention on these individuals.

NOTE

This program was provided during 1980–1983 by staff from the San Fernando Valley Child Guidance Clinic, thanks to a grant from Project Heavy, San Fernando Valley, administered through the State of California Office of Criminal Justice Planning.

REFERENCES

Berkovitz, I. H. 1987. Value of group counseling in secondary schools. *Adolescent Psychiatry* (in this volume).

Berne, E. 1973. *What Do You Say after You Say Hello?* New York: Grove.

Gordon, T. 1970. *Parent Effectiveness Training.* New York: Wyden.

Lange, A. J., and Jacobowski, P. 1979. *Responsible Assertive Behavior.* Champaign, Ill.: Research Press.

McCormick, P. 1971. *Guide for Use of a Life-Script Questionnaire in Transactional Analysis.* Berkeley, Calif.: Transactional Publishing Co.

Yochelson, S., and Samenow, S. 1977. *The Criminal Personality.* New York: Aronson.

36   TOBACCO AND ALCOHOL PREVENTION: PRELIMINARY RESULTS OF A FOUR-YEAR STUDY

WILLIAM B. HANSEN, C. KEVIN MALOTTE, AND JONATHAN E. FIELDING

The problems associated with smoking tobacco and misusing alcohol are well known and have been extensively documented. The purpose of this chapter is to examine why young people smoke and drink abusively and what can be done about it. A major focus will be on the Tobacco and Alcohol Prevention Project (TAPP). This project was originally designed to answer two questions. First, Why do young people use such substances as tobacco and alcohol? Second, How can the use and abuse of these substances be prevented?

Why Children Use Tobacco and Alcohol

PREVALENCE, AGE OF ONSET, DEMOGRAPHY, DISTRIBUTION, AND RECIDIVISM

Tobacco and alcohol are the two most commonly used nontherapeutic drugs in the United States today. As young people enter the teenage years, nearly all try smoking and drinking. Large proportions of those who experiment with these substances become regular users as adults.

Between 1968 and 1974, there was a dramatic increase in the proportion of youth who reported regular smoking (USDHEW 1972, 1974, 1976a). Since 1974, there has been a significant reduction in the proportion of male adolescent smokers (Green 1979). However, between

1974 and 1979, the proportion of seventeen- and eighteen-year-old female smokers increased to an all-time high of 27.2 percent. Recent
surveys of high school students (Johnston, Bachman, and O'Malley
1982) indicate a nearly one-third drop in daily cigarette smoking among
high school seniors from 1977 to 1980—a leveling off in the early 1980s
and a further decline in 1984 to 18.7 percent. While these trends are
encouraging, the proportion of youth who continue to experiment with
cigarettes and eventually become regular smokers remains at an unacceptable level.

A key matter in smoking prevention involves the age at which young
people begin to smoke. In 1976, the average age at which an adolescent
smokes his or her first cigarette was between twelve and thirteen years
(Johnston, Bachman, and O'Malley 1977). It appears that cigarette
smoking is irregular and experimental up until the adolescent is around
fifteen years old, when relatively large increases in the number of
adolescents who are regular users have been observed. For example,
in 1979, only 3.2 percent of twelve- to fourteen-year-old males smoked
on a regular basis, compared to 13.5 percent of fifteen- to sixteen-year-
old males (Green 1979). Our own data (see table 1) suggest that nearly
half the seventh graders in a nonrandom sample have tried smoking,
while 17 percent have smoked more than once. Thus, it seems that
early adolescence is a high-risk period for smoking onset.

Cigarette smoking varies according to a number of demographic variables other than age. In adults, it is more prevalent among males than
females (USDHEW 1979). Smoking is more prevalent among less educated adults, except the individuals who have had less than high school
education (USDHEW 1973a, 1973b, 1976b). Only 8 percent (Johnston,
Bachman, and O'Malley 1982) of high school seniors who are planning
to complete four years of college smoke at least half a pack of cigarettes
a day, compared to 21 percent of those not planning to attend college.
For males, the prevalence of smoking decreases as family income increases. For females, the opposite trend can be observed, with a higher
proportion of females from high socioeconomic backgrounds (Bonham
and Leaverton 1979).

Cigarette smoking has had a high rate of recidivism among former
users (Hunt and Bespalec 1974). On the average, less than 25 percent
of adult smokers who try to quit are successful—based on a single
attempt—for longer than six months (Moss 1979). Similarly, high rates
of recidivism after smoking cessation attempts have been found among

adolescents who have smoked for only a short time (Hansen 1983). Interestingly, nearly 75 percent of all current high school smokers report having tried to quit and failed. These data lend support to a strategy of prevention rather than treatment, since treatment is not only costly but relatively unsuccessful.

The use of alcohol is also a widespread phenomenon among adults and youth in this country. It has been reported that over 10 percent of all alcohol consumers have some alcohol-related problem (Clark and Midanik 1982). Incidents of intoxication are especially prevalent among youth, and the proportion of those who report drinking more than two drinks per day peaks in the eighteen to twenty-five age group and declines thereafter (Noble 1978).

A comprehensive analysis of 120 surveys of American teenage drinking practices from 1941 to 1975 indicated that the proportion of drinking teenagers rose steadily from World War II until approximately 1965 (Noble 1978). This review also reported that the age at which teenagers had their first drinks decreased from 13.6 to 12.9 years between 1969 and 1975. A more recent study (*The Nation's Health* 1985) indicates that the use of alcohol has remained roughly constant since 1975.

Alcohol use is more widespread than cigarette smoking among youth, although the period of onset is roughly the same. A national survey conducted by the National Institute on Alcohol Abuse and Alcoholism in 1974 reported that 63 percent of boys and 54 percent of girls in the seventh grade had tasted alcohol at least once. The percent increased every year for both sexes—to 93 percent of boys and 87 percent of girls in the twelfth grade (Noble 1978). These data corroborate our own survey of seventh graders (see table 1), which suggests that a significant proportion have experimented with alcohol by the seventh grade.

It is apparent that smoking and drinking—particularly problem drinking—are highly interrelated. Previous research by us and by others (Gould, Berberian, Kasl, Thompson, and Kleber 1977; Hansen, Malotte, and Fielding, in press; Johnson, Graham, and Hansen 1981; Kandel 1975; Malotte, Hansen, and Fielding 1983) has shown that cigarette smokers are very likely to drink alcohol and that heavy alcohol users are more likely to smoke cigarettes. Further, the use of one substance (either tobacco or alcohol) is a risk factor leading to later adopting the use of the other substance. Teenage, heavy drinkers have smoked about seven times the number of cigarettes as both light drinkers and nondrinkers on the average (Malotte et al. 1983). By the time they are in

TABLE 1
LIFETIME TOBACCO AND ALCOHOL EXPERIENCE OF SUBJECT:
SEVENTH-GRADE STUDENTS

Lifetime Experience	Smoked Cigarettes	Drunk Alcohol	Been Drunk
Never	695	207	1,053
	(56.8)	(16.9)	(86.1)
Once	316	732	101
	(25.8)	(59.8)	(8.3)
Two to four times	90	99	44
	(7.45)	(8.1)	(3.6)
Five to ten times	33	74	13
	(2.7)	(6.1)	(1.1)
Eleven to twenty times	45	46	8
	(3.7)	(3.8)	(.7)
Twenty-one to 100 times	32	48	4
	(2.6)	(3.9)	(.3)
100 or more times	12	17	. . .
	(1.0)	(1.4)	

NOTE.—N = 1,223. Numbers in parentheses are percentages.

the seventh grade, smokers have had three times the number of drinks as nonsmokers.

Together, tobacco use and alcohol use constitute a serious national problem. Reducing the proportion of youth who use one or both substances will be of significant value for the health and quality of life of the nation. Because of the difficulties associated with helping those who smoke and abuse alcohol to stop, developing effective prevention strategies appears to be a very important alternative.

PSYCHOSOCIAL FACTORS INFLUENCING ONSET

Why children begin using tobacco and alcohol is of central concern to the development and proper implementation of prevention programs. If we do not understand the process through which one becomes a substance user, our prevention efforts will be of limited value.

During the past twenty years, hundreds of published surveys and reports have examined the role of various theoretical models of substance-use onset. From these, the contexts within which young people begin smoking and begin abusing alcohol are becoming clearer.

A number of researchers (Flay, d'Avernas, Best, Kersell, and Ryan 1983; Hirschman, Leventhal, and Glynn 1984; McCarthy 1985) have

559

noted that there are several steps from nonsmoker to confirmed-smoker status. Factors that influence the adolescent at the various steps appear to be different as well. The same could probably be said for alcohol abuse. Our interest is in the influences that are related to initial onset. In the case of both substances, early use and abuse are strongly associated with use by same-age friends and family. In fact, of all correlates of tobacco use and drunkenness, use by one's close friends is clearly the dominant variable that discriminates users from nonusers (Hansen et al., in press; Malotte et al. 1983). While other variables (e.g., personality characteristics such as rebelliousness, need for affiliation, and achievement motivation or cognitive/belief measures) correlate with both tobacco and alcohol use, they are less important than peer use. In other words, the onset of smoking and drinking has less to do with what young people believe will happen to them or what kind of people they are and more to do with what their friends are doing. Initial use of substances is a social phenomenon.

There are several relevant explanations of how peers influence the early use of tobacco and the early abuse of alcohol. When young people enter adolescence, they feel intense pressure to fit in and be liked by their fellows. It is apparent, even from a nonobjective examination of different generations of groups of young people, that conformity in dress, speech, and behavior is common. This need to be accepted is generally heightened during adolescence and becomes acute when young people are put into situations in which they need to make new friends, as typically happens when they leave elementary school and enter junior high school. In seeking social approval by trying to establish a presumably accepted social image (Barton, Chassin, Presson, and Sherman 1982; Chassin, Presson, Sherman, Corty, and Olshavsky 1981; McCarthy 1985), young people are willing to adopt the practices of their peers in exchange for inclusion into a group. Indeed, we have observed that many adolescent friendships seem to form around substance use. It is likely that groups composed of users solidify their bonds through substance use, with tobacco and alcohol serving as symbols and rituals that reinforce group cohesion.

When trying to establish new friendships or maintain old ones, friendly offers, which adults find easy to refuse, may be very difficult for young people to say no to. Situations in which the pressure is more threatening—such as when an individual is ridiculed—are, of course, more difficult still. In a recent survey (Chewing and Lindner 1984), over 30 percent of students reported pressure to smoke and drink. For male seventh graders who reported pressure, the most important sources of pressure to drink were their friends—52 percent reported this pressure. For females, 65 percent felt pressure from friends. It is quite likely that, even in the absence of overt approval or disapproval, many young adolescents develop strong beliefs about what others think of them. Thus, even presumed or imagined approval or disapproval may have a strong influence on what they do.

Young people's understanding of what is actually practiced and what is acceptable to their friends is typically vague and frequently found to be inaccurate and distorted. For instance, it is not at all uncommon for young people to overestimate grossly the proportion of the population that gets drunk or smokes tobacco (Duryea and Martin 1981). In many cases, adolescents misjudge what others actually feel to be acceptable and assume risk-taking behaviors to be highly prized when, in fact, this may not be the case. Thus, when they are offered a cigarette or a drink, the misperception that "everyone else is doing it" implies nonuse to be strange and atypical. Since fitting in is highly important, this misperception increases the likelihood of a young person's trying tobacco or alcohol.

In addition to being susceptible to peer influence, young adolescents are also striving to become independent of parental influences. Rebellion against parents and authorities is quite common and, not surprisingly, is fostered by peers who are similarly engaged and who frequently reinforce each other's rebellious tendencies (Jessor and Jessor 1975). Smoking and getting drunk are ideal behaviors for gaining such peer reinforcement.

In the final analysis, it appears that early smoking and early alcohol misuse are primarily attributable to social influences to which young adolescents find themselves to be uniquely susceptible.

Prevention Efforts

Numerous programs aimed at reducing the acquisition of smoking and drinking habits have been developed. Traditionally, these have been based on the knowledge-attitude-behavior model of change (Botvin and McAlister 1981; Wittman 1982). This model assumes that, by increasing the level of students' knowledge about the hazards of smoking and alcohol abuse, they will develop rational attitudes, and appropriate behavior (nonsmoking and nonuse or nonproblem use of alcohol) will follow. Many of these programs stress long-term health consequences almost exclusively. Unfortunately, this approach has had little effect on levels of consumption. This is not too surprising, since most children, even without formal education, early in their lives develop a belief that smoking and drinking are harmful behaviors. While some of these programs have had success in changing attitudes positively (Schaps, DiBartolo, Palley, and Churgin 1978), even attitude-change results are generally discouraging. By increasing levels of knowledge, some early programs in fact seemed to increase experimentation with drugs (Stuart 1974).

More recent programs have emphasized psychosocial approaches to dealing with factors related to initiation and have adapted both content and teaching approaches based on the research findings noted above. Much of the work that has been well evaluated has come from tobacco-prevention efforts.

Evans and his colleagues were among the earliest to apply knowledge of psychosocial processes to tobacco prevention (Evans, Rozelle, Mittlemark, Hansen, Bane, and Havis 1978). The Houston smoking-prevention project refocused discussion from long-range consequences of smoking to short-term consequences likely to be more salient to a young audience (Hansen and Evans 1982). For example, bad breath, increased heart rate, and hand tremor were emphasized rather than lung cancer and heart disease. Based on McGuire's (1964) ideas of social inoculation, the Houston group also introduced videotapes and role-playing exercises that dramatized students attempting to influence their peers to engage in smoking behavior. This component of the program was designed to inoculate the students so that they would be more able to resist pressures to smoke.

The approach initiated in Houston has been replicated and expanded in various sites throughout the nation, notably at the University of Minnesota, Stanford University, Cornell University, and the University of Waterloo in Ontario, Canada. These various programs, for the most part, maintained a focus on teaching resistance skills but added a number of features to increase the effectiveness of the programs.

In early work at Stanford University (McAlister, Perry, and Maccoby 1979), high school students were trained to act as peer counselors for junior high school students. These peer counselors taught skills relevant to resisting pressure in small groups. In Minnesota (Hurd, Johnson, Pechacek, and Luepker 1980), same-age peer leaders were trained to assist in program implementation. Both programs made an attempt to make programs more active and to include behavioral rehearsal sessions. Work directed by Botvin at Cornell (Botvin, Eng, and Williams 1980) extended basic resistance techniques to include also various other life skills, including training in decision making.

Despite methodological problems, results from these studies suggest that, compared to traditional approaches and nontreatment controls, these programs were all moderately effective in reducing the onset of cigarette smoking. The effects have persisted for up to three years. Most effective have been programs that emphasized using peers as counselors.

In the most rigorously designed evaluation conducted to date—the Waterloo Smoking Prevention Program—Best and his colleagues (Best, Flay, Towson, Ryan, Perry, Brown, Kersell, and d'Avernas 1984; Flay et al. 1983) studied students at twenty-two schools in Ontario, Canada. Complex results were found, but overall the program proved to be moderately successful; its greatest effect was on those thought to be at highest risk for smoking since they had parents, siblings, and friends who smoked. In an insightful review of many of the social influences of smoking-prevention programs (Flay 1985), one of the principal investigators of the Waterloo study also notes that the program appeared to be successful in some schools but not in others.

Recent additional research, for which results are currently not available, has been initiated at the University of Southern California (Johnson, Flay, and Hansen 1982). In this research, the psychosocial prevention approach has been expanded to include multiple drugs as well as a comparison of the resistance-skill-training approach with a self-management approach. Preliminary findings support the social-pressure-resistance-training approach for preventing tobacco, alcohol, and marijuana use. Self-management-skills training was not successful in preventing onset. A second study has tested a psychosocial program for high-school-aged populations with similar results (Johnson, Hansen, Collins, and Araham, in press).

The UCLA Tobacco-Prevention Project (TAPP) Curriculum

The original TAPP curriculum (Alvarez, Hansen, Malotte, and Fielding 1982) was an attempt to combine successful tobacco- and alcohol-abuse prevention strategies in order to integrate many of the previously discussed approaches in a package that could be implemented by the classroom teacher with only minimal in-service teacher training. It consisted of fifteen lessons. There were three basic components of the curriculum. The first was both the identification of the various social pressures to smoke and drink abusively and the teaching of skills that enable the students to resist these pressures. The second was the teaching of decision-making skills. The third was the teaching of the consequences of tobacco use and alcohol abuse, with an emphasis on immediate physical, behavioral, and social effects.

As was discussed, early adolescence appears to be the period during which the greatest increase in the initiation of smoking and drinking occurs. In addition, seventh grade, for many students, marks the transition from elementary school to junior high school. For these reasons, the TAPP curriculum was designed to be used with seventh-grade students.

The TAPP curriculum was activity oriented; each lesson utilized at least one student work sheet. Much of the work was done in small groups. It was designed to take advantage of the naturally existing peer-opinion leaders in each class. In every class, four or five individuals who seemed to be able to influence their classmates' opinions and attitudes more than others were elected. These students served as leaders for small group activities.

OVERVIEW OF LESSONS

Prior to the first lesson, the teacher met with the group leaders in a separate group either at lunch or after school. The qualities of good group leaders were discussed. Several of the group leaders were allowed to practice their new roles, the group leaders' responsibilities and tasks were spelled out, and students were assigned to groups. One possible source of influence that can be readily identified is that presented via advertising, movies, and television—via the media. The first lesson was designed to demonstrate to students how they may be influenced by advertising even without being aware of it. Students were asked to analyze cigarette or liquor ads for the appeals used and then to make fun of the ads by drawing or writing on the ads some of the "bad" things about cigarettes or alcohol.

The next lessons of the curriculum presented information and asked questions specific to either alcohol or tobacco. Material on the chemical ingredients of cigarettes and the short-term health effects of smoking were presented. Student work sheets and a videotape showed how cigarettes affect the body right away—not just at some time in the future. Students were encouraged to visualize the bad effects of smoking and drinking that were personally relevant. In addition, the traditional, basic information on the long-term health effects of smoking was also covered. A nongraded oral quiz format was used to facilitate student participation and to identify myths and misconceptions about smoking. Discussion of the behavioral and health effects of alcohol followed, again with an emphasis on immediate effects, such as impaired coordination, behavior and mood changes, and blood vessel dilation.

The idea that inappropriate use of alcohol can lead to many social problems—the most serious of which, for teenagers, is an increased likelihood of having an accident—was also emphasized. Articles about accidents involving alcohol that the students had previously collected were discussed. Situations where it might be dangerous to drink were explored. Students discussed and completed a work sheet about how drinking alcohol might affect their relationships with friends and families, their work at school, and so forth. An optional lesson that reviewed the health and social effects of alcohol and tobacco using a quiz-show-type name and crossword puzzle was also included.

The next section of TAPP focused on having each student examine how alcohol and tobacco may interfere with his life's priorities, and it encouraged students to make rational decisions about tobacco and alcohol use. In particular, students became aware of those things in life that are most important to them and then calculated how the consequences of smoking and drinking might interfere with these values.

The process of making carefully reasoned decisions often is not undertaken, even by many adults. Adolescents are particularly prone to taking action without exploring alternatives or contemplating the consequences associated with the action. Students learned and practiced decision making by using a simplified decision-making process. They first practiced using these skills in situations not involving alcohol and tobacco. Then, using information they had previously learned from TAPP, students applied the decision-making process to situations involving these two substances.

Using student-generated lists, the next lesson covered both the motivation that leads to smoking and drinking and alternative behaviors to satisfy each motivation. Students were encouraged to be creative in searching for alternatives. Training in the identification of peer pressure and in techniques to refuse pressure was covered next. Students first identified the pressures to smoke and drink they may experience. A videotape showing peer pressure and resistance to it was presented. Peer pressure was defined and discussed and students were asked to estimate the percentages of their peers and of adults who smoke and drink. In almost all cases, students overestimated both smoking and drinking. Reasons for overestimation and true figures were discussed.

Following this, students learned techniques that may be useful for resisting peer pressure. Students practiced resisting pretend offers to smoke or drink. In addition, the small groups were each given a scenario and asked to prepare a skit showing resistance techniques and to present it to the class. The overall goal was to encourage students to master appropriate techniques to say no to substance offers.

Students got further practice in solving problems, making decisions, and dealing with pressure situations by responding to "Dear Abby" letters. Each wrote his own "Dear Abby" letter, traded with a fellow student, and responded to that student's letter.

The final two lessons covered communication and self-management skills. Students discussed how to make new friends. They also teamed up with partners and practiced getting to know others by trying to find out how they and their partners were alike. Finally, students learned the steps necessary to change a habit, and the curriculum concluded with the students' writing a self-contract with their code of conduct regarding tobacco and alcohol.

EVALUATED TRIAL

To assess the effectiveness of the TAPP curriculum, two school districts in the greater Los Angeles area were selected to participate in an evaluated trial of the program. In the first school district (district A), there were three junior high schools. Two were chosen at random to implement the program; the third served as a nontreatment control.

Teachers from the treatment schools were selected by district administrators and principals. District A initially selected science teachers to implement the program. Because of the program's nonbiological approach, social studies teachers were ultimately given the responsibility of implementing the program. In the second district (district B), health-education teachers were selected to deliver the program. Teachers were trained to deliver the program in a two-day seminar. In district B, two schools—one treatment and one control—were selected.

Students in all five schools were tested using a 102-item questionnaire. Items on the questionnaire assessed tobacco and alcohol use as well as beliefs, knowledge, and attitudes about tobacco and alcohol. Saliva specimens were collected in conjunction with the administration of the questionnaire in an attempt to increase the accuracy of self-reports of behavior (Evans, Hansen, and Mittlemark 1977; Luepker, Pechacek, Murray, Johnson, Hund, and Jacobs 1981). Students were tested immediately prior to delivery of the program—six months later, one year later, one and a half years later, and two years later. Thus, students were measured twice in the seventh grade, twice in the eighth grade, and once in the ninth grade.

TRIAL RESULTS

Baseline rates of smoking in the two districts differed greatly. In district A, 5.7 percent of seventh graders smoked at pretest, compared to 11.7 percent of students in district B (χ^2 = 13.24; $p < .0001$). Drinking statistics differed only slightly; 38.5 percent of district A students reported having had a drink during the month prior to the pretest, and 35.9 percent of students in district B so reported (χ^2 = .75; NS).

Because baseline smoking was different, because the program was implemented under different circumstances in each district, and because there appeared to be vast differences attributable to socioeconomic status among districts, data for each district were analyzed separately.

SMOKING

There was pretest nonequivalence of smoking when comparing treatments and controls in each district. These were more smokers among students assigned to the treatment condition in district A (7.3 percent vs. 2.9 percent; χ^2 = 6.36; $p < .05$). In district B, there were more smokers among controls (13.3 percent) than among treatment students (9.9 percent; χ^2 = 6.23; $p < .02$). The same general pattern held at the immediate posttest conducted during the spring of students' seventh-grade year. Overall, there does not appear to have been a strong immediate impact of the program on smoking.

567

By the second posttest, the rate of smoking dropped from 9.8 percent to 5.1 percent for treatment subjects in district A. Where there had been more smoking among treatment students in this district at the immediate posttest ($\chi^2 = 7.07$; $p < .03$), at the fall of the eighth-grade test there were no differences ($\chi^2 = 1.43$; NS). Nor were there differences at the third posttest ($\chi^2 = .15$; NS). By the time of the final posttest, the rate of smoking among subjects receiving treatment in district A was 22.3 percent, whereas 30.1 percent of controls had smoked in the past thirty days. While not statistically significant ($\chi^2 = 2.96$; $p < .10$), this lends encouragement to the effectiveness of the program in district A.

In district B on the other hand, no such evidence of program effectiveness occurred. In fact, the controls used less tobacco at the fall of eighth-grade measure (13.7 percent) than at the spring of seventh-grade measure (15.6 percent). This pattern of reduced use among the controls held through the spring of eighth grade, at which time use was down to 13.5 percent. Treated subjects used more at each point. By the spring of eighth grade, more treatment students than controls (21.6 percent and 13.5 percent, respectively; $\chi^2 = 3.31$; $p < .07$) were smoking. By the spring of the students' ninth-grade year, however, there were no differences between treatments and controls.

DRINKING

For the pretest and the first three posttests, there were no differences between treatment and control students in district A. The final posttest approached significance ($\chi^2 = 2.96$; $p < .09$), with controls having an increase in the proportion of drinkers from 54.4 percent at the spring of eighth-grade measures to 61.2 percent in the spring of ninth grade. During the same period, drinking in the treatment group remained constant at about 52.2 percent.

In district B, rates of drinking for treatment and control students were significantly different at pretest ($\chi^2 = 12.93$; $p < .001$) and at immediate posttest ($\chi^2 = 7.46$; $p < .01$), with more control students drinking. Groups remained somewhat different in rates of alcohol use at the fall ($\chi^2 = 3.19$; $p < .08$) and spring ($\chi^2 = 2.94$; $p < .09$) of eighth-grade measures. What appeared to be happening was a gradual increase in drinking among treatment subjects (from 27.9 percent to 34.7 percent), while controls had very little change overall (43.0 percent at pretest to 41.4 percent at final posttest).

INTERPRETATION OF FINDINGS

Results of this study are to date ambiguous. Considering only district A, we may conclude that the program was marginally successful at limiting the overall proportions of smokers and drinkers. There appeared to be modest short-term effects on tobacco use among these subjects (between seventh and eighth grades) and the end-point rate of smoking was 25 percent lower among treated students. The effects of programming on the prevalence of alcohol use was also modest and confined to the end-point measure. No short-term results for the program on alcohol were observed.

Results of district B are even more difficult to interpret. There appeared to be no suppression in onset of cigarette smoking among students who received the program in this district. During the middle part of the study, it even appeared that controls were benefiting from their nontreatment status. In fact, it is likely that they may have benefited from an alternative program since a reduction over time in control-group smoking is not typically found in most studies and is certainly not expected. Unfortunately, our ability to document competing interventions that may have been implemented was poor. Given end-point results, there appears to have been no difference in smoking due to the TAPP curriculum.

The effects of the program on the prevalence of drinking in district B students are not interpretable. While the rate of increase appears modest for treatment students, there is noncomparability with controls from the outset.

Conclusions

The results of this study neither confirm nor disconfirm the approach adopted in the TAPP curriculum. Other studies that have included similar components have apparently been moderately successful at reducing the onset of smoking. In one case, TAPP appeared successful; in the other, success was either not achieved or at least not discernible. While this is disappointing, one of the best-designed, most successful studies also had negligible results in some schools (Flay 1985). All programs have limits in terms of their effectiveness. It is clear that further research is needed to document under what conditions programs such as TAPP will be and will not be successful.

Perhaps one explanation of the differential effectiveness of the program lies in the nature of the program providers. Most studies have had programs delivered by teachers who were part of the research staff. In this study, the programs were delivered by regular classroom teachers. There are likely to be significant differences between these two groups. Research staff tend to be highly specialized individuals who are also highly motivated to deliver the program as designed. Regular classroom teachers, on the other hand, may have less motivation to deliver the program effectively and, despite efforts to instill some expertise through training, are likely to be less skilled at program delivery. Researchers come into a setting and are immediately recognized as outsiders who have a special program to present. Teachers may fail to gain such attention when the program is delivered as part of their routine teaching load.

At the end of teaching, teacher feedback allowed us to identify several flaws in the mechanics of the program that may have contributed to its ineffectiveness. Furthermore, a critical analysis of the program as presented revealed that peer-pressure-resistance training was downplayed. Overall, the TAPP curriculum guide as tested in this program may have been a relatively weak version. (The curriculum guide has subsequently been altered extensively. Among other things, the emphasis placed on peer-pressure-resistance training has been greatly heightened. With the inclusion of marijuana as a target drug, the name of the curriculum guide has been changed to *Well and Good*.)

Our experience has also led us to conclude that most experimental designs utilized in the testing of tobacco, alcohol, and other drug-abuse prevention programs are relatively weak. In many cases, the results may be due as much to the selection of appropriate populations as to program effectiveness. It seems quite reasonable to find programs to be effective under some conditions and in some environments and not others. In our case, school district A may have been a hospitable environment, whereas district B may have been less friendly to the cause. Anecdotally, there is some evidence for this. For example, district A had a strong parent group that formally encouraged the adoption of the program. No such support was observed in district B. Other examples of differences include socioeconomic status, community activity against drug abuse, and community cohesiveness. While firm conclusions cannot be reached, future studies should attempt to control for such variation in their designs, including alternative programs for districts in which competition is likely to be a major source of confounding.

Additional data are being collected as part of this project, when students reach the tenth grade. With these data, prevention effects, especially in district A, may be more concretely displayed.

REFERENCES

Alvarez, L. C.; Hansen, W. B.; Malotte, C. K.; and Fielding, J. E. 1982. *Tobacco and Alcohol Prevention Program: A Curriculum for Adolescent Health Promotion*. Los Angeles: University of California.

Barton, J.; Chassin, L.; Presson, C. C.; and Sherman, S. J. 1982. Social image factors as motivators of smoking initiation in early and middle adolescence. *Child Development* 53:1499–1511.

Best, J. A.; Flay, B. R.; Towson, S. M. J.; Ryan, K. B.; Perry, C. L.; Brown, K. S.; Kersell, M. W.; and d'Avernas, J. R. 1984. Smoking prevention and the concept of risk. *Journal of Applied Social Psychology* 14:257–273.

Bonham, G. S., and Leaverton, P. E. 1979. *Use Habits of Four Common Drugs: Cigarettes, Coffee, Aspirin, and Sleeping Pills, United States, 1976*. Washington, D.C.: Vital and Health Statistics, Ser. 10. National Center for Health Statistics.

Botvin, G. J.; Eng, A.; and Williams, C. L. 1980. Preventing the onset of cigarette smoking through life skills training. *Preventive Medicine* 9:135–143.

Botvin, G., and McAlister, A. 1981. Cigarette smoking among children and adolescents: causes and prevention. In C. B. Arnold, L. H. Kuller, and M. R. Greenlick, eds. *Advances in Disease Prevention*, Vol. 1. New York: Springer.

Chassin, L.; Presson, C. C.; Sherman, S. J.; Corty, E.; and Olshavsky, R. W. 1981. Self-images and cigarette smoking in adolescence. *Personality and Social Psychology Bulletin* 7:670–676.

Chewing, B., and Lindner, F. 1984. Middle and high school student attitudes and perceived pressure to smoke, have sex, and use alcohol.

Paper presented at the 112th annual meeting of the American Public Health Association, Anaheim, Calif., November.

Clark, W. B., and Midanik, L. 1982. Alcohol use and alcohol problems among U.S. adults: results of the 1979 national survey. In *Alcohol and Health Monograph* 1: *Alcohol Consumption and Related Problems,* pp. 3–52. Publication no. (ADM) 82–1190. U.S. Department of Health and Human Services. National Institute on Alcohol Abuse and Alcoholism. Washington, D.C.: Government Printing Office.

Duryea, E. J., and Martin G. 1981. The distortion effect in student perceptions of smoking prevalence. *Journal of School Health* 51:115–118.

Evans, R. I.; Hansen, W. B.; and Mittlemark, M. 1977. Increasing the validity of self-reports of behavior in smoking in children investigation. *Journal of Applied Psychology* 62:521–523.

Evans, R. I.; Rozelle, R. M.; Mittlemark, M. B.; Hansen, W. B.; Bane, A. L.; and Havis, J. 1978. Deterring the onset of smoking in children: knowledge of immediate effects and coping with peer pressure, media pressure, and parent modeling. *Journal of Applied Social Psychology* 8:125–135.

Flay, B. R. 1985. Psychosocial approaches to smoking prevention: a review of findings. *Health Psychology* 4:449–488.

Flay, B. R.; d'Avernas, J. R.; Best, J. A.; Kersell, M. W.; and Ryan, K. B. 1983. Cigarette smoking: why young people do it and ways of preventing it. In P. McGrath and P. Firestone, eds. *Pediatric Medicine.* New York: Springer.

Gould, L. C.; Berberian, R. M.; Kasl, S. V.; Thompson, W. D.; and Kleber, H. D. 1977. Sequential patterns of multiple-drug use among high school students. *Archives of General Psychiatry* 34:216–222.

Green, D. E. 1979. *Teenage Smoking: Immediate and Long Term Patterns.* Washington, D.C.: Department of Health, Education, and Welfare, National Institute of Education.

Hansen, W. B. 1983. Behavioral predictors of abstinence: early indicators of dependence on tobacco among adolescents. *International Journal of the Addictions* 18 (7): 913–920.

Hansen, W. B., and Evans, R. I. 1982. Feedback versus information concerning carbon monoxide as an early intervention strategy in adolescent smoking. *Adolescence* 17:89–98.

Hansen, W. B.; Malotte, C. K.; and Fielding, J. E. In press. Alcohol behavior patterns and psychological correlates of adolescent alcohol use. *Journal of Alcohol and Drug Education.*

High school seniors' use of drugs, alcohol, cigarettes declining. *The Nation's Health* (February 1985), p. 6.

Hirschman, R. S.; Leventhal, H.; and Glynn, K. 1984. The development of smoking behavior: conceptualization and supportive cross-sectional survey data. *Journal of Applied Social Psychology* 14:184–206.

Hunt, W. A., and Bespalec, D. A. 1974. An evaluation of current methods of modifying smoking behavior. *Journal of Clinical Psychology* 30:431.

Hurd, P. D.; Johnson, C. A.; Pechacek, T.; and Luepker, R. V. 1980. Prevention of cigarette smoking in seventh-grade students. *Journal of Behavioral Medicine* 3:15–28.

Jessor, R., and Jessor, S. L. 1975. Adolescent development and the onset of drinking. *Journal of Studies on Alcohol* 36:27–51.

Johnson, C. A.; Flay, B. R.; and Hansen, W. B. 1982. Prevention of multiple substance abuse—youth. Proposal submitted to the National Institute on Drug Abuse, Washington, D.C.

Johnson, C. A.; Graham, J. G.; and Hansen, W. B. 1981. Interaction effects of multiple risk taking behavior: the relationship between tobacco, alcohol, and marijuana use among high school students. Paper presented at the 109th meeting of the American Public Health Association, Los Angeles.

Johnson, C. A.; Hansen, W. B.; Collins, L. M.; and Araham, J. W. In press. High school smoking prevention: results of a three year longitudinal study. *Journal of Behavioral Medicine*.

Johnston, L. D.; Bachman, J. G.; and O'Malley, P. M. 1977. *Drug Use among American High School Students, 1975–1977*. Washington, D.C.: Department of Health, Education and Welfare, Public Health Service, National Institute on Drug Abuse.

Johnston, L. D.; Bachman, J. G.; and O'Malley, P. M. 1982. *Highlights from Student Drug Use in America 1975–1981*. Washington, D.C.: Department of Health and Human Services, Public Health Service, National Institute on Drug Abuse.

Kandel, D. 1975. Stages in adolescent involvement in drug use. *Science* 190:912–914.

Luepker, R. V.; Pechacek, T. F.; Murray, D. M.; Johnson, C. A.; Hund, F.; and Jacobs, D. R. 1981. Saliva thiocyanate: a chemical indicator of cigarette smoking in adolescents. *American Journal of Public Health* 71:1320–1324.

McAlister, A.; Perry, C.; and Maccoby, N. 1979. Adolescent smoking: onset and prevention. *Pediatrics* 63:650–658.

McCarthy, W. 1985. Date the cognitive developmental model and other alternatives to the social skills deficit model of smoking onset. In C. Bell and R. Battjes, eds. *Prevention Research: Deterring Drug Abuse among Children and Adolescents*. National Institute of Drug Abuse. Washington, D.C.: Government Printing Office.

McGuire, J. W. 1964. Inducing resistance to persuading: some contemporary approaches. In L. Berkowitz, ed. *Advances in Experimental Social Psychology,* Vol. 1. New York: Academic Press.

Malotte, C. K.; Hansen, W. B.; and Fielding, J. E. 1983. Predictors of smoking and drinking in adolescents. Paper presented at the 111th annual meeting of the American Public Health Association, Dallas, Tex., November.

Moss, A. J. 1979. Changes in cigarette smoking and current practices among adults: United States, 1978. *Advance Data* 52:1–16.

Nobel, E. P. 1978. *Third Special Report to the U.S. Congress on Alcohol and Health from the Secretary of Health Education and Welfare*. Washington, D.C.: Department of Health, Education, and Welfare, National Institute on Alcoholism and Alcohol Abuse, June.

Schaps, E.; DiBartolo, R. L.; Palley, C. S.; and Churgin, S. 1978. *Primary Prevention Evaluation Research: A Review of 127 Evaluations*. Walnut Creek, Calif.: Pacific Institute for Research and Evaluation.

Stuart, R. B. 1974. Teaching facts about drugs: pushing or preventing? *Journal of Educational Psychology* 66:189–201.

U.S. Department of Health, Education, and Welfare (cited in text as USDHEW). Public Health Service. National Clearinghouse on Smoking and Health. 1972. *Teenage Smoking, National Patterns of Cigarette Smoking, Ages 12 through 18, in 1968 and 1970*. DHEW Publication no. (HSM) 72–7508. Washington, D.C.: Government Printing Office.

U.S. Department of Health, Education, and Welfare (cited in text as USDHEW). Public Health Service. National Clearinghouse for Smoking and Health. 1973a: *Use of Tobacco, Practices, Attitudes, Knowledge, and Beliefs: United States, Fall 1964 and Spring 1966*. Washington, D.C.: Government Printing Office.

U.S. Department of Health, Education, and Welfare (cited in text as USDHEW). Public Health Service. National Clearinghouse for

Smoking and Health. 1973b. *Adult Use of Tobacco 1970*. Washington, D.C.: Government Printing Office.

U.S. Department of Health, Education, and Welfare (cited in text as USDHEW). Public Health Service. National Clearinghouse on Smoking and Health. 1974. *Patterns and Prevalence of Teenage Cigarette Smoking: 1968, 1970, 1972 and 1974*. Washington, D.C.: Government Printing Office.

U.S. Department of Health, Education, and Welfare (cited in text as USDHEW). Public Health Service. National Clearinghouse on Smoking and Health. 1976a. *Teenage Smoking: National Patterns of Cigarette Smoking, Ages 12 through 18, in 1972 and 1974*. DHEW Publication no. (NIH) 76–931. Washington, D.C.: Government Printing Office.

U.S. Department of Health, Education, and Welfare. Public Health Service. National Clearinghouse of Smoking and Health. 1976b. *Adult Use of Tobacco, 1975*. Washington, D.C.: Government Printing Office.

U.S. Department of Health, Education, and Welfare (cited in text as USDHEW). Public Health Service. National Center for Health Statistics. National Center for Health Services Research. 1979. *Health: United States 1978*. Washington, D.C.: Government Printing Office.

Wittman, F. 1982. Current status of research and demonstration programs in the primary prevention of alcohol problems. In *Alcohol and Health Monograph*, no. 3. *Prevention, Intervention and Treatment: Concerns and Models*. U.S. Department of Health and Human Services. DHHS Publication no. (ADM) 82–1192. Washington, D.C.: Government Printing Office.

THE AUTHORS

DENNIS ANDERSON is Staff Child Psychiatrist, Pryme Community Health Center, Medical and Health Research Association of New York.

ROBERT ATKINSON is Research Fellow in Adolescent Psychiatry, University of Chicago and Michael Reese Medical Center.

HOWARD S. BAKER is Clinical Assistant Professor of Psychiatry, University of Pennsylvania.

SADI BAYRAKAL is Clinical Associate Professor of Psychiatry, University of British Columbia.

IRVING H. BERKOVITZ is Clinical Professor of Psychiatry, University of California, Los Angeles; Senior Psychiatric Consultant for Schools, Los Angeles County Department of Mental Health; and a Special Editor of this volume.

LUIS BRIONES is a paraprofessional clinical aide, San Fernando Child Guidance Clinic, Northridge, California.

AARON H. ESMAN is Professor of Clinical Psychiatry, Cornell University Medical College; Director of Adolescent Services, the New York Hospital; Faculty Member, New York Psychoanalytic Institute; and a Senior Editor of this volume.

CARL B. FEINSTEIN is Assistant Professor and Director, Program in Developmental Disabilities, Emma Pendleton Bradley Hospital, Brown University Program in Medicine, Providence, Rhode Island.

NAME INDEX

Abraham, A., 488, 498
Abraham, J. W., 563, 573
Abraham, K., 210, 217
Achenbach, T., 395, 405
Ackerman, N., 113, 117
Adamczyk, J. S., 538, 543
Adams, G. R., 233, 258
Adams, J., 38, 41
Adams, R. F., 271, 277, 294
Adelson, J., 10, 25, 33, 35, 39, 59, 62, 378, 393
Adler, A., 159, 161
Adler, G., 320, 329
Aguado, D. K., 506, 510, 532, 544
Ahn, H., 429, 439
Aichhorn, A., 280, 294
Alexander, F., 215, 217
Altschul, S., 218, 229
Altshuler, K., 538, 544
Altshuler, K. Z., 461, 476
Alvarez, L. D., 563, 571
Anderson, D., 136
Anderson, G., 492, 498, 537, 541
Anthony, E. J., 113, 118
Appolone, C., 538, 540
Apter, S. J., 489, 498
Ariès, P., 9, 25
Arkowitz, H., 539, 544
Armstrong, T. D., 538, 541
Arnold, L., 395, 400, 405
Arroyo, W., 498
Atkins, L., 430, 439
Atkinson, R., 135, 149
Austin, J., 92, 109
Awerbuch, W., 523, 540

Bachman, J. G., 557, 573
Bachrach, L. L., 139, 145
Baird, H. W., 429, 439
Baker, H. S., 425, 441, 450, 459

Bane, A. L., 562, 572
Bank, S. P., 218, 227, 229
Bardill, D. R., 535, 540
Barnhart, D., 350, 356
Barnhart, F. D., 138
Barton, J., 560, 571
Basch, M. F., 128, 130, 131, 444, 459
Bates, M., 492, 498, 535, 541
Bayrakal, S., 5, 112, 538, 541
Beaber, J. D., 538, 544
Beavers, W. R., 261, 269, 351, 356
Begoin, F., 301, 306, 314
Begoin, J., 301, 306, 314
Beisser, A. R., 494, 498
Bell, A. P., 162, 178
Bergin, T., 119, 131
Berkovitz, I. H., 425, 481, 483, 492, 498, 500, 503, 509, 511, 515, 520, 522, 527, 529, 532, 537, 541, 542, 546, 547, 555
Berkowitz, D. A., 196, 205, 206, 207, 362
Berlin, I. N., 361
Berne, E., 549, 555
Bernfeld, S., 214
Bespalec, D. A., 557, 573
Best, J. A., 559, 563, 571, 572
Bettleheim, B., 320, 330
Biegel, A., 342, 357
Blackwell, Elizabeth, 29, 30
Blackwell, Emily, 30
Blanchard, P., 427, 434, 439
Blatt, S., 183, 184
Bloch, A., 488, 498
Block, J. H., 9, 25, 33, 39
Blomquist, K. R., 507, 509
Blos, P., 9, 23, 25, 84, 109, 112, 118, 128, 129, 131, 214, 216, 217, 379, 392, 493, 498
Blotcky, M. J., 144, 145
Blumberg, S., 351, 356
Bodley, R., 30
Bonham, G. M., 538, 541

Bonham, G. S., 557, 571
Bonham, H. E. E., 538, 541
Bonier, R. J., 318, 319, 320, 329, 330
Bonime, W., 214, 217
Book, H. E., 320, 321, 330
Borowitz, G., 368, 377, 380, 393
Botvin, G. J., 561, 563, 571
Bourne, E., 233, 257, 258
Bowlby, J., 365, 377
Brady, J. P., 139, 145
Branch, J. D., 16, 26
Braslow, J. B., 31, 32, 33, 39
Brenner, M. H., 22, 25
Bretagne, A., 72, 74, 78
Briones, L., 362, 529, 542, 546
Brooks, P., 123, 130, 131
Brown, C., 60, 62
Brown, C. H., 16, 26
Brown, H. S., 259, 269
Brown, K. S., 563, 571
Brown, L. J., 139, 146, 329, 330
Brumback, R. A., 431, 439
Bruner, J., 92, 109
Buhler, C., 158, 160, 161
Buie, D. H., 192, 206, 317, 330
Bullough, B., 29, 39
Burns, B. J., 26
Burrus, G., 413, 416

Campbell, R. J., 317, 330
Caplan, G., 361
Carr, E., 492, 498, 537, 541
Carroll, L., 39
Carson, D. I., 138, 147
Cartwright, J. D., 427, 439
Casper, R. C., 13, 25
Catanzaro, R. J., 332, 335, 340
Chadwick, O., 62, 376, 377, 403, 406, 408, 416
Charone, J. K., 179, 184
Chassin, L., 560, 571
Chernin, K., 179, 184
Chess, S., 137, 148, 449, 460, 462, 476
Chewing, B., 560, 571
Chick, J., 413, 416
Choras, T. P., 320, 331
Churgin, S., 562, 574
Chusmir, L. H., 35, 39
Clark, D. B., 527, 541
Clark, W. B., 558, 572

Cleckley, H., 279, 294
Cline, D., 272, 294
Coen, S. J., 226, 229
Cohen, J., 370, 377
Coleman, J. C., 379, 392
Colish, H., 514, 520
Collins, G., 332, 340
Collins, L. M., 563, 573
Colonna, A. B., 218, 229
Conners, C., 405
Corner, G. W., 28, 39
Corty, E., 560, 571
Costello, J., 351, 357
Crabtree, L. H., 137, 138, 146
Cravioto, J. R., 435, 439
Crawford, J. D., 34, 39
Cremerius, M., 13, 26
Crohn, J., 259, 269
Csikszentmihalyi, M., 9, 25
Curtis, H., 441, 459
Curtiss, G., 293, 295

Dalle-Molle, D. M., 280, 295
Dalsimer, K., 84, 110
Darwin, C., 407
d'Avernas, J. R., 559, 572
Davidson, J., 83, 111
Davies, M., 391, 393
Davis, M., 325, 330
DeCecco, J. P., 487, 489, 498
Deigh, M., 532, 543
Deisher, R. W., 163, 178
Del Gaudio, A. C., 408, 416
DeMartino, M., 538, 545
Demeny, P., 69, 72, 73
Deutsch, H., 23, 25
Dewey, J., 159, 161
DiBartolo, R. L., 562, 574
Diller, J., 512, 520
Dilthy, W., 150, 161
Domash, L., 83, 110
Donovan, E., 342, 357
Douvan, E., 10, 25, 33, 34, 35, 39, 59, 62, 378, 393
Downey, T. W., 138, 148
Driver, H. I., 522, 541
Dube, W. F., 30, 40
Dumas, R., 494, 499
Dunbar, C., 36, 40
Durrell, V. G., 538, 542
Duryea, E. J., 561, 572

616

Greenacre, P., 67, 81
Greenberg, B., 490, 498
Greenberg, J. R., 83, 110
Greenberg, L., 300, 316
Greenberg, M. T., 379, 392, 393
Grinker, R. R., 141, 143, 146
Grinker, R. R., Jr., 143, 146
Grove, S., 38, 41
Grumet, G. W., 332, 340
Grunert, U., 308, 314
Gundlach, R. A., 4, 82, 99, 110
Gurman, A. S., 536, 542

Hafez, H., 414, 416
Haiman, S., 300, 316
Haley, J., 141, 146
Hall, G. S., 407, 416
Halliday, M. A. K., 93, 110
Halperin, D. A., 4, 63, 73, 81, 316, 317, 319, 320
Hamburg, B. A., 505, 509, 538, 543
Hamelberg, L., 536, 543
Hammersmith, S. K., 162, 178
Hansen, D. B., 42
Hansen, W. B., 362, 558, 560, 562, 563, 571, 572, 574
Hardin, J. W., 189, 271–94, 295
Harding, C. M., 135, 137, 414, 416
Hardy-Fanta, C., 536, 543
Harootunian, B., 489, 498
Harper, G., 320, 330
Harris, D. B., 379, 393
Harris, M. B., 536, 543
Harrison, C., 350, 356
Hart, J., 514, 520
Hart, N. A., 507, 509
Hartmann, E., 351, 357
Hastings, L., 461, 476
Hauser, S. T., 379, 393
Havis, J., 562, 572
Heald, F. P., 501, 510
Heins, M., 31, 32, 33, 39
Heir, D. B., 430, 439
Hendin, H., 22, 25
Hendrickson, W. J., 138, 146
Hennig, M., 34, 35, 37, 40
Hesiod, 48
Hickler, H., 191, 197, 206
Hinsie, L. E., 317, 330
Hirschman, R. S., 559, 573

Hofmann, A. D., 83, 110
Holdsworth, L., 429, 439
Holinger, P. C., 21, 22, 25, 208, 217, 512, 521
Hollister, L., 361
Holmes, D. J., 138, 146
Hong, G. K., 500, 509
Hopkins, L., 233, 258
Horney, K., 115, 118
Houser, B., 34, 40
Howard, B. L., 135, 137, 138, 146
Howard, K. I., 10, 13, 19, 26
Howard, J. L., 489, 498
Howze, B., 514, 521
Hudgens, R. W., 408, 415
Humes, C. W., Jr., 538, 543
Hunt, H. K., 29
Hunt, W. A., 557, 573
Hurd, P. D., 562, 573
Husain, S. A., 501, 509

Ilchman, A., 38, 40
Inhelder, B., 87, 90, 110, 194, 206
Isay, R. A., 220, 227, 229
Izambard, Georges, 68, 69, 70, 71, 72, 75, 78

Jacobowski, P., 549, 555
Jacobs, J., 211, 217
Jacobs, S. M., 532, 543
Jacobsen, L., 50, 62
Jacobson, A. M., 379, 393
Jacobson, E., 82, 83, 110
Jacobson, M. D., 538, 544
Jacobziner, H., 512, 521
Jardim, A., 34, 35, 37, 40
Jaureguy, B. M., 332, 340
Jessor, R., 561, 573
Jessor, S. L., 561, 573
John, E. R., 429, 439
Johnson, A. V., 533, 542
Johnson, C. A., 558, 562, 563, 573
Johnson, P., 38, 40
Johnston, L. D., 557, 573
Jones, G. F., 491, 499
Josselson, R. L., 188, 230, 234, 242, 253, 258
Jung, C., 157, 161

Kacerguis, M. A., 233, 258
Kael, P., 128, 131

Witmer, H., 361
Wittman, F., 561, 575
Wolf, E., 446, 447, 452, 459, 460
Wolff, S., 413, 416
Woodall, C., 136, 179, 184
Woods, N. F., 114, 118
Wright, R., 320, 330

Yalom, I. D., 164, 178
Yankelovich, D., 49, 62, 490, 499
Yasser, A. M., 332, 341

Yochelson, S., 549, 554, 555
Yoder, J., 38, 41
Yule, W., 376, 377, 403, 406, 408, 416

Zegans, L. S., 494, 499
Zinkus, C. B., 430, 440
Zinkus, P. M., 430, 440
Zinn, L. D., 138, 147
Zinner, J., 196, 197, 205, 206, 207
Zuckerman, S., 500, 510
Zweig, P., 72, 81

SUBJECT INDEX

Intake phase, in hospitalization, 352
Intentional phase, in development of purpose, 154–55
Intentionality, and development of purpose, 160
Internalization of objects, failure of, in identity diffusion, 253
Intimacy, failure of, in identity diffusion, 240
Intimacy *vs.* isolation, development in young adults and, 141

Juvenile delinquents, underachievement and, 430–31

Language, play with in adolescence, 90–91
Leadership roles, women's, 4, 28–39, 42–46
  career choices and, 34
  cultural factors and, 36–37
  current status of, 31–33
  developmental issues and, 34–35
  father-daughter relationships and, 35
  group experiences and, 37–38
  history of women physicians, 28–30
  roles women play, 35–36
  socialization and, 33–34
Learning disabilities, suicide and, 512
Limits, need for, 59–60
Long-term treatment needs, 300, 342–56
  aftercare phase, 353–55
  case examples, 348, 352, 354
  diagnostic categories in study of, 344–45
  hospital therapeutic phase, 353
  intake phase, 352
  outcome classifications in study of, 345–50
  phases of treatment, 351–56
  resistance phase, 352–53
  stable, long-term relationship, 342–43, 350–51, 356
  subjects in study of, 343–44
  termination phase, 355–56
Loss
  remarriage situations and, 264
  underachievement and, 433–34
  see also Sibling loss

Loss reactions, and school group counseling, 546–55
  assertion training in, 548–49
  career planning in, 549–50
  case examples, 551–54
  communication skills in, 548
  junior high groups, 550–51
  program for, 547–50
  senior high groups, 551

Maintenance of identity, 369
Manifest phase, in development of purpose, 155
Meaning
  search for, 115
  see also Purpose
Mental health professionals, perception of adolescents as in turmoil, 13–14
Mental health utilization, of psychiatrically ill youth, 15–19
Middle adolescence
  described, 378
  defensive style of, 389–90
  see also Personality functioning
Minimal Brain Dysfunction (MBD), underachievement and, 429, 431
Mirroring, 443–44
Missing children, myth of, 57
Mothers
  relationship with, of identity diffusions, 243
  see also Parents
Mourning, sibling loss, 219, 226
Movies, as myths, 5, 119–20
  see also Purple Rain
Myth, of the Western hero, 271
Myths
  about adolescents, 4
  films as, 5, 119–20
  see also Purple Rain
Myths, of adolescence, 48–58
  drug and substance abuse, 53
  fear of nuclear annihilation, 55–56
  generation gap, 49
  history and, 48–49
  identity formation, 52
  it's a stage theory, 51–52
  most difficult period of life, 51
  sexuality, 54
  suicide epidemic, 52–53

early poems, 67–69
family of, 65–67, 68
father issues of, 66–67, 68
father surrogates, 67, 68–69, 78
final poems, 75–76
influence of, 63–64
mother of, 67, 69, 75, 79
Paris years, 70
personal themes of, 65, 71–73, 78
relationship with Auguste Bretagne, 72, 74, 78
relationship with Georges Izambard, 68–69, 70, 71, 72, 75, 78
relationship with Paul Verlaine, 74–75, 76, 78
therapeutic value of poetry, 79–80
turning point in development of, 70–71
Role assumption, 370
Roles, played by women in the workplace, 35–36

Safe School Study, 484
Schizoid personalities, 280
Schools
aggression in, 483–97
behavior at, 399–400
group counseling in, 522–40, 546–55
loss reactions, school counseling for, 546–55
problems with, in our culture, 115
suicide prevention in, 500–509
tobacco and alcohol prevention programs, 557–70
see also Underachievement
Self-image
disturbed adolescents, 13–14
normal adolescents, 11–13
results from Offer Questionnaire, 11–14
Self psychology, 441–49
academic underachievement and, 449–53
case examples, 453–58
defining "self," 447–49
idealizing, 444–45
mirroring, 443–44
parental failures, 442, 448–49
self-object relations, 445–46
therapeutic alliance and, 449
twinship needs, 445
usefulness of, 458–59

Self-esteem, 369
studies of, 379
Self-object relations, 445–46
Sensorimotor period, interference in and underachievement, 431
Separation anxiety, underachievement and, 433
Separation issues
borderline adolescents' suicide attempts and, 197
bulimia and, 179–80
Sexual behavior
deaf students acting out through, 471–72
and familial factors, 19–20
and school performance, 20–21
Sexual self, of normal adolescents, 12
Sexuality
confusion about, 114
myths about, 54
Sibling loss, 188, 218–29
case reports of, 220–25
homosexual panic and, 219, 225–28
incapacity to mourn and, 219
lack of writing about, 218
theories about, 225–28
Smoking. See Tobacco and alcohol use
Social forces, identity diffusion and, 255
Social self, of normal adolescents, 12
Sociocultural factors, psychopathology and, 112–17
Socioeconomic status, underachievement and, 434, 435
Splitting, 422
Stepfamilies. See Remarriage families
Story, defined, 123
Structural defects, 419–20, 422
Structural discontinuity, 420–21
Substance abuse, underachievement and, 433
Suicidal behavior, 187, 191–205
borderline adolescents and, 195–96, 197
case examples of, 197–99, 200–203
family dynamics and, 192–95, 196–97, 202–5
mismanagement of bodily care for child and, 192–95
narcissistic adolescents and, 195, 196–97
parental ambivalence and, 192–93
suicide notes, 191